Who's Fit to Be a Parent?

D1073396

In recent years parenting and parenthood have increasingly come under examination from the media, professionals and, in particular, government and politicians. More and more, parents are being held to account by society for their failure to deliver the sort of citizens it wants. But what are parents supposed to be doing? Are there some people who are inherently unfit to be parents and does there exist a body of knowledge that defines fit parenting?

Who's Fit to Be a Parent? conducts a thorough and wide-ranging investigation into how society currently judges parents by looking at the professionals who assess parenting and by examining the charges made against certain 'unfit' groups who are, nonetheless, becoming more widespread as parents (for example, those who are single, gay, disabled or drug-addicted). Bringing together professional and academic research which challenges traditional views of how to assess parenting with the personal experiences of a wide-range of 'non-conventional' families, Mukti Jain Campion also examines the role of the media in guiding public opinion and opening up the boundaries of what is considered 'normal'. The book concludes with a challenging proposal for a new framework by which to understand and assess parenting in the future.

This unique combination of information and ideas provides a sound basis to promote broad debate about the job of parenting as well as the job of assessing parenting. It is essential reading for any professional or student of social work and social policy, those working in the voluntary services concerned with the family, social policy makers and for anyone interested in understanding what it means to be a parent today.

Mukti Jain Campion is a writer and a mother of two children. She is a former BBC television programme maker, currently working as an independent producer.

Who's Fit to Be a Parent?

Mukti Jain Campion

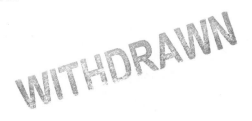
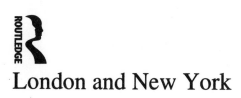

London and New York

First published 1995
by Routledge
11 New Fetter Lane, London EC4P 4EE

Simultaneously published in the USA and Canada
by Routledge
29 West 35th Street, New York, NY 10001

Typeset in Times by LaserScript, Mitcham, Surrey
Printed and bound in Great Britain by
Mackays of Chatham PLC, Chatham, Kent

British Library Cataloguing in Publication Data
A catalogue record for this book is available from the British Library

Library of Congress Cataloging in Publication Data
A catalog record for this book has been requested

ISBN 0–415–06683–2 (hbk)
ISBN 0–415–06684–0 (pbk)

Contents

Preface

The idea for this book came to me during a period when I was approached for advice in a succession of cases of parents with disabilities whose fitness to parent was being called into question. I had written a book on pregnancy and disability (Campion 1990) which had brought me into contact with hundreds of parents with disabilities, many of whom reported increased professional scrutiny and surveillance due to the fact of their disability. I began to wonder how professionals made their assessments of whether parents were fit to care for their own children or not and whether there existed a body of knowledge which objectively defined what comprises fit parenting.

As I began to explore the area it became apparent that there are many books on the practical aspects of caring for children which seem to take for granted that everyone knows the norm to which all parents should be aspiring. Aspects of parenthood have variously been researched and explored by sociologists, doctors and psychologists who have proposed certain models of what good *parenting* should contain. None seemed to have directly tackled the question of *who* is fit to be a parent. Yet this is a question that is becoming increasingly important in western societies. The notion of 'fitness' (as opposed to 'goodness') suggests selection criteria that have to be met before someone will pass the parenting test and be allowed to care for children. Who is allowed to adopt? Whose children are removed and taken into care? Who 'gets' the children after the parents split? Who is allowed fertility treatment? More and more professionals are exercising power when deciding who will be permitted to be a parent. So it seemed timely to examine what criteria different practitioners are using to assess fitness and to see whether a consensus view emerges that all parents should be aspiring to fulfil.

But it is not just professionals who determine who is considered fit to be a parent. The media, politicians and religious leaders regularly pass judgement on certain groups of people and assert that it is their unfitness as parents that is responsible for all of society's problems. Parents nowadays appear to be under siege both from their children's demands and from society at large. So it also seemed timely to examine exactly what it is that society expects parents to be doing.

This book is a chronological account of my own personal investigation which took in a wide swathe of opinion and ideas. In exploring the nature of what is deemed fit parenting and how it is assessed, I looked to the following sources:

- Professional and academic research
- The media
- Parents and children from a wide variety of backgrounds
- Professional practitioners.

In writing this book I have tried to avoid using any professional or academic jargon and have also chosen not to feign academic detachment in my writing style. Both these seemed to constitute a more honest and accessible way to present what I have uncovered.

Acknowledgements

This book was researched and written over a period of three years, beginning just after the birth of my second child. It has therefore been a major part of the lives of both my husband and our two young children, an exciting and at times challenging presence that has brought new ideas into our own daily parenting. My greatest thanks go to them for participating in this journey and for providing a constant source of ideas on how to view the material I was uncovering.

My sincere thanks go also to all the parents and children living in a very wide variety of circumstances whose experiences have profoundly informed the direction of the research in this book.

Acknowledgements are also due to all the professionals and academics whose work I have quoted, particularly those at the leading edge who have dared to question orthodox views of family life. This book is a tribute to their work.

Finally, I would like to acknowledge the excellent library staff at the National Children's Bureau whose endeavours have provided me with much support in my research for this book.

Introduction

Who's fit to be a parent? Few people stop to think about this before embarking on parenthood. In the democratic world, no one can stop the vast majority of men from having the capacity to impregnate and of women to become pregnant, so the question may have seemed superfluous in the past. But a number of social and medical advances are changing this:

1 The recognition of the rights of a child.
2 The demands for equal rights to parenthood by groups previously excluded or discouraged.
3 The increase in break-up of parental relationships which leads to the decision about who looks after the children.
4 The advance of medical knowledge which now gives doctors the ability to offer children to many people previously incapable of unassisted reproduction.

Until a century ago, children were regarded as mere possessions of their parents to be sold off, used, cared for or not – just as the parents pleased. The rights of parents were paramount and their responsibilities minimal. The state did not intervene to protect children or consider them to have any rights worth safeguarding. (In fact, a society for the Prevention of Cruelty to Animals existed before one to protect children.)

Within the space of little more than a hundred years, there has been a gradual recognition of the importance of children's welfare, with progressive moves to prevent children from suffering at the hands of their own parents. In Britain the Children Act 1989 has now arrived on the statute books, asserting the position of children as individuals with rights and emphasising parents' responsibilities towards their children.

What has significantly changed our attitudes in the developed world is that we are having fewer children (for example, because we can count on them surviving), and the length of time we are responsible as parents for looking after them (before they are permitted by the state to entertain the notion of independence) has risen to a minimum of eighteen years – the longest time in history that parents have been expected to financially support their children. We are therefore required to invest more (financially, emotionally and practically) in fewer children for longer than ever before.

The other major influence has been the academic and professional research in mental and physical health, emphasising the connection between childhood care and adult well-being. As this body of knowledge has grown, more and more responsibilities have been laid at the door of parents. It has become unarguable that both the state and individual parents therefore need to invest more considered effort in bringing up children who develop into socially well-adjusted, healthy and productive adults. This seems fine in theory, except that no one seems certain of how to achieve acceptable standards of parenting, and even well-intentioned parents find themselves wondering whether they are getting it right and, if not, to whom they should turn for advice.

Everyone, however, seems to have an opinion on what bad parenting is. Most people would now agree that serious physical or sexual abuse of a child is not acceptable but everything else is open to discussion. In the United States of America cases are coming to the courts where children are suing their parents for depriving them of health or happiness by their irresponsible abuse of alcohol or drugs either in pregnancy or while the children were young. Throughout the western world psychotherapists are uncovering what they consider to be suppressed memories of childhood abuse – which has led to a spate of attempts by adults to sue their elderly parents for damages. In Britain as well as the USA, a few well-publicised cases of young children 'divorcing' their parents has caused a flurry of anxiety and speculation about the progress of children's rights.

This path is a potential minefield: will children be able to sue their parents for divorcing and thus causing them mental trauma? Or for passing on a genetic condition or illness such as HIV that could have been avoided by not having children? Is it the law that will determine the rights of the child through cases such as these and hence define who is fit to be a parent? Will all parents come to live in fear of such scrutiny?

We have reached a dramatic point in the history of children's rights in relationship to their parents, and the way forward is littered with ambiguities and dangers which we need to address. What does society want for children and what does it expect of parents? The time is ripe for an open and wide-ranging debate to take place not only amongst professionals working within their own particular areas. The issues affect everyone and cannot be resolved by laws alone. It is in this belief that I have chosen to write this book.

I intend to try and answer the question of who is fit to be a parent by looking first at how the state currently determines fitness to parent in those areas where it becomes involved. Second, I wish to examine some of the groups which have hitherto been regarded by society as unfit to parent and to show how the traditional objections to them are being challenged – and what these tell us of society's expectations of fit parenting. In the final section I hope to draw these perspectives together to build a portrait of the 'fit' parent. Once this is made explicit, I will consider the issue of children's rights and whether they can be accommodated at the same time as allowing the unfettered freedom for all people to become parents.

I am not a professional who has to tangle with the practicalities of assessing parents and have not been a target for any particular procedure of selection myself. To that extent this investigation is by a disinterested bystander – I did not know where the investigation would lead before I started to research this book and have no ulterior motives to find fault with any particular professional groups or to promote any political ideology. As a full-time parent of two young children, however, I do have a personal interest in what this examination will reveal about society's expectations of a 'fit' parent. The 1989 Children Act embodies a central principle that has been promoted with the slogan: 'Parenthood – a job for life'. Well, I would like to know more about the 'job description'.

Part I
Parents on trial

There are now a growing number of people who require the approval of others to be allowed to become, or to remain, parents. Over the past century, the state has been drawn increasingly, but somewhat reluctantly, into family life, driven by the public's conscience to protect children's right to minimum care but also by the economic expediency of trying to prevent delinquency, crime and adult ill health. As more children become the responsibility of the state, a body of welfare professionals has developed – notably doctors, social workers, health visitors, child psychiatrists and court welfare officers. These act as a buffer zone between the state and the family, carrying out family intervention under the state's legal and political guidance, but largely defining their own guidelines.

One of their key roles has become that of assessing families, in particular whether certain adults are able to provide the right sort of parenting to their existing children or to children in the future. In Part I, I will examine the four key situations in which the assessment of parents takes place: child protection, adoption, childcare after the break-up of the parental relationship, and the provision of treatment for medically assisted reproduction. These four areas may be likened to the four facets of a pyramid-like edifice, constructed piecemeal by the state to regulate parenthood, at least to the extent of protecting some children. I would like to examine the exposed faces of this pyramid but also try and uncover any common ideological base on which it rests. Thus in each of these four 'practical' areas, I will examine who carries out the assessment of parents, what criteria they use and what they tell us about the expectations of all parents. The aim is to see how much consensus exists about who is fit to be a parent and to see how consistently and effectively the assessment processes safeguard the interests of children – and their parents.

1   The state versus parents
Children into care

The British media recently reported the case of a reclusive mother and son who were found living in a squalid house in suburbia, surrounded by neglected and dying pets. The 11 year old boy was described as never having attended school and as having no contact with other children, but

> despite her problems, the mother seems to have lavished attention on him acting as a teacher as well as a mother and friend. Social workers were astonished to find him articulate, literate and numerate. Poised and well-spoken, he has not necessarily suffered lasting damage from his strange childhood.
>
> (Margaret Driscoll, *Sunday Times* 1/12/91)

The media also pursued the question of who was to blame for not intervening to save the boy from his circumstances.

> The social workers argued that no one had reported his predicament to them, so how were they supposed to help? – 'We rely heavily on intervention by schools or the community to trigger our work'.
>
> Neighbours saw no reason to pry: 'The boy looked plump and healthy. If he had been starved or bruised, well, that would have been different. But people live the way they want to live. You can't interfere'.
>
> (Margaret Driscoll, *Sunday Times* 1/12/91)

The media reports focused on the boy as a victim of his mother's irrational behaviour, describing him as a captive in their relationship. An independent social worker summed up her initial assessment of the boy thus:

> It will certainly have done him some harm, in that he does not seem to have had peer relationships or the ability to play. The crucial thing is the relationship with his mother, if she had managed to keep it unintense, then he may develop quite normally. The problem is that it is probably a very intense relationship because there was just the two of them.

At the time of writing this chapter, the mother and son were 'being kept under observation at a special unit while social workers gently try to prise apart the roots of their mutual dependency'.

The way the story was reported highlights some of the expectations western society currently has of normal parents and the normal childhood to which all children should be entitled – parents should adequately nourish and physically care for their children, they should send them to school, the children should mix and play with children of their own age and have non-intense relationships with sociable parents who conform to society's standards of normal behaviour. The reports also highlight the role of the 'community', e.g. neighbours, teachers and social workers, in monitoring parents so that 'unfit' parenting can be identified and dealt with in order to protect children. It assumes they have the knowledge and skills to do so.

This monitoring of parents is notoriously haphazard and this is what I would like to examine in this chapter. The state's role in protecting children reveals the most about the minimum standards that 'fit' parents are expected to meet. The assessment of children at risk in their own families is concerned with identifying whether the parents are good enough to keep their children. So the question is: *At what point do good enough parents cease to be good enough?* The answer seems to be: at the point when their fitness to parent is called into question, observations made and criteria applied to see whether they pass the parenting test, and then a decision is taken as to whether they can retain possession of their children – or whether the children should be 'taken into care' (the very phrase emphasises the notion that parents have been *care-less* towards their children to have reached this point).

What criteria are applied in assessing whether parents are fit to care for their own children? Are these criteria based on widely accepted knowledge? Are they applied consistently and fairly? Are parents aware of how they are being assessed? Are they offered appropriate resources to improve their abilities to be fit parents? How much freedom should the state have to come between parents and their children? What are the underlying philosophies that are being represented when professionals intervene?

These are all questions which have not been openly explored or debated in the public arena. The result has been that society makes ill-considered demands on those professionals at the sharp end of policy implementation. Perhaps even more significant, we may not be giving all children an equal opportunity to be helped when their own families are unable or unwilling to care for them. For professionals to be seen to be getting the balance right, there needs to be a clearer consensus from society at large about what defines adequate parenting and what justifies state intervention.

To understand the state's current attitudes to who is fit to be a parent we need to begin by looking back into the brief history of state intervention into family life.

A HISTORY OF CHILD PROTECTION BY THE STATE

Children embody all that is pure, innocent and hopeful in our society. Whether or not we are parents, when this is corrupted it undermines all that gives stability, meaning and purpose to our own adult lives. It offends our sense of what is right and just. Modern society is easily horrified by the extremes of physical and sexual abuse of young children, particularly when it is inflicted by parents. Yet society has conflicting expectations of the professionals that intervene. The almost daily reports of battered children whom the social workers could not protect focus on the plight of the vulnerable young suffering at the hands of hapless dregs of adult society, because the social workers have been too optimistic about their parents' natural love.

In contrast, the British media coverage of the social workers' responses to the alleged sexual abuse of children in Cleveland, Rochdale and the Orkneys in recent years focused almost exclusively on the plight of the parents and the horror of having children removed. Public sympathy see-saws between parents and children with little consistency because there exists an underlying conflict of social philosophies about whether children are the property of their parents or whether they are individuals with rights.

Freedom of the individual is paramount, and that extends to bringing up children as that individual wishes. This is endorsed by the European Bill of Human Rights, Clause 8:

1 Everyone has the right to respect for his private and family life, his home and his correspondence.
2 There shall be no interference by a public authority with the exercise of this right except such as is in accordance with the law and is necessary in a democratic society in the interests of national security, public safety or the economic well-being of the country, for the prevention of disorder or crime, for the protection of health and morals, or for the protection of the rights and freedoms of others.

The state should protect those who are vulnerable. Children cannot determine and safeguard their own interests, and since the young are the builders of future society we all share a responsibility to protect them.

All too often it becomes a case of parents versus children. In the past there was no doubt whom the state backed: children were regarded as the property of the father. The father was even entitled to compensation for loss of the child's earnings if the child died in the hands of his employer or foster parents.

Even the principle that parents are responsible for every child born to them is a relatively recent one. As John Boswell described in his book *The Kindness of Strangers*, the abandonment of children was a common and acceptable feature of life over most of western history. For example, in his discussion of the wide-spread practice of abandonment in Roman times he writes:

Even Hierocles' ideal parent might only bring up 'most' of his children and hence would abandon some. Most ancient moral writings evince indifference toward or acceptance of abandonment. Gellius, who excoriates abortion as an act 'worthy of public contempt and general hatred' and even rails against the evils of mothers not nursing their own children, mentions abandonment as a common or normal occurrence without any suggestion of disapproval.

(Boswell 1991)

The only reason children came into the public arena in the past was because they were abandoned, usually as a method of family planning (for reasons of poverty or desire to maximise the inheritance for a few offspring).

> Their fate was left to the whim of individuals: they were exposed in public locations in the central city without any supervision or civic intervention, and no effort was made to regulate their treatment or to guarantee their well-being. But they were gathered up, generally survived to adulthood, reared as children as often as kept for slaves and frequently achieved considerable success in life, often marrying into their adoptive families. Society relied on the kindness of strangers to protect its extra children, a kindness much admired and prominent in the public consciousness.
>
> (Boswell 1991)

There was no suggestion of the state intervening to remove children from their parents for the welfare of the children themselves, but none the less, Boswell argues, the children did better than when, 1,500 years later, the state,

> too conscientious to leave the fate of unwanted children to chance, and too preoccupied with family ties and lineage to admire affective solutions, intervened to establish an orderly public means of handling them. . . . In Renaissance cities the infants disappeared quietly and efficiently through the revolving doors of state-run foundling homes, out of sight and out of mind, into social oblivion, or more likely death by disease.
>
> (Boswell 1991)

This was the fate of unwanted infants. The move away from agricultural communities to urban isolation and poverty considerably increased the problem of child exploitation and of child destitution and it was these abandoned children who prompted philanthropic individuals and church groups to set up schemes providing such children with homes where they could be corrected by strict moral guidance and vocational training. There was a strongly moralistic line pursued against those parents who allowed their children to become destitute, as poverty and criminality were still seen by many as self-inflicted – a sign of weakness of character and poor stock.

But what of the children who were inadequately cared for by parents who had chosen to keep them? It seems that the beginning of state intervention into family life did not occur until the mid-nineteenth century when individual philanthropists revealed the horrors to which children were subjected in factories and workhouses. Pressure from individuals and voluntary groups led to laws making it illegal for children to work more than a certain number of hours and required them to receive a certain amount of schooling. That the prospect of such laws met with considerable opposition at the time reflects the economic importance of children to parents and to the state (as cheap labour for the factories and mines) but also the strong belief in parents' ownership of their children. This was further emphasised by the acknowledgements of many reformers of the need to protect the sanctity of the family.

In a quotation that has chillingly taken on new significance in the light of modern stories of nannies abusing children of working mothers, Ruth Inglis writes:

> Another 'reformer', Whately Cooke Taylor in 1874 invoked the sanctity of family life when questioned by followers as to why strong legislation had not been passed to help reduce the high infant mortality rate. While he conceded that there was a connection between the high death rate and the phenomenon of mothers leaving their babies unsupervised while they went out to work, he proclaimed, 'I would far rather see even a higher rate of infant mortality prevailing . . . than intrude one iota further on the sanctity of the domestic hearth'.
>
> (Inglis 1978)

This reluctance to interfere with the authority of parents was an indication of how irrelevant the notion of children's rights was at the time. Much of the initial support for children had been driven by the desire to wipe out destitution, but in the last three decades of the nineteenth century there appears to have been a distinct shift towards considering children as individuals with some rights in terms other than simply preventing them from turning to crime or prostitution.

The media played a role even then; for example, in reporting the widespread neglect of illegitimate babies who had been adopted for a fee by those exploiting the stigma of illegitimacy for unmarried mothers – and then left to die. Public sentiments were thus harnessed and led to a rapid succession of reforms. In 1871 a Select Committee on the Protection of Infant Life proposed a compulsory registration of births and deaths as a way of publicly monitoring the existence of children, and this became law in 1874. Soon came laws which undermined the notion of children as possessions of their parents. In the 1889 Prevention of Cruelty Act, for the first time the state empowered the police to enter a home (if they had the sworn evidence of a witness that children were suffering at the hands of parents) and gave powers to the courts to take children away from parents convicted of wilful cruelty or neglect. The state emphasised the parents' continued responsibility by making them liable to pay for the child's maintenance. The 1891 Custody of Children Act gave charitable organisations such as the homes run by Dr Barnardo the right to rescue children from neglect or cruelty and permitted judges to prevent their parents from demanding them back.

At the turn of the century, research into poverty and its effects on children, particularly the high rates of infant mortality, shifted the emphasis away from blaming parents for poverty. The large numbers of young men rejected by the Army for fighting in the Boer War on the grounds of poor physical health also highlighted the importance of child-rearing practices to adult well-being. The movement for public health and state education had already begun and now addressed children as prime targets: how could parents be supported in rearing healthier children? This led to the provision of school meals, health check-ups at school, and the notification of births to a local medical officer to involve a health visitor as early as possible in the child's development. Education too was being emphasised as something which needed to address the individual child's needs and aptitudes and to make the best use of them. This was the first time in history that a child-centred approach was being promoted and reflects the considerable shift in attitude which led to the first ever Children Act in 1908.

This Act was the culmination of a number of simultaneous changes in thinking that had been taking place with regard to the position of children as social beings separate from adults with specific needs for development and protection. As well as increasing the level of protection, the Act stopped the imprisonment of under-16s and instead put in place the plans for remand homes where children would be kept separate from adult offenders and given opportunities for reform.

In 1924 research led to the discovery of the extent of sex offences against young people, apparently because they did not have adequate supervision from their parents. The 1933 Children and Young Persons Act extended the range of situations in which children could be protected by the state:

> A child or young person who, having no parent or guardian, or a parent or guardian unfit to exercise care and guardianship, or not exercising proper care and guardianship, is either falling into bad associations or exposed to moral danger, or beyond control or is ill treated or neglected in a manner likely to cause his unnecessary suffering or injury to health.

The responsibility to protect children now lay with the local authority health and education departments. Overall, there was a reduction in the correctional stance the state had previously taken towards destitute children and a more generous, supportive one – as unfortunate victims of parental inadequacy. For the first time in history, the law was stating that the welfare of the child was paramount.

The economic depression of the 1930s led to many break-ups of families and a rise in the sort of problems which would have required state intervention. It was soon realised that the state did not have the resources to deal with every unsuccessful family situation that was coming to light in the way that it had previously hoped, i.e. by removing the child to other carers or educational establishments until the age of 18. A gradual shift to exploring more preventive approaches within the family started to take place.

The influence of psychoanalysis had begun to underline the importance of family relationships. The impact of the Second World War on family life strengthened this view – the experience of evacuation showed that the family preferred to cling together as a fundamental unit in the face of every obstacle. The recognition of the family's strengths led to some new changes in the Children Act in 1948. For the first time since the state had started to intervene in family life, the Act emphasised a need to restore the child to its natural family.

This led to the rise in casework by which skilled social workers could examine each family situation with a view to helping that family solve its problems which otherwise would result in the child being received into care. The intention was to prevent children from becoming indefinitely left in the care of the state. This emphasis on individual therapeutic casework was only possible because it went hand-in-hand with other aspects of the newly founded welfare state, namely, the provision of minimum financial security, healthcare and education. The Act evoked the notion of the best interests of the child in a way which perhaps reflects the general optimism of the times:

> Where a child is in the care of a local authority it shall be the duty of the authority to exercise their powers with respect to him so as to further his best interests, and to afford him opportunity for the proper development of his character and abilities.
>
> (Section 12.1)

It emphasised the need to use the resources of the community to support a child within his family rather than to segregate him.

The 1948 Act was also significant in that it brought into central control of the Home Office and the Secretary of State all work relating to deprived children. Local authorities now had an inescapable duty to receive into care as a voluntary measure children whose parents were temporarily or permanently unfit or unable to care for them, and to supervise fostered children, to oversee adoptions, to supply information to magistrates about children appearing before the courts and to be responsible for all children taken into care by the courts.

There followed in the 1950s the heyday of the 'traditional' nuclear family – a golden era for social workers and a time of tremendous confidence in the sanctity and merit of family life. Those researching the origins of deprivation and mental illness increasingly pointed to the need for more preventive work with families to act before neglect had occurred.

In the course of the 1950s local authorities were given more and more powers to intervene in family life – ostensibly to promote the strength of the family and so prevent crises and deprivation from occurring. Such laudable aims were so in line with public perceptions of the child's need for the right sort of family life and the need to avoid future costs of delinquency and deprivation that they proceeded virtually unchecked. The caseworker's policing role to protect the child was now combined with a therapeutic assessment of the family as a whole. Thus by 1952 a child for the first time was able to get protection of courts when there was other than wilful neglect or wilful cruelty.

The advent of this preventive approach of the state's representatives has arguably given rise to the most controversy over the years. The power for more or less such intervention has been given, reined in, extended and reined back in response to public outcry over alternating stories of child battering and infringement of family privacy.

From 1952 to the present there have been many new laws relating to childcare but these seem to have largely been to restructure the mechanics by which state intervention is carried out. The most significant shift in attitudes towards children had already taken place fifty years ago.

During the 1960s and early 1970s the discovery of the extent of modern-day child battering shattered the post-war myth of the natural family as the ideal place for all children. By the time the Children Act of 1975 was drawn up, the emphasis on the importance of the family was diluted and the child's welfare became the dominating factor in all proceedings concerning children. The rights of children were no longer seen as complementary to those of the parent and steps were taken to allow the child to be independently represented in court hearings. Severance of parental rights was taken a step further, allowing courts to dispense with parents' consent if they had mistreated the child. The notion of parental authority was to be ignored in favour of the child's best interests.

This paved the way for local authorities to assume draconian powers to remove children and to ignore the wishes of parents for access to their children and involvement in decisions concerning their future. Stories of social workers 'playing God' with families abound and there is considerable evidence that 'innocent' parents have had their children removed when all they needed was short-term support. Stories of the abuse of children in residential care and the fact that so many enter adulthood with few qualifications or job opportunities also highlighted the inability of the state to provide a better alternative to that of many of the parents that it had deemed unfit.

The point of presenting this history is to show the relatively rapid progress of the recognition of children's rights, but also to show the oscillations between the state's attitudes to parents and children over the course of the last 150 years. The pendulum has swung back and forth between public perceptions of the state as intervening too much and public outcries for the state to do more to protect innocent children. It is generally accepted that too much state intervention is undesirable (both for ethical and economic reasons) but at the same time there is no consensus on what constitutes adequate state intervention.

The practical approaches to state dealings with family life have shifted over the decades in the light of different types of research and political thinking. The underlying areas of debate (Bebbington and Miles 1989) have been:

1   The origin of deprivation (social malaise or parental inadequacy?).
2   Who should take responsibility for a child becoming delinquent?
3   How important are the bonds between a child and his natural parents?

At the heart of all three of these issues is the question, how important is the parent to how the child turns out? None of these debates has yet been resolved conclusively but there is an ever-growing body of research which is more or less helpful to practitioners and those they monitor.

A number of other points emerge from looking back:

- The poorer families in society have always been most targeted for state intervention in the belief that they offered the greatest potential for future gain (i.e. avoiding delinquency, crime, unemployment, etc.).
- There has been a strong emphasis on promoting physical health and protecting children's physical welfare because of the historical origins of state intervention through public health departments. There seems to have been a haphazard progression from recognising the need to protect a child from life-threatening behaviour towards the recognition that his emotional welfare is also important.

- Family life is vulnerable to the economic shifts between recession and growth – it appears most under stress in times of economic depression (with higher rates of divorce and family break-up and children requiring welfare support), and at its strongest in, for example, the 'you've never had it so good' 1950s.
- Repeated Children Acts have promoted aspirations which have been laudable for their times but which have subsequently not been fulfilled.

As we approach the end of the twentieth century there is increasing, but hesitant, support for the notion that the rights of children are more important than the rights of parents to their children. In Sweden this has already resulted in giving the social services unprecedented rights to remove children from their parents. In the UK there has even been a call by judges to amend Clause 8 of the European Bill of Human Rights in recognition of this change in attitudes as displayed in our legislation and judicial thinking (Graham Hall and Martin 1991).

An addition to Art 8(2) is suggested: '*subject to any question arising concerning the upbringing of a child in which the child's welfare must be the paramount consideration.*'

The UN Convention on the Rights of the Child has recently been ratified by Britain. The Children Act 1989, while restoring a belief in the need for children to be cared for in their own families, endorses the paramountcy of the child's welfare and goes further in terms of some recognition of children as having legal rights of their own.

All these measures to protect children depend on professionals applying criteria to assess whether children are being adequately treated in the care of their parents. The issues surrounding child protection today are very complex and have been the subject of a considerable amount of professional literature. It is not my intention to deal with all of them here but to examine only those which might contribute to an understanding of society's current expectations of fit parents.

Parents rule, OK? Why society still has a prevailing bias against intervention

Despite the historical shifts towards recognition of children's rights, there are a number of prevailing ideological and practical constraints to state intervention into family life:

- The biological bond invests parents with rights and responsibilities and should not be broken without good reason.
- The family is better than any alternative environment for bringing up children.
- The state cannot afford to prop up families – most have to be self-reliant.

Our family lives are private and increasingly territorial: all who live within the four walls of a western home are ideally seen as being self-sufficient and answerable to no one unless they or their children are caught breaking the law. Parents (preferably two of the opposite sex) are expected to take full responsibility for the welfare of their children – after all (the thinking seems to go), they chose to bring them into this world and they should be able to build and maintain the support structures necessary to bring them up. Schools, health and social services should be there to support and inform parents but the responsibility for the emotional and physical well-being rests with one or two adults. This is the freedom we so wish to guard.

Yet, paradoxically, this freedom – the right to be self-determining – can become oppressive when given to those who are not equipped to handle it or when external crises arise which renders the self-sufficient position untenable. Extended family and community cannot be relied on to support parents or to protect children. Those who make assessments only become involved when someone alerts them to a serious problem. With a few notable exceptions, there is little interest or continuity of personnel to enable relationships between professionals and parents that are supportive and which are able to pre-empt crises.

Thus the vast majority of children who suffer neglect and emotional abuse are never likely to receive help. There is a tacit acceptance that there will always be some children who are luckier than others – not just financially, but in terms of how their parents bring them up. It is a lottery. So to judge whether a child is just unfortunate or actually 'at risk' is necessarily subjective. A further difficulty is recognising the difference between short-term disturbances and long-term effects on children of parental behaviour – particularly versus the alternatives if the children are taken into care. Resources for alternative childcare are limited and there is much debate over whether the state can really offer a better alternative future for the children whom it takes into care. Everyone wants problems to solve themselves and hopes that time will resolve everything. So there may be an inherent bias towards inactivity in all but the most life-threatening cases.

But even if alternative resources are available, there is still the practical problem of when and how intervention should take place. As individual citizens, it is easy to criticise other parents and not feel obliged or able to do anything to help the child who seems at risk. For professionals it is important to be seen to have taken action when a severe problem has been brought to their attention but also to feel confident that intervention is going to improve prospects for the child. Between these private and public positions there is a great swathe of blurred responsibility where children continue to suffer and adults continue to turn a blind eye, justifying their inaction by pointing to the right to privacy of the parents. This is written with no scorn towards those professionals who hesitate to intervene. As individuals, we all have our own personal concern 'switches' which flick on when we see adults exposing children to unnecessary danger. Our sympathies are almost always focused on the child, yet we remain helpless in most situations because we respect the parent's right to autonomy.

Danger signals flash all around us. This morning I watched from a car window as a boy of no more than 4 years old stood in the middle of a busy road trying to do up his flimsy anorak, apparently unaware of the traffic swerving around him. I looked around for signs of a responsible adult and saw a woman idly window-shopping a few yards away. As a car sounded its horn she turned and, showing apparently little concern, just said, 'Get back here you little bastard'.

The boy strolled back to the pavement with a chilling lack of acknowledgement of his mother. The mother was young, immaculately made up and well-dressed. Beside her was a pushchair with a toddler asleep, clutching a canned drink and a packet of sweets. The two children may be loved and cared for, but this thirty-second street theatre display made me fear for them both. As I drove away, I wondered what I could have done – perhaps I should have said something to the mother. But then I imagined her response to what she would no doubt see as interference. And perhaps I would have aggravated the situation by drawing attention to her neglect – perhaps she would take it out on the children later. I did nothing.

Whether we are professionals or private individuals, we all find that prevailing social attitudes and our own personal value systems do affect the way in which we assess parents. The neighbours who did not intervene over the 11 year old boy did not believe his living in a squalid house justified their intervention. The above account reveals as much about my expectations of good parenting as it does about the mother and children involved, but it also spells out the very central dilemma of when *can* a parent's fitness be called into question? Given these ambiguous social attitudes, accurate diagnosis of child abuse and neglect through fair and skilled assessment of parents and their children is a challenging task.

WHY ARE CHILDREN REMOVED FROM THEIR PARENTS?

Tens of thousands of children are taken into care each year. By examining the reasons why children have been removed in the past from their parents we get an outline of what constitutes inadequate parenting. Children may be removed when there is evidence of or significant risk of:

- Abandonment
- Neglect
- Physical abuse
- Sexual abuse
- Criminal behaviour of child/parent
- Poor home environment
- Failure of attendance at school
- Failure to protect child's health, e.g. by withholding medical treatment to an ill child
- Inadequate parenting arising from parental illness/disability.

There are some parents whose behaviour towards their children makes them very clearly unfit to be parents in the eyes of society. To that extent there is some consensus over how society should judge parents who abandon their children (as in the recent well-publicised 'home-alone' cases), who continuously neglect their children, who have a diagnosed mental illness which poses a threat to the well-being of their children and those who are unable to stop themselves from violent physical or sexual abuse of children in their care. The consensus is absent over the majority of cases where children suffer or are deemed in danger of suffering harm through occasional acts of neglect or abuse by their parents; that is, in situations which are undesirable but not obviously life-threatening. Then the issue becomes more problematic.

WHO CAN INITIATE INVESTIGATION OF PARENTAL FITNESS?

The answer is that anyone who suspects or witnesses abuse or neglect of children can notify the child protection authorities. Investigation usually arises when a professional (e.g. teacher, police, health visitor, doctor, social worker) notices or is alerted to a particular child's appearance or parent's behaviour. The National Society for the Prevention of Cruelty to Children (NSPCC) is regularly alerted to suspected child abuse by anonymous phone calls. The fact that so many callers choose to remain anonymous shows how ambivalent feelings are towards 'telling on' parents.

Any suggestion of neglect or physical abuse can prompt an initial investigation by social workers. If the initial investigation confirms the need for concern, the seriousness of it will determine whether the child is removed immediately or allowed to remain at home while a detailed assessment is set up. This may result either in planning a course of treatment or, in the beginning, of care proceedings whereby the state is effectively deciding that the parents are unable to meet the child's needs at the time. Courts may ask for expert witnesses such as paediatricians or child and adult psychiatrists to provide independent assessments of the child and/or his parents. The court will then decide whether there is sufficient evidence to justify taking the child into local authority care.

HOW DO PROFESSIONALS ASSESS PARENTAL FITNESS?

Parents whose fitness has been called into question may be assessed by a wide range of professional experts such as social workers, child psychiatrists, paediatricians, teachers, health visitors, magistrates and judges to determine whether they are providing their children with an adequate environment and adequate care.

In the course of the last one hundred years three principal professional frameworks have developed to assess parents and their children; these may be described as legal, social work and medical. The *legal* is governed by the laws of a state and is supposed to provide a general framework applicable to every member of society with equal fairness. It concerns itself with whether parents are breaking any existing laws and how children can be protected by recourse to the courts. The *social work* (as practised by social workers and court welfare officers) is that based on observation of whether a family is conforming to the minimum standards of legally acceptable behaviour and is concerned with looking at the social and economic context of the parenting with a view to alleviating the stresses on families. The *medical* framework (as used by, for example, paediatricians and psychiatrists) concerns itself with clinical appraisal of one or several members of the family in terms of their physical and mental state with a view to seeking out pathology.

In applying these various frameworks it is impossible to know all the criteria that are actually used by professionals but by surveying the literature it is possible to highlight the criteria that are recommended to practitioners as being important in assessment.

The legal framework

Laws are based on assertions of right and wrong and seek to lay down openly available rules on what is deemed by the state to be unacceptable conduct. In the area of family relationships, however, the assessment of right and wrong is far from easy because of the problem of asserting certainty of outcome.

The legal framework endorses the privacy of the parent–child relationship unless there is firm evidence that intervention is required to protect the child. The law is generally reactive – laws are only made when it is felt that without regulation there is the risk of harm and with regulation there is the possibility of minimising the likelihood of harm. It is a relatively blunt instrument of change – to recognise the limitations of the legal framework it is important to remember that the law cannot predict the future; nor can it enforce good family relationships, though it can break them (Goldstein *et al.* 1973).

Professionals have the legal right to intervene whenever there is evidence that a child is likely to have suffered or will suffer significant harm. The extent of the intervention can vary from supportive advice to the parents through to severance of parental access to the children by taking them into care. Before 1991, children coming into care of local authorities in Britain did so under a variety of pieces of legislation, principally:

Section 2 of the Child Care Act 1980 – whereby their parents requested or were persuaded to put them into voluntary care – usually as a temporary measure because of illness, homelessness, death or desertion by parents.

Children and Young Persons Act 1969 – a compulsory court order because the child needed protection or better care or as a result of a criminal offence by the child.

The Children Act 1989 replaced all the previous legislation concerning children coming into care. It is underpinned by the belief in the paramountcy of a child's welfare but also in its endorsement of the family as the best environment for children. It thus urges local authorities to do more to keep children in families and prevent them coming into care. It requires local authorities to do this by safeguarding and promoting the welfare of children who are in need. The details of preventive duties include identifying and catering for the needs of disabled children, taking reasonable steps to prevent neglect or abuse, providing home help, holidays, family centres, counselling, etc. – all to keep children in their families. All this sounds very promising. It remains to be seen whether the resources will be provided to effect such changes and how the definition of 'in need' will be interpreted.

Clause 19 empowers a local authority to provide accommodation for children in need when the person caring for the child 'can no longer do so for any reason' and parents can ask for their children back at any point. This is a significant change to the previous notion of voluntary care, whereby parents frequently lost their rights of access to their children. For compulsory admissions, the local authority or authorised persons (e.g. NSPCC) have to persuade the court that the child has suffered significant harm or is likely to suffer such harm, and the harm is attributable to the standard of care given to the child – being below the standard of care which is reasonable to expect of the parent of a similar child. The court also has to be satisfied that making a compulsory order would be better for the child than making no order at all.

The impact of the new legislation on the challenge of protecting children within their families remains to be seen, but there seems to be a definite move by the state to withdraw from claiming responsibility for all children and to urge and support families to care for their own. The process by which new laws come into being is an interesting combination of political expediency, the particular background of those charged with drawing up a Bill and seeing it through parliament and the influence of lobbyists (e.g. representing child protection and family rights groups). The clauses which receive support and those which disappear before the Bill becomes an Act also reflect the particular composition of the House of Commons in terms, not only of party politics, but personal interests that come from one's own experience of life. Nigel Parton's fascinating account of the passage of the 1989 Children's Bill reveals many such factors; for example, the clause giving more rights to grandparents was at least in part a reflection of the number of grandparents in the House of Commons. It is a salutary reminder that the laws of the land are determined by the subjectivity of a relatively small number of people.

The Children Act 1989 along with other laws (e.g. those relating to divorce) lays down the legal framework within which parents should be assessed when state intervention is required. How individual professionals (social workers as well as lawyers and judges) actually interpret the laws and the courses of action they recommend still remain subject to their individual professional discretion.

The social work framework

State social workers collaborate with health visitors, teachers and others in operating a child protection service for a local authority. It is social workers who take prime responsibility for assessment of parental fitness when there is concern over the welfare of a child, and who preside over case conferences on particular families. Of the three frameworks the social work is the most difficult to describe, as it is not based on any single theoretical or practical body of knowledge. Instead it is a complex mixture based on:

- Psychoanalytically derived theories of normal family relationships.
- Academic, statistically based research into different aspects of family life.

- Various sociopolitical theories.
- Current legislation.
- Previous experience (of the individual practitioner and of the profession as a whole).
- Peer expectations (sometimes described as the particular agency 'culture').
- Society's expectations.
- Values of the individual practitioner.

It is a subjective framework that has been remarkably resistant to attempts to make it more objective. Over the years a number of different instruments for assessing parents have been devised, using scales to measure different aspects of parental functioning. Their names are usually pseudoscientific, e.g. The Heimler Scale of Human Social Functioning, the Conceptual Level Paragraph Completion Test (this measures the way the parent views the world, in particular how they respond to being told what to do and how they react when someone tells them they are doing something wrong, the aim being to find out what degree of structure the parents respond to best). There are other tools which have been used in Britain over the years, some locally, some nationally. It is difficult to know exactly how important these tools are to social workers in building up their individual frameworks.

The social workers' importance lies in their personal involvement with each case and their profession's belief in the possibility of rehabilitation for people in stressed situations. Unlike most other practitioners (such as solicitors or psychiatrists) social workers can get to know families in their own homes, over a period of time. They are thus better able to observe the context in which parenting is taking place as well as the actual relationships. They are usually the only professionals who are responsible both for assessment and 'treatment' in the context of parenting problems and this can give rise to difficulties as to whom they are serving – the state, the parents or the children. There exists an inherent confusion of loyalties which each social worker has to tackle.

Social workers themselves have come to the job from a variety of different routes. Despite their profession's great powers, as individuals they do not enjoy the same status as lawyers and doctors. Yet lawyers and doctors rarely become the target of public inquiries when their decisions result in mishaps – it is the social workers who are publicly called to account, alternately being criticised for being too ineffectual or too powerful.

The individuality of their responses is at once what is recognised as important and simultaneously feared for not being transparently consistent or objective. The deaths of numerous battered children such as Jasmine Beckford, Kimberly Carlile and Tyra Henry in the mid 1980s, and the ensuing public inquiries have led to considerable attention to procedures. The motivation has been as much to protect professionals from accusations of incompetence as to protect vulnerable children. It was the media outcry over the abuse of parents' rights in Cleveland and the subsequent public inquiry that prompted the Department of Health to publish guidelines for social workers carrying out a comprehensive assessment of families where they have been alerted that the children may be at risk (DoH 1989). It is a detailed document which stresses the need for objective information gathering as a check against the social workers jumping to hasty conclusions based on personal prejudices. It is clear that the Department of Health consulted widely amongst professionals in social work, child development and child protection in drawing up this document, so it does represent a professional consensus on assessing minimum levels of parental fitness required by the state.

The document underlines the state's position on intervention:

> It is accepted that the basic needs of children in our society are best met within the family structure

and the state should become involved only when children

> come to the attention of the helping professions because of difficulties they or their families are experiencing.

It also acknowledges the difficulty of assessing parental fitness:

> defining what is unacceptable in parental behaviour presupposes a common understanding of what is normal in terms of parent–child interaction . . . judgement as to what constitutes abuse is therefore in part a matter of degree, opinion and values.

And it warns:

> a balanced assessment must incorporate a cultural perspective but guard against being oversensitive to cultural issues at the expense of promoting the safety and well being of the child.

The guidelines lead the social worker through well over a hundred questions to record information on the following key areas:

- The causes for concern.
- The child (parents' perceptions, daily routines and care, history, physical and emotional development, child's perceptions).
- The family composition.
- Individual profile of parent(s) (background and history, personality and attitudes).
- The couple's relationship (including sex lives) and family interactions.
- Networks.
- Finance.
- Physical conditions.

The professional skill of the individual social worker carrying out the assessment is crucial to how the guidelines are tailored to the individual situation but the emphasis is on observing, not just recording answers. The guidelines also emphasise careful phrasing so that they do not ask leading questions which suggest a right or wrong answer. There are no clues as to what would be considered right answers, but the nature of the questions gives a clear indication of which areas are considered important for the social worker to scrutinise.

It is up to the social workers to assess whether the problem is short term (precipitated by a crisis such as redundancy or bereavement) or an ongoing one with little likelihood of improvement. They may be able to effect service provision such as nursery care for children, home helps or improved housing to help a family through a crisis. The relationship a social worker builds with particular families may in itself help improve the confidence and coping skills of the parents.

In many ways the approach advocated for use by social workers with parents mirrors prevailing beliefs about how parents should behave with their children. For example, the DoH guidelines state:

> They have a right to expect careful assessment of any problems prior to long term decisions being taken. Their views should be sought and taken into account, although engaging them in assessment and planning does not mean a total sharing of responsibility for decisionmaking.

And elsewhere:

> Child protection work inevitably involves the use of authority . . . the positive use of power and authority can be a helpful tool in the therapeutic process as well as a means for protecting a child . . . authority should not however be exercised without responsibility or to excess. An authoritarian and punitive approach will ultimately be destructive.

Another recent DoH publication, *Working Together* (DoH 1988), urges professionals to involve parents more in decisions regarding their children's futures, for example, by including them in case conferences. This has been regarded as good practice for some time but the guidelines appear to be a way of emphasising that it should become more widely practised. The DoH guidelines are still relatively new and it is difficult to assess how widely they have been taken up and prompted more rigorous and fair assessment of families.

The medical framework

This concerns itself with the physical and psychological aspects of children's well-being and occasionally with those of the parents. It has grown out of a large body of research and clinical experience which prides itself on being based on scientific objectivity. It is the growth of medical knowledge that has led the development of child protection law and practice over the past one hundred years and is likely to continue to do so in the future. The medical framework has hitherto provided the most objective means of identifying the parameters of children's physical health and development and relating it to environmental conditions and parental style. (I say 'most objective' but that does not been it has been infallible. Many pieces of medical advice given out to parents in the past have been and continue to be overturned or revised.)

The development of medical diagnostic techniques has been critical to the recognition of the extent of modern child abuse. In the early 1960s, X-ray characteristics were recognised which enabled professionals to distinguish injuries caused by accidents from those caused by deliberate beating. In the 1980s, the 'sudden' recognition of the extent of child sex abuse was at least partly prompted by the discovery of medical techniques to diagnose it. (Not all these have been accepted; the most notable controversy surrounded the technique of anal dilatation used by the paediatricians in Cleveland.) Doctors (such as GPs, those working in casualty hospitals and orthopaedic surgeons) are often the first to notice signs of non-accidental injury or they may be asked to examine a child with a view to providing medical evidence of abuse.

In the future, medical knowledge will be able to show the link between specific maternal behaviour in pregnancy and its long-term effects on the adult health of the foetus. A growing body of literature is already taking shape regarding the effects of what pregnant women eat, what jobs they do, whether they are addicted to drugs, and so on. The more medical science tells society about the importance of the foetal and neonatal period, the more responsibility the mother will shoulder for her child's future well-being.

The bottom line for the medical framework is the prevention of death. Prevention of ill health is a more nebulous aspiration. The World Health Organization definition of health encompasses more than an absence of illness and describes it as a state of optimal physical and psychological well-being. This is an objective which medical knowledge and expertise alone cannot fulfil. It requires a consensus from society as to the values which should be promoted by the state. It is also important to note that the experience of most medical practitioners (with the exception perhaps of health visitors) is not of healthy people but of ill people – nor do most doctors have much experience of seeing people in the context of their normal daily lives. Recognition of the boundaries of the medical framework is thus important in understanding the role of medical practitioners in assessment of families.

The medical framework itself is split between physical and psychological. Society is more alert to the physical aspects of well-being for children, and the state, through its provision of antenatal care, dental check-ups, inoculations and free healthcare, takes reasonable steps to promote children's physical well-being. In cases of suspected abuse or neglect, paediatricians may be asked to give an assessment of the physical development of the child as an indicator of whether or not the child is thriving under his current parental care. There are held to be close connections between quality of parental care and environment and the child's physical appearance and behaviour. Over thirty years ago Dr Mary Sheridan produced a chart describing normal developmental progress for young children from birth to 5 years of age and this is still much used by paediatricians today. I will not reproduce it here, as it forms the basis of much of what appears in childcare books readily available to parents and the public and which is monitored by health visitors and school medical inspections. To a large extent it deals with objective measures that can be considered within the range of 'normal', and is simply a tool for alerting parents and professionals to the presence of significant physical problems or developmental delays.

But how does one measure psychological well-being as an aspect of the quality of parenting a child is receiving? The answers are thought to lie in the powerful legacy of Sigmund Freud. His identification of the subconscious as a stage where the emotions act out the powerful dramas that dictate human behaviour laid the foundation for a psychoanalytical framework by which adults could be understood in terms of their childhood experiences. His particular ideas have been taken and adapted by hundreds of different psychiatrists and psycho-therapists over the decades, but all share this view of childhood emotional experience as being of paramount importance to adult behaviour. Since the 1950s the popular uptake of these ideas has led to an apparent consensus amongst the middle classes throughout western society – it seems so all-pervasive that it is difficult to stand aside from it and wonder how parent–child relationships would look from outside this framework. But the specific theories about how exactly to view family relationships are as varied as the practitioners – professionals such as child psychiatrists, developmental psychologists and psychotherapists. All share the essential difficulty of distinguishing between fact and interpretation.

Child psychiatrists may be asked by social workers or by the courts to provide assessments in certain cases. Their expertise is believed to lie in being able to assess whether a child's emotional and psychological needs are being met and if not, which of the available options is most likely to be the most successful for the child's future development. Occasionally assessments take place at home, but usually (as with other practitioners of the medical framework) they take place at the hospital or clinic.

While the contribution of the psychiatrist is becoming more and more signi-ficant to assessment of parental fitness, many have pointed out that it needs to be used with caution (Black *et al.* 1989, Steinhauer 1983). The specific expertise only can be used – it remains for others to assess whether the child's physical and intellectual needs are being met by the parents. Unlike doctors concerned with physical signs of abuse, their opinions may often be treated with more circum-spection in the courts. Providing evidence of emotional abuse is less easy than producing X-rays showing broken bones (Furnell 1991).

Child psychiatrists look at a number of the same areas as social workers, but from their different perspective. They concentrate on the current emotional state of the child and on the parent–child relationship. They use their clinical experi-ence and their profession's frameworks and ideas about children's emotional needs to assess whether these are being adequately met by the parent(s) in the home environment.

Do the parents view the child age appropriately, or are their expectations un-realistic? Can they tolerate immature behaviour (wetting, crying, demanding)? Do they demand parenting from the child (reversal of roles)? Can they demon-strate empathy with their child? Are their discipline, guidance and comfort techniques appropriate and effective? Do they use distance controls too freely with young children (shouting commands rather than physical removal or distraction)? Are they aware of what can be expected of their child? Can they understand and tolerate normal attachment behaviour? Do they prepare the child for their departure? Do they enjoy the child's company, her development and achievements? Can they meet the child's needs before their own?

Is the child thriving physically and emotionally? Or is she physically and cognitively impaired, fearful, frozen, withdrawn or sustainedly sad, anxious or destructive? When stressed to whom does she turn for comfort?

(Black 1990)

The work of American psychotherapist Vera Fahlberg has been prominent in providing professionals with guidelines to measure the strength of the attachment relationship between child and parent. She has produced checklists of observations to be made for children of different ages and of their parents:

Birth to 1 year

Does the parent

- respond to the infant's vocalisations?
- change voice tone when talking to the infant or about the infant?
- show interest in face to face contact with the infant?
- exhibit interest in and encourage age-appropriate development?
- respond to the child's indications of discomfort?
- show the ability to comfort the child?
- enjoy close physical contact with the child?
- initiate positive interactions with the child?
- identify positive or negative qualities in the child that remind the parent of another family member?

1–5 years

All of above plus:

Does the parent

- use appropriate disciplinary measures?
- accept expressions of autonomy?

Primary school children

Does the parent

- show interest in the child's school performance?
- accept expression of negative feelings?
- respond to child's overtures?
- give support for child in terms of developing healthy peer relationships?

- handle problems between siblings equitably?
- initiate affectionate overtures?
- use appropriate disciplinary measures?
- assign age-appropriate responsibilities to the child?

Adolescents

Does the parent

- set appropriate limits?
- encourage appropriate autonomy?
- trust the adolescent?
- show interest in and acceptance of adolescent's friends?
- display interest in adolescent's school performance?
- display interest in adolescent's outside activities?
- have reasonable expectations of chores and or responsibilities the adolescent should assume?
- stand by adolescent if he gets into trouble?
- show affection?
- think this child will turn out ok?

(Fahlberg 1985)

These checklists are suggested as a basis for observing and understanding the quality of the parent–child relationship. While encouraging a systematic approach to assessment, they clearly leave much room for subjective interpretation; for example, what constitutes appropriate disciplinary measures or equitable handling of sibling problems?

If there is any question of mental instability, adult psychiatrists may be invited to assess parents' mental fitness to care for their children by examining their histories and their relationships with their partners as well as with their children. Mental illness covers a wide spectrum of conditions, some of which are temporary and some of which are permanent, some are treatable with drugs and/or therapy, some can be improved by improving the external circumstances (e.g. better housing or social support) and so on. There is much confusion about which forms of mental illness preclude good enough parenting and the adult psychiatrist may play a significant role in clarifying this with regard to a particular family. As Oates (1984) highlights, there may sometimes be a conflict of interests, in that the adult psychiatrist might put those of his client (i.e. the parent) before that of the child and thus perhaps encourage a family to stay together when a child psychiatrist might recommend that the child be removed. These are issues which cannot be resolved in general terms, other than to reiterate that the state's policy of 'the best interests of the child' is paramount.

There has been a suggestion (Steinhauer 1983) that after such expert assessment parents fall into three categories, each of which implies a certain course of action.

Group A

Providing adequate care and need no further intervention unless specifically asked for.

Group B

Parenting has been adequate until recently although there are serious problems at present.

   The profile that describes most of such situations is:

1 Evidence of basically sound child development with minimal developmental interference on the part of parents.
2 Recent onset of problem causing reduction in parents' abilities to meet child's developmental needs.
3 Absence of a chronic parental psychiatric diagnosis that is untreatable or has a markedly poor prognosis.
4 Evidence of cooperation and openness and a history of being able to seek, accept and benefit from help for a family problem.
5 Ability of parents to accept significant responsibility for their contribution to the development of the problem or their past failures to deal with it.
6 Family members have maintained adequate relationships with extended family, neighbours, or community agencies from whom they can accept advice and support.

The more of these factors that are present, the greater the likelihood of improving parenting capacity by appropriate therapeutic intervention.

Group C

Parents in this group are most at risk of losing their children. The general profile that describes their situation is:

1 Evidence of widespread disturbances in physical, cognitive, language, academic, emotional or social development of children.
2 Problems in development and adjustment have been present for years.
3 One or both parents suffer from a psychiatric illness which significantly affects their parental ability and which has associated with it a poor prognosis.
4 Past attempts to provide help have consistently failed.
5 Parents cannot accept even partial responsibility for the problem.
6 The family is isolated from and unable to accept help or emotional support from friends, neighbours, extended family or appropriate mental health professionals.

The more of these factors that are present, the less likely the chances of improvement by therapeutic involvement.

   This type of assessment of a parent by a psychiatrist can significantly affect the course of action that is then taken by other professionals and/or the court.

Often treatment is recommended (e.g. family therapy, regular visits to a child psychologist) as a condition for the parents to be allowed to keep their children.

The relationship between the three professional frameworks

Over the century, there has been a continuous shifting in balance between the importance attached to the three professional frameworks. For example, post-Cleveland, an increasing emphasis was placed on social workers and police working together:

> While the police and social services became the primary agencies, particularly at the point of investigation, the health experts took on a much more second-ary role and level of responsibility. If child abuse had previously been con-stituted as a disease, and thus a sociohealth problem, the focus now was child protection, which was constituted as a sociolegal issue.
>
> (Parton 1991)

All three frameworks require information to be gathered from professionals asking questions and making observations, informed by their expertise: in a passive sense, by observing the interactions as they happen and, in an active sense, by asking parents and/or children to carry out tasks which gives the assessor an opportunity to see what parenting skills the parent can demonstrate and how the child responds. Having gathered all the information and different professional opinions, the decision whether to take a child into care still remains at least partly subjective, based on assessment of relative risks and availability of resources for treatment and alternative care.

HOW FAIR ARE THESE ASSESSMENT CRITERIA?

There is no doubt that assessing parental fitness is a very complex task because of the huge variety of factors involved. It is rarely an ideal situation to begin with – professional interventions usually begin because a child is already believed to be experiencing unsatisfactory care; thus intervention is to improve on this rather than to find an ideal solution. There is also the awareness that no one can definitely predict the future outcome of any childcare decisions – it is always a matter of assessing relative risks and opting for what appears to be the least detrimental to the child given the evidence available. Whether the criteria are seen as fair has to take into account this uncertainty.

The greatest bar to fairness appears to be the lack of openness about the criteria that are being used. As Adcock and White (1985) wrote:

> The criteria that are used are often not explicit. Professionals have their own standards based on a combination of values, knowledge and case law but these standards are not usually shared. They are not clearly described in text books on the law, medicine or social work. It is uncertain whether there is any consensus of public opinion about a minimum sufficiently good level of

parenting. Consequently parents and children who come under professional scrutiny are very much at a disadvantage. Parents do not know how they will be judged or what they can challenge. It is often unclear what changes they have to make for standards of care to be acceptable.

A bar to openness is the vocabulary and professional status of each group – they both combine to make their expertise virtually impenetrable to an outsider. Fairness also depends on consideration of the parent's perspective in addition to that of the child. That assessments should be therapeutic in their aim is a point stressed by many professionals writing on the subject. They talk of the need not only to protect children but also to protect inadequate parents from the consequences of harming their own children. Thus there seems to be an aspiration to treat the 'unfit' parent as much as the child through intervention – even if such intervention results in permanently removing the child from the parent. The extent to which this aspiration is fulfilled is not clear, but it appears to be subject to the whims of the individual professionals involved. The fairness of the criteria thus rests on:

- To whom they are applied: whether certain groups are more likely to be discriminated against by the professional criteria.
- Why they are applied: the extent to which the professionals are able to make their knowledge, frameworks and value judgments transparent to outside scrutiny.
- How they are applied: to what extent procedures are followed in a professional manner and monitored carefully and the opportunities parents have to be involved in decisions concerning their children's future.

Where those acting in a professional capacity should differ from the average person in the street is in the level of information and experience they bring to their assessments and in the resources they can summon up to effect improvement. How able they are to do this effectively depends on their understanding of the many personal influences that contribute to the way they look at others of a different race, sex, class, age and so on. Their values about how society should ideally function, how mothers, fathers and children should behave, how children should be treated, are all significantly coloured by their own upbringing and life experiences. These cannot be denied but need to be explored, discussed and made explicit so that they do not confuse fact with prejudice. This appears to be little recognised in the training and ongoing education of every social worker and psychiatrist or lawyer.

Another aspect of fairness depends on professionals understanding the needs of children, particularly with reference to their close relationships and their experience of time. This is something that was highlighted by Goldstein *et al.* in 1973 and emphasises the need for judges, social work professionals and parents to have a better understanding of child development and the needs of children at different ages and stages, but this body of knowledge is far from comprehensive and many are questioning the psychoanalytical base on which it rests.

The most important common thread that emerges from a survey of the literature and by talking to practitioners is that fair and accurate assessment depends on the *total* picture, built up by applying a number of tools and employing a number of areas of expertise. The question then is how many different tools are necessary before it becomes a total picture and this depends on the individual case and the individual practitioner, but it is clearly desirable to have more than one person making such momentous judgements.

The total picture means understanding:

- the needs and demands of the particular child (e.g. with regard to the child's age, health, gender, history, relationship with parent, the child's wishes) and informing this with knowledge about what the normal ranges are for children of a similar age.
- the particular circumstances of the parent(s), their physical and mental health, their ability to understand and respond to the child's needs appropriately, their desire and motivation to care for their children, their relationships, and their financial and domestic situation. Again, this needs to be informed by a wider knowledge of adult needs and how good enough parents behave with their children.
- the particular environment of the family, e.g. housing, neighbourhood, family and friend support networks. This needs to be informed by how different aspects of the environment affect parents' and children's behaviour so that other solutions (e.g. finding new housing) are considered to effect improvement.

The three professional frameworks (legal, social work and medical) obviously overlap and need to be used together in assessing a family and building up such a total picture. However, to an outsider, there appears to be little success in doing this in any consistent and planned way. For example, numerous public inquiries into the deaths of battered children repeatedly identified social workers as lacking a full understanding of the necessary legal and medical criteria. The Cleveland Inquiry highlighted the social workers' collusion with the paediatricians in ignoring the legal framework within which child protection had to be seen to work. The inquiry report, referring to the failure of the paediatricians to produce reports for legal purposes, suggested that 'If a doctor does not understand the importance of the report for the police then he or she should leave the recognition and management of child sex abuse to others.'

Social workers have been criticised for not making ready use of unproven 'scientific' medical knowledge (e.g. Jasmine Beckford) and then for using it too readily (e.g. Cleveland). There often appears to be a degree of animosity between the practitioners of the different modes of assessment and a lack of clear guidance on who should be consulted and when. One of the dominating media themes of the Cleveland affair was the lack of unison between the various professionals and state agencies:

Not only were there significant differences between professions, particularly paediatricians, social workers and the police, but there were important differences within professions. This was most evident in the medical profession, where there were heated disputes between two paediatricians, and the police surgeon and subsequently other sexual abuse medical 'experts'.

(Parton 1991)

How consistently are the procedures applied?

All professionals are expected to follow certain procedures in carrying out assessments. The procedures may be underpinned by laws or by codes of good practice but will be affected by the prevailing workloads and external pressures. Previous studies (DHSS 1985, quoted in Parton 1991) have shown that a large proportion of children are removed at times of crisis, often the decision being taken only a matter of days or hours before. This suggests that considered assessment prior to removal has not been the principal procedure experienced by many families. In fact, consistency and fairness of approach are not measured in any rigorous way by the social work profession or by lawyers or psychiatrists.

The Children Act 1989 has made some attempt to make the procedures more consistent. It has simplified the many legal procedures by which the state can intervene and prevent parental access to children. It has also restored the balance of power to parents by demanding that the burden of proof of parents' unfitness should rest with the state agency that has intervened and, if this is not done within a short period of time, the child should be returned to its parents. The hope is to avoid past trends of indefinitely severing parent–child relationships while gathering evidence during which period parents were assumed guilty and often lost their children because they had been 'settled' into new families. (For social workers who suspect that children are being abused, protecting them while getting firm evidence can be hampered by bureaucracy and lack of resources, so the outcome of the new Act may, in fact, offer less protection for children at risk.)

The DoH 1989 guidelines also reflect a serious attempt to make the procedures fairer not just to parents but to children and, to some extent, the individual social worker. They also stress the need to involve other professionals in the 'multidisciplinary network' – presumably to inform their judgement and to make inappropriate subjectivity more transparent.

What sort of parents are considered high risk?

Children taken into care are more likely to come from atypical families (Bebbington and Miles 1989) – to come from poor neighbourhoods, be on Income Support, live in rented accommodation and be living with only one parent. Other factors which appear to increase risk of entry to care are if the mother is under 21 or if the family is large (i.e. over four children), or if the child is of mixed race.

The *reasons* why such families are at higher risk are open to debate and have been the focus of much research. Common sense tells us that security of income, home and marital relationship are likely to make a family more resilient to stresses. Often an improvement in external circumstances is all that is needed to allow people to become fit parents. But there is clearly more involved – not all poor families abuse their children, for example.

Many observers (e.g. Rutter and Madge 1983) have noted the repetition of poor parenting through generations: abused children growing up to be abusing parents – parents who cannot distinguish what is acceptable behaviour because they have not experienced it themselves as children. In surveying the literature regarding the typical characteristics of 'unfit' parents certain terms recur: 'emotional immaturity', 'low self-image', 'unreal expectations of children', 'social isolation' and so on. Abusing or neglectful parents are often depressed and lack a sense of control over their lives – they often lack competence at dealing with the day-to-day aspects of living such as running a home or keeping a job. They tend to have poor support networks within the community and are more likely to move house frequently. Social isolation seems to be a key factor. Being single and poor does not preclude adequate mothering, but being isolated from family and/or community support networks as well seems to tip the scales dangerously in the wrong direction.

The prevalence of stepfathers as abusers has also been noted, though this seems anecdotal rather than proven. Again and again reports of battering and sexual abuse identify the mother's boyfriend as the perpetrator. What is striking is how often the mother colludes. Social workers describe how mothers literally turn a blind eye, sometimes deliberately leaving the house when they know that abuse is about to occur. Their emotional dependency on men who are often immature and jealous implies mothers with unmet needs unable to do what society expects of them – i.e. to put their children first.

But looking at the parental characteristics alone is inadequate: the child's character plays a role too. In the case of child battering, a 'difficult' child is often singled out for abuse while others are not. A child who was born prematurely and/or cries a lot seems especially vulnerable – perhaps because he makes more demands which parents cannot meet.

These recurring characteristics provide, by extrapolation, some of the key features of fit parenting. The overwhelming point of note is that being a fit parent does not always come naturally. A poignant reminder was a recent report of a woman who had stabbed her 6 month old baby to death. In her defence, her lawyer said, 'She wanted the baby and loved it, and did all she could to bring him up properly. . . . She went round Mothercare believing she would become part of motherhood and get close to other mothers' (*Evening Standard* 23/3/92).

It is a sad fact that there have always been and continue to be a large number of parents who do not fall within the socially acceptable end of the spectrum of parenting behaviour. But labels such as 'inadequate' and 'unfit' can add to their social isolation and low self-esteem with further implications for their capacity to care for their children. This is particularly dangerous if one child has been removed but others are allowed to remain with the parent.

Families which are poor and socially isolated predominate as far as child protection teams are concerned. It would be interesting to know how much conscious and unconscious targeting of certain types of families goes on. For example, a family that is living close to the edge is more likely to have contact with welfare professionals. Their professional experience is likely to mean that they are more alert to the possibility of children from such families being at risk and therefore act more readily to intervene. Middle-class families are less likely to come into contact with social services professionals, so any maltreatment of the children is less likely to come to light.

The much reported story of the battered 6 year old Lisa Steinberg, who finally died at the hands of a wealthy Manhattan couple who had illegally adopted her, was a chilling reminder that articulate, middle-class parents are not subject to the same sort of scrutiny as those from poor backgrounds. Despite Lisa's bruises and withdrawn behaviour, nursery teachers and friends did not 'see' the warning signs: 'Child protection agencies were contacted more than once and visited Steinberg's apartment but were fobbed off by his bluster, his class and his status' (Beatrix Campbell, *Guardian* 2/1/89). This is perhaps an indication that professionals find surveillance of groups that they see as different easier to carry out – it is much more uncomfortable to scrutinise your own kind in the same way.

Recent research (Higginson 1990) on decision making in assessment of child abuse cases highlights the distortion of social workers' judgements by their stereotypical ideas about abusers. There is undoubtedly increased public surveillance of parents exhibiting deviancy against community values (e.g. alcoholism, drug addiction, violence and criminality).

> Parents thought to wilfully transgress community values became the subject of heightened concern unwarranted by evidence. Deviant behaviour became confused with abuse. Those parents judged to be unintentional in breaching community values had their behaviour excused and justified. Serious risk was minimised.
>
> . . . The combination of perceptual distortions, deprivation being confused with abuse and inadequate assessments has led to child protection services being overloaded. There was a loss of direct work with families as a result of the cumbersome procedures. Limited resources are squandered when universally applied. There was no prioritisation of cases on the basis of seriousness of risk.
>
> It is not surprising that there is a lack of confidence in the system's ability to offer constructive solutions. This has led to political pressures but the fear of an inquiry adds pressure to complex decision making. This negative social pressure then creates the environment in which perceptual distortions are likely.
>
> (Higginson 1990)

This is a hard-headed plea for society to recognise the limitations of what state agencies can do, given only limited resources and an open-ended brief:

> The current use of the terms 'the child's interests are paramount' and the well being of the child are good principles but they may also encourage unrealistic

attitudes as to what is considered abusive when they are applied to parental behaviour. The best interests of the child can cover almost every non-positive parental action. Inadequate parents who fail to put the child's needs first are in danger of being classified abusive. This encourages the confusion of child care issues with serious abuse. It also encourages personal value judgements about what is 'best' for the child, rather than focusing on the evidence presented.

(Higginson 1990)

In Part II of this book I will be looking at some of the groups that have traditionally been the targets of increased public surveillance and examine how far this is justified. For now, suffice it to note that the surveillance system is predominantly geared to certain sections of the population.

PREDICTION AND PREVENTION OF PARENTAL UNFITNESS

Understanding the characteristics of abusing parents obviously has implications for prevention. If social isolation, poor self-esteem, a premature or handicapped child, unfamiliarity with normal child development and inability to cope with daily living are such crucial factors then these clearly need to be addressed before a parent abuses.

By looking at the sort of families that are over-represented on their caselists, social workers are more alert to targeting the same types of families prior to any abuse occurring. This is particularly true of families who get welfare support prior to having children, e.g. adults who are disabled or single mothers. The most obvious families for concern are those who have previously had a child removed. Various methods for prediction in the postnatal ward have also been proposed by observing how mothers handle their newborn babies. Whether these methods are regarded as sensible precautions or unacceptable intrusions of privacy depend on how openly and sensitively they are carried out as well as on how successful they are at supporting families labelled as risky.

Prediction is no guarantee of prevention but can help welfare agencies to plan longer-term strategies rather than simply deal with crises. It is also a pragmatic response to stemming the expensive flow of welfare-dependent children of the future. There is therefore considerable interest in prediction and prevention. A number of projects around Britain and in the USA have pioneered such approaches and found that the most successful are those that are based on partnership with parents rather than policing or nannying parents. The buzz-word is empowerment.

I was particularly struck by one such project started in 1980 by the Bristol University School of Applied Social Studies and described as the most radical and ambitious parenting scheme in Britain.

'Tackling low self esteem in mothers is the key to providing effective child-care' says the programme director Walter Barker. He aims to intervene in the way that children are brought up not by offering more welfare services but by supporting the mothers' own childrearing skills. By such an approach he hopes to foster self reliance, which he predicts will achieve deeper and more permanent change.

(*Community Care* 14/6/90)

The project has had considerable success using health visitors as the key professionals to build partnerships with parents at an early stage and provide ongoing ideas and feedback on child-rearing and child development. It seems so obviously a good idea, underpinned as it is by a belief in supporting parents rather than scrutinising them. Using health visitors who straddle the social work and medical traditions and work within the family's homes seems particularly valuable, and so far twenty-eight local authorities have taken up the scheme.

WHAT DOES THE ASSESSMENT OF PARENTS OF CHILDREN 'AT RISK' TELL US ABOUT THE EXPECTATIONS OF FIT PARENTS?

Ideal

- Parents love their children and naturally do what is in the best interests of each child.
- Parents conform to the professional expectations of their behaviour with regard to their children.
- Once a fit parent always a fit parent – to any child.
- Parents put their children's needs and happiness before their own.
- Parents do not become over-involved in their children to the point of preventing the children from forming other relationships with their peers.
- Parents conform to the common standard of normal behaviour.
- Parents create their own support networks to ensure their children are adequately cared for.
- Parents have a knowledge of child development.
- Parents know how to run a household, keep a job.
- Parents ensure their children attend school regularly and comply with laws such as those relating to child labour.
- Parents show affection, interest and trust in their children.
- Parents provide a home environment which promotes the physical, emotional and intellectual development of their children.
- Parents know how to set appropriate limits on their children's antisocial behaviour.
- Parents know how to deal fairly with sibling disputes.
- Parents supervise and protect their children from danger.
- Parents bring up their children in such a way that they are not a burden or threat to society.
- Middle-class parents are better than lower-class parents.

Actual

- Parents' behaviour towards their children is affected by their own childhood experiences.
- Parental love does not always come naturally and does not always lead to the protection of a child's best interests.
- Parents have needs which are as important as children's needs – these must be met to enable good enough parenting.
- Parents may be good enough parents some of the time but may also fall below what is considered acceptable at other times.
- Parents may be fit for one child but not another.
- Children have no entitlement to happiness though it may be a desirable goal.
- The nature of the individual child, the individual parents or their particular external circumstances may be such that they need extra support to enable them to be fit parents most of the time. All three need to be considered – it is rarely possible just to look at a person in isolation and say whether or not s/he is fit to be a parent.
- Parents may need to be taught those skills which are deemed necessary for good enough parenting (e.g. running a home, child development, playing responsively, using appropriate discipline).
- Good enough parenting is made more possible by the availability of continuous and familiar support with child-rearing.
- Parents of lower socioeconomic status are more vulnerable to stresses in parenting, but they are also less powerful in their relationship to those who assess fitness. (Middle-class parents are likely to share the values and home backgrounds of the professionals who assess.)
- A sense of control and choice over one's life is important to being able to be a good enough parent.

2   Other people's children
Who's fit to adopt?

In 1989 the *Daily Mirror* reported the case of a 40 year old married man whose application for adoption had been turned down on the grounds that, at seventeen stone, he was too fat. He was quoted as saying:

> 'What a cheek. We have brought up three children of our own as well as fostering twelve others. Now I am told that I am not fit enough to be a father. Not only is it ridiculous, it is also insulting and hurtful'. The Barnardo's spokesperson involved explained the agency's position thus: 'This is certainly not a reflection of his ability to cope as a parent. It is just that in putting a child in long term care we seek parents likely to be of good health for the next 15 years – and his weight could be a risk to the welfare of a child who may have already suffered loss. That is a risk we cannot take. The interests of the child are foremost.'
>
> (Clive Crickmer, Daily Mirror 18/5/89)

The story highlights a number of issues about the selection of who is fit to be a parent:

- There often appears to be a conflict of interests: those of the children versus those of would-be parents.
- There is a gap in understanding between those selecting and those offering themselves for selection as to what the selection criteria should be.
- When selection is being carried out, demands can be made of would-be parents that would not be made of other parents.

In a similar story reported by the *Independent*, an Australian couple who had also been told to lose weight if they wanted to adopt protested: 'They're saying that being overweight might affect our health in the future. But how can anyone guarantee they'll be healthy for the next 15 or 20 years?' (Reuters Report 4/12/86).

One thing is clear: whereas assessment of parents in child protection work is governed by whether *minimum* standards of parenting are in operation, selection of parents for adoption is concerned with finding the *maximum*. Thus adoptive parents need to be not just ordinary parents but extra-ordinary parents – with an emphasis on the 'extra'. Many studies have shown that adoptive parents give their children an advantage over what they would have had with their biological parents (Tizard 1977). This appears to be because adoption generally brings an improvement in socioeconomic status to that of the child's birth parents and also because adoptive parents are generally highly motivated to being parents and therefore invest more attention in making a success of their role. This is what agency workers want to achieve for children by way of compensation for the loss of the blood bond.

While the Australian couple's story deals essentially with the issue of physical fitness for parenthood, selection for adoptive parenthood involves many other fitness criteria – emotional, moral, financial and cultural. The full range of criteria are not legally defined but depend on the availability of children and on the policies of the numerous different state and private agencies. The criteria that are in operation now have their roots in the history of state-controlled adoption, so that is where I will begin.

A BRIEF HISTORY OF ADOPTION

Adoption is probably as old as civilisation itself and has existed in many forms in many ancient cultures. In Roman society, for example, it was considered legal for parents to abandon their children (usually because of poverty) and for wealthier families to adopt them into their own homes, perhaps as slaves. Sometimes they were treated with affection and may have become heirs to a childless couple's property. More commonly throughout the centuries there has been a trade in children for cheap labour and for sexual exploitation. Those adults who chose to take in other people's children were regarded as kindly benefactors whose motives needed no further examination.

For example, in his Declamationes 372, the Roman philosopher Quintilian depicts a foster father who, having severely punished the child he reared, defends himself by arguing that the son 'could not deny that I was his father':

'You were not', he might say, 'my biological father'.
So much the worthier was I then: while others were abandoning their own I was taking in someone else's.

(quoted in Boswell 1991)

The history of adoption is closely linked to the history of children taken into state care. In the Middle Ages, institutional care became the predominant way for the state to deal with abandoned or illegitimate children and the state made no attempt to regulate private arrangements that individuals made over children.

The shifts in attitudes to children during the latter part of the nineteenth century as described in Chapter 1 led to a recognition that abandoned children were better reared in family environments than in institutions. The boarding-out system by which deprived children were sent to live and work for families in return for board and lodging developed the idea of substitute parents as a resource for children separated from their own parents. Some attempt was made to regulate the standards of care that these homes offered by means of inspection:

The choice of home is no doubt a matter of the highest importance. An improper selection is inexcusable as showing either want of care or of judgement. But selection is not the only thing necessary, supervision should come afterwards and it is neither safe nor right to trust even the best selected foster parents.

(Heywood 1978)

The availability of babies for adoption as opposed to children for fostering has been closely linked with attitudes to and prevalence of illegitimacy over the past century. On the whole adoption remained a stigma – the child was tarnished by his illegitimate origins and there was a prevailing belief in the idea that children inherited their parental traits such as criminality and immorality. Adoption was limited to the lower socioeconomic classes until the importance of nurture rather than nature came to be understood in the 1940s – and then it became an increasingly middle-class process.

Adoption as a legally recognised procedure which gave security to adopted children and to their adoptive parents only came into being in 1926, prompted by the large number of children born illegitimate during, or orphaned by, the First World War. The 1926 Adoption Act prescribed certain conditions regarding those who could adopt and specifically stated that any adoption authorised by the court should be for the welfare of the child.

Voluntary societies sprang up everywhere and carried out placements in their own individual fashion, answerable to no one. Eventually a committee was appointed to investigate the methods used by adoption agencies and to recommend on whether their activities needed to be regulated.

The committee, which reported in 1936, gave a number of examples of hastily and poorly contrived adoptions. Some children had been placed with blind, deaf or mentally unstable people or with families that wanted to exploit them. The committee reported that some societies were doing their selection through correspondence without adequate investigations to satisfy themselves of the suitability of the applicants. In outlining the duties of adoption agencies the committee firmly stated that 'the first duty of an adoption society is beyond question to the child'. They added that the child's future was at stake and society therefore should take every reasonable step to satisfy itself as to the suitability of the prospective adopters on all grounds before the child is handed over.

(Triselotis 1970)

The findings and recommendations of the Horsburgh Committee led to the Adoption of Children (Regulations) Act in 1939. This included compulsory registration for all adoption agencies and an obligation that every applicant should be interviewed by suitably qualified people. The modern approach to adoption had been launched and defined the basis of adoption practice for the next fifty years.

In the period following the Second World War, adoption became increasingly seen as a solution to the problem of infertile couples, not simply a problem of finding homes for illegitimate babies. Thus the interests of the adoptive applicants were carefully considered – only babies that were medically fit were placed and if a medical problem emerged after placement it was considered quite acceptable for the couple to return them rather as one would return damaged goods to a shop. There was a great emphasis too on matching children to their adoptive parents in terms of appearance and social background, and this idea of matching has persisted to the present day.

Until the late 1970s most of the children available were babies; the difficult-to-place older, handicapped or ethnic minority children were small in number and most were relegated to institutional care. As the social climate shifted to de-stigmatise adoption, the demand soared and agencies applied very strict rules as to who could adopt – they could afford to be choosy and favoured almost invariably the traditional 'ideal' couple where the husband was the wage earner and the wife the homemaker. This couple was probably in their early thirties, white, able-bodied, with a secure income, no criminal record and no outlandish pursuits – and proven to be infertile. There were plenty of such ideal couples around.

In the past twenty years another shift has taken place. There are now few 'easy-to-place' children (i.e. white babies under 2). As a result of more effective contraception methods fewer unwanted babies are now born and of those that are, fewer are put up for adoption (because of the de-stigmatisation of single parent-hood). If you are fat, a smoker, over 35, a career woman, single, gay or disabled, your chances of adopting a white baby in most western countries are now virtually zero. Those few babies who are available still tend to go to the traditional 'ideal' couples. Nowadays most of the available children are older, many are from ethnic minorities and most have very troubled backgrounds.

At the same time there has been increasing awareness of children's emotional and physical needs and the long-term importance of taking care to see that their best interests are served. These needs are seen primarily as: the need for a stable and affectionate relationship with care-givers within a family environment rather than in an institution; minimum disruption to this relationship, particularly at certain ages; the need to make speedy, but not hasty, decisions concerning their future so that they are not left in limbo; and a growing recognition of the need to maintain links with the birth family wherever feasible. This has caused institutional care to fall from favour and there is now a prevailing desire to get children into families.

It is increasingly difficult, and often inappropriate, to look for the traditional 'ideal' couple for many of the children now available for adoption. Suitable parents are becoming a scarce resource for these sorts of children, so those responsible are having to cast their nets more widely and to look afresh at groups that they would previously have ignored. The need to find 'unusual parents for unusual children' means that assessment criteria and procedures have to be examined more closely so as not to exclude anyone who might be able to provide a secure future for the available children.

Family life is also changing in style and expectations. It is increasingly difficult to make generalisations or long-term predictions and it may be argued that it is more of a lottery now than ever before, because children are dependent on just one or two people to make it work. In the US there is a worrying trend of adopted children being returned when the parents find they cannot cope with them. In Britain the first case of this kind has recently come to light.

ADOPTIVE PARENTS SUE OVER BOY'S HIDDEN PAST

A Midlands couple who adopted a child who proved violent and impossible to manage are planning to sue a local authority and adoption agency for allegedly failing to disclose that he had been seriously abused. The case is believed to be the first of its kind in Britain.

The boy now 12 is back in council care and seems unlikely to be able to lead an independent life. The parents argue that if they had known the boy's history they would not have adopted him. They say their five years of ignorance meant that he was denied the correct treatment which might have saved him.

(Stephen Ward, *Independent* 22/2/93)

All in all there is clearly a greater need for more careful assessment before, and appropriate support after, a child has been placed. Most people today – including would-be parents – can see the importance of selection so that the child will not be endangered or disadvantaged with his new parent/s. But how is it possible to predict which people are fit to be parents and what does this tell us about the expectations of what makes good parents generally?

AN OUTLINE OF THE PROCESS

The vast majority of those seeking to adopt for the first time have been through a period of trying to give birth to a child of their own. In the minds of the would-be adopters the process has thus begun even before their initial approach to an adoption agency. The agency they contact may be chosen because of a personal recommendation or in response to a media piece advertising needy children available for adoption. In Britain there are about 150 adoption agencies, run both by the state through local authorities, and by private, often religiously inspired, organisations.

Nowadays many agencies run informal introductory group sessions open to anyone interested in adopting. These meetings are designed to show the sort of children that are available, to explain the agency procedures and to help people decide whether adoption really is for them. During this time social workers may detect unsuitable attitudes towards adoption and suggest that some applicants withdraw; others will drop out voluntarily. By the time formal assessment for fitness to be an adoptive parent begins quite a lot of self-selection will have taken place – as few as one in ten applicants remains to the assessment stage – perhaps because their circumstances change or because the full impact of what is involved begins to dawn.

Those who remain interested fill out an application form giving basic details about themselves. Posting the application form is often a momentous transition in the lives of those applying to adopt. It launches a period of uncertainty, vulnerability and loss of control while a literally life-changing decision is made – will they become parents to an existing child?

Adoption agencies, however, do not exist to solve the problems of the childless or those who want more children to complete their families. They are there to solve the problem of displaced children who cannot live with their own birth parents for whatever reason. Their task is to place such children in homes where they are at minimum risk of being disadvantaged in the future. The ideal is to find homes where children's particular needs are matched to what the adoptive parents are known to be able to provide.

The assessment itself is carried out in different ways by different agencies. Some depend entirely on interviews and observations by an agency worker in the applicants' homes over a period of time, others use a combination of home visits and outside group work with several applicants together. Triselotis (1970) identified four different types of assessment approaches:

1 *Administrative* (which focused on tangible criteria such as age and socio-economic circumstances).
2 *Investigative* (influenced by insights from psychoanalysis and dynamic psychology).
3 *Educative* (which depended more on self-learning and self-selection).
4 *Scientific* (which relied on elaborate tests and graded results).

Most agencies use some combination of these, but the scientific has fallen from favour and the educative has gained the most amongst the more progressive agencies in the last few years. Little work has been done to evaluate the long-term significance of the different approaches so there is an element of fashion and personal preference that influences different agencies' methods. All assessment procedures require the agency worker to get to know the applicants on a personal level because the parent–child relationship itself is such an intimate one.

In trying to understand the process it is important to appreciate the practical nature of the task facing those whom we charge with tidying up the lives of displaced children. Society expects them to do what it does not expect anyone to do for 'ordinary' children: to predict with which strangers a child will fare best and then launch the child into a new family. It is also important to recognise that the process is driven by different expectations of parents and agencies. The child's own expectations can often be lost in all this – all too often they are kept in a state of limbo while waiting, perhaps in short-term foster care, perhaps in a children's home. The child's own birth parents may or may not be involved in the decisions about where the child is placed. The social worker has to concern herself with 'the best interests' of the child while weighing up all the conflicting risks.

Whether it is state or private agencies who are responsible, they will err on the side of caution for two reasons. The first is to do the best for the child and the second is to be free of any criticism of their decision with regard to the child's welfare. Unfortunately the latter reason may sometimes appear to predominate and may result in more disruption for the child than necessary. It has also prevented willing and suitable parents from being given a chance to show their abilities. At the same time children need to be found homes, so a collision of two processes is now occurring (i.e. having to make selections that will not attract criticism, yet having to cast the net more widely) that seems to have thrown up many dilemmas in who is deemed fit to be a parent. Age, sexuality, race, religion, health, employment, marital status, have all become moveable goalposts for those trying to adopt. Public outcry at unusual placements (often media-incited, such as recent stories involving children placed with gay or strongly religious substitute parents) can create moral dilemmas for those trying to find creative solutions that serve the best interests of specific children. It often encourages them to be conservative and nervous of attempting anything new because they cannot be seen to be taking risks.

The opinions of the agency workers carrying out assessments are rarely called into question if they do not recommend particular applicants. Each agency has to put its recommendations to an adoption panel of independent assessors (a mix of professionals, politicians and representatives of the community, whose names are kept confidential) who have the final say in whether or not applicants are approved as fit to be adoptive parents. These panels have access to training from BAAF (the British Agencies for Adoption and Fostering) to inform their judgements on who should be approved, but they are not obliged to take this training. They may reject a social worker's recommendations, particularly about the suitability of 'unusual' applicants such as those who are gay, single or disabled. If they do so, the people applying have no automatic right to an explanation of the reasons for rejection. (The Children Act 1989 may change this, making all those in local authority responsible for children more answerable.) For those who are approved by the panel, there is still no guarantee of getting a child. Thus even if the assessment hurdles have been successfully surmounted, some parents will be deemed less suitable than others for the particular children available. Some will never become adoptive parents.

If a suitable child is matched with approved parents, the legal step of adoption is usually a formality. Judges rarely question the suitability of adoptive parents unless there is a formal objection by the birth parents. All in all, the social worker carrying out the assessment is deemed to be able to take the major responsibility of deciding who is fit to be a parent and who is not.

CRITERIA FOR ASSESSMENT OF WOULD-BE PARENTS

In the past the assessment criteria were designed to exclude all groups that were unknown quantities as far as parenting ability was concerned. The basis for selecting applicants has been that they must closely resemble society's perception of successful parents – with the best possible future in terms of health, security and material comforts. The argument seemed to be that a child will be best placed in a setting that conforms to society's previous experience of what is normal and therefore most ideal. The unspoken rule is that the child will be placed with parents who will most closely adhere to the conventions of what society considers desirable and will improve on his previous home background.

In 1966, in an important and highly regarded book aimed at adoption agency workers entitled *Parents, Children and Adoption*, Jane Rowe wrote:

> Certain factors are total disqualifications for adoptive parenthood. They are obvious and usually quite easily discovered. Briefly they are: criminal or antisocial behaviour; communicable illness or a disease or disability which seriously affects life expectancy or physical activity; mental illness or severe neurosis; a standard of living too low for the safety, health and normal development of the child.
>
> (Rowe 1966)

In selecting families she pointed out the need to find couples (rarely could spinsters be considered) of good moral standing who had been married for at least three years, who were lacking in any obvious neuroses (e.g. she states that very houseproud women rarely make good mothers), and who would be able to provide financial and emotional security to the adopted child. She indicated a preference for a wide geographical separation between birth and adoptive parents to minimise the possibility of their paths crossing in the future.

Rowe emphasised the need to discover the true motives of the applicants' desire to adopt and not merely to accept at face value their own explanations. On the whole, she prescribed a flexible approach that depended on the agency worker getting to know the applicants in their homes by talking to them and observing them. She did not mention the suitability of wives or single women who go out to work, or of gays – presumably because at that time such people would not have tried to apply.

A quarter of a century later, most agencies still employ most of these criteria in assessing who is fit to adopt a baby and many of these criteria for who is fit to adopt an older child. The only legal requirements in Britain are that the applicant be over 21, resident and domiciled in this country – everything else is left to the adoption agencies to decide who is suitable. Each agency has its own way of working and particular criteria that may be peculiar to it – thus would-be adopters who are rejected at one may not be at another. For example, most agencies have a policy about age (not more than forty years' difference between child and parent), some specify geographical boundaries, some are restricted to applicants of particular religious denominations and so on. For non-baby adoptions there is a slowly increasing flexibility towards non-traditional applicants, e.g. women who work, older people, people who are single, gay or disabled – factors which would have previously entailed outright rejection. The criteria employed are also underpinned by the growing recognition of the nature of the many differences between 'ordinary' parenthood and adoptive parenthood.

Adoptive parents are different. There is much that substitute parents will have in common with parents who care for their own children: the desire for a satisfying family life and for the position this brings in society, the need to love and be loved by children, the desire to contribute to children's well-being and to help them make the most of their opportunities for success and happiness. However, the prospective adoptive parent is different from most birth parents in a number of respects (and this is acknowledged by agency workers when making assessments); most adoptive parents have had a particular type of emotional history associated with not being able to give birth to their own children. Many will have undergone the stresses of medical investigations and treatment, perhaps over several years. The motives and feelings about becoming parents may be confused, and the relationship between a couple may have become skewed by the overwhelming desire to found a family. The arrival of a child may be seen as the solution to a whole host of problems.

Becoming an adoptive parent is hard – there is no pregnancy in which to prepare but instead a tumultuous period of uncertainty preceding the placement. There are additional stresses associated with adoption that do not arise with children who are produced through birth; for example, there is no automatic sense of authority, affection and lifelong commitment that the biological bond usually confers. For those who are ill-prepared, these differences can produce overwhelming stresses and could result in a disastrous situation for child and parent if an adoption were allowed to happen. So ultimately the interests of the would-be adoptive parent and the adopted child are the same – and it is for the social worker to help all applicants realise this.

Children needing substitute parents are different. In the days when most adoptions were of babies, the issue of the child's needs was limited to his future security. Little attention was paid to the child's pre-adoption history beyond his health and likely inherited traits. The work of Bowlby and others had alerted social workers to the need to place the baby as early as possible and to avoid disruption thereafter. The job of the social worker was a relatively straightforward one of finding a good home from a selection of many hundreds and then leaving the chosen parents to get on with it.

Today, things are very different because most of the children are older. Any child other than a newborn baby who has been separated from his first care-giver will be 'different' to a greater or lesser extent and need special attention from all those subsequently responsible for his welfare to adjust to a new relationship and a new life.

Past experience has shown that the chances of successful adoption are best when a newborn baby is placed with a highly motivated and well-prepared couple. The earlier the adoption, the more closely it simulates the desirable parent–child relationship.

> Under ideal conditions adoption provides the child with continuity of affection and care, stimulation and protection leading to trust and confidence in the new parents. It provides the adoptive parents with satisfying responsibility, fulfilment and permanence in their relationship to the adopted child.
>
> (Nordhaus and Solnit 1990)

This mutual satisfaction of needs is easiest when the demands of both adoptive parent and adopted child are of a measure that can be accommodated. The older the child, the more he will remember of his past life, the more ingrained will be his habits and the more it will take for him to trust a new relationship. Much work is being done on trying to understand exactly what the needs are of such children which make them different from children living with their birth families. One of the obvious differences is brought about by the simple fact of the failure of the biological bond with the birth parents which is so highly regarded by society. The experience of rejection is a great knock to a child's sense of self-worth. Most of the children will have suffered emotional disturbance prior to their placement.

Many of the children may have been abused by previous caretakers. Their physical, emotional and intellectual welfare is likely to have been jeopardised: the all too common pattern of rejection and repeated upheaval soon leads to anxiety and distrust in the future – substitute parents need special skills to restore a sense of security and optimism. It is estimated that 50 per cent of teenage placements fail. Given the scale of the necessary adjustments for both adoptive parents and children, it is impressive if 50 per cent succeed.

The adoptive parents' acknowledgement of difference and their preparation to deal with it are vital to the success of a placement. The social worker, whether working in a state or private agency, is expected to be trained to be aware of the different nature of the adoptive family and to avoid merely trying to replicate a 'normal' family of parents and their natural offspring. All these factors affect the criteria employed for selecting would-be adoptive parents.

THE FORMAL BASIS FOR SELECTION

In Britain, filling in Form F with the social worker is the formal stage of outside assessment. The British Agencies for Adoption and Fostering (an umbrella organisation for state and private adoption agencies) originally designed Form F, and the 1983 version has recently been updated (1991) to reflect shifts in general attitudes and in the circumstances of children available for adoption and fostering. Obviously, the mere issue of a new Form F will not change assessment processes overnight but it does herald a change in approach and aspiration which is significant.

The most striking aspect of revisions is that they reflect a greater under-standing of the variety of modern family life-styles and have dropped or revised questions which seemed to reflect too narrow a vision of what is ideal; for example, there are more references to disability and ethnicity and to the wider support structures available to a household. The new Form F also appears to reflect the changes in understanding in wider society (e.g. awareness of sexual abuse, recognition of importance of contact with birth family, wider acceptance of different types of families) as well as much more specific acknowledgement of the particular types of children available (i.e. disabled/from ethnic minorities/ older). There appears to have been an attempt to minimise value-laden language, e.g. the new form has dropped references to whether applicants are 'cuddlers or touch-me-nots', and refers to 'birth' parents rather than to 'natural' parents.

There is also a significant shift to getting applicants to think about their own views, behaviours and expectations rather than just for the agency worker to investigate them – so there appears to be a firm intention for the process to be a preparation as much as an assessment. This is very different from the assessment processes of the not-so-distant past, where the intention seemed to be to weed out and exclude anyone on the slightest whiff of doubt. (Helen Caine (1990) quotes Shaw: 'Church going couples in their mid-thirties with proved infertility and otherwise blameless lifestyles might even in the late sixties still ruin their chances by indulging in a weakness for garden gnomes.')

Different agencies may use different forms, but almost all are looking at the same areas that Form F covers. Part I of the form asks for factual information concerning age, marital status, ethnic origin, religion, occupation, income, hours of work, health, type of accommodation and neighbourhood – and who already lives in the household. It gives no clue to what is acceptable in the eyes of the agency with regard to the responses to these factual questions. It is stated that a check of criminal records will be carried out but does not state what would happen if past offences were found. It also asks for two personal references for the applicant/s and asks the agency worker to comment on each referee's views of the applicants' ability to understand and relate to children, to perform the tasks involved, whether they think the applicants will be able to ask for help/support and whether they have any reason to believe that the applicants might physically or sexually abuse a child.

It is Part II that is the descriptive report which calls on the agency worker's experience to formally assess the applicants as to their suitability to be adoptive parents. This is effectively a structured way of observing what are deemed to be the important aspects of the applicants' lives. The final assessment does not strictly take place until Form F is submitted to the panel, although, since the applicants do not usually meet the panel, the observations of the social worker are all important to the final assessment of suitability. A lot of thought obviously went into designing the checklist for this and it makes fascinating reading – it indirectly tells a lot about the expectations of how successful family life happens. I am going to examine this in some detail for two reasons: to show what criteria are deemed relevant, and to see what they tell us about the expectations of all parents.

FORM F PART II

(*The asterisks are mine and denote sections which are new to the 1991 Form F.*)

1 Individual profile on each applicant

a) Background of each prospective parent (family of origin, childhood experiences, significance of culture/ethnicity, religion and language in upbringing. *Attitude to own disability/experience of people with disabilities. Assessment and feelings of and feelings towards own upbringing and family relationships).

b) Education – type of school, views on own experience of own education, qualifications.

c) Employment – work experience, attitude to work, present job and plans for future. *Views on work/unemployment as it relates to family life/ family roles.

d) Interests/talents: what? when? who with? amount of time involved.

e) Personality: self-presentation – how do the applicants see themselves – include ethnic identity.

*2 Support networks

Asks for a general picture of the support systems used by the applicants including extended family, friends, godparents, neighbours, religious activities, community groups, clubs, etc. It then asks for an indication of the most significant systems and their importance for the applicant/s in relationship to the proposed child placement.

*3 Children in household

A description of each child is requested (general impression of personality, how they see themselves – including ethnic identity, temperament and any special talents and needs). How much they have understood and been prepared for the proposed placement. It also asks for a description of any special relationship between a particular child and a parent or between children.

*4 Other adult members of the household

(Including grown-up children living at home or in regular contact; and any significant person not living in the house.) For each adult, a description is suggested of: how much time they spend within the home, their role/ relationship to the applicant/s and family members. Whether they are likely to remain part of the household long term and what their attitudes are to the proposed placement.

5 Previous relationships

The form asks for a description of previous significant relationships and their outcome. It also asks about any children of previous relationships, what difficulties they experienced and details of the contact that now exists. *It also asks if these children know about the proposed placement and, if so, what their attitude is.

6 Present relationships

This asks for a description of the strengths and resources of the applicant/s and for details of the most significant relationship, how it developed and what makes it stable and satisfying to the applicant/s. Within the relationship it asks how they deal with problems/stress/decision making/ disagreements/anger, and what the possible areas of strain are. It asks too how the roles are distributed and *how this relates to the applicants' culture/ upbringing and how they support each other.

7 Description of family life-style

*This suggests the agency worker should outline what the family considers important (e.g. how important are religion, cultural customs or practices as these relate to everyday life?). How the family shows affection, whether there exist special roles in the family, whether gender roles are stressed (e.g. a stress on femininity for girls/toughness for boys), *their attitude to food/awareness of nutrition. *It asks how important educational achievement and homework are, and whether this is linked to a wish for the betterment of a child.

With regard to special occasions it asks how they are celebrated, *and whether there are any hobbies or leisure activities that the family undertakes as a whole group. *It also asks what languages are spoken at home.

*This section also deals with race and racism and asks questions about family attitudes to race and how they will ensure an anti-racist approach to parenting.

8 Parenting capacity

Description of the applicants' experience of caring for or working with children, their adjustment to parenthood, their understanding of child development (*and how children in care may differ); use of own childhood experience – what would be repeated and what would be changed? *Experience and understanding of adapting parenting skills to meet the needs of individual children.

* Applicants (including those with disabilities) are asked for an assessment of their own parenting strengths or potential, or if they have only limited or no direct experience of caring for children.

* Whether this is an open or relatively closed family unit in relation to other people involved in the parenting of children.

* With reference to physical and sexual abuse: how will the applicants ensure that a child will be safe in their family and wider support networks? It also points out that family attitudes to nudity /who baths a child may be of significance to a child who has been sexually abused.

* Behaviour management: what are the rules of the household, what sort

of punishments are there and who decides them? How do the applicants show approval/disapproval?

 * What consideration have the applicants given to their proposed form of discipline (e.g. sending a child to his bedroom may have a more detrimental effect than envisaged, dependent on the child's previous experiences and expectations).

9 Childlessness/limitation of family size

This is an exploration of the history, experience and attitudes of the applicants to being childless. In particular it asks to what degree they have come to terms with their childlessness/inability to have further children and asks whether they are aware that they may never come to terms with this fully. It also asks for details of applicants who are choosing to adopt rather than to give birth to their own children: why and how they have come to this decision.

*10 Agency support/financial considerations

This asks about the applicants' attitudes to and management of money – if they give up work how will they cope with loss of income? If the applicant/s does not have the choice/wish to give up work, who will be involved with the care of the child? If the employer is not sympathetic to applicants and unpaid leave has to be taken during introductions, what can the agency do to provide financial assistance? This section also deals with what the agency will be able to provide in the way of support after a placement.

11 Placement and post-placement considerations

a) Background factors: *what understanding do applicants have of social pressures contributing to children coming into care? What is their appreciation of the effects of separation/loss/lack of attachments upon children? What are their feelings about heredity? What is their attitude to mental health? Do they have an understanding of the social pressures contributing to mental ill-health? Can they accept a child where little is known about the father and/or the mother?

 b) Child as *she/he is: this section lays out in detail those factors likely to arise in the adoption of children and asks the applicants' attitudes to these:

Identity problems
Sexual abuse
Puberty/adolescence
Medical problems
Physical disabilities/learning difficulties

c) Contact with birth family/people from the child's past.

It asks about the social worker's assessment of the applicants' willingness and capacity to maintain links with the natural family or other people from the child's past.

*12 Post-adoption

This deals with the issues of how applicants will deal with the adopted child's future attitudes to being adopted.

Social worker's assessment

Finally, Form F asks for the social worker's assessment of the applicants – in particular, the expressed motivation to adopt/foster the skills they have in relating to/working with children and what sort of children the applicants would probably do best with; how they will work with the agency and with other officials, with birth parents and other contacts of importance to the child; the strengths and resources of the applicants and the areas where they may experience difficulty.

It also asks the worker to record any point of disagreement between herself and the applicants. *For minority ethnic applicants, it asks for a statement about the type and involvement of minority ethnic professionals in the assessment.

(Details of Form F reproduced with the kind permission of BAAF)

DISCUSSION OF FORM F AND THE ASSESSMENT PROCESS

'No adult has the right to a child but every child has a right to as stable and happy a home as it is possible to achieve.'
(The then junior Health Minister Virginia Bottomley in 1991, announcing a tightening of controls on foreign adoptions)

This belief underlies all assessment procedures – the adoption agency, whether private or run by the local state authority, owes its first duty to the children on its books, not to would-be parents. Agencies have to look at the particular children they have and try to match these with the best homes possible. The selection process is thus not just a matter of finding people who would be fit to look after children, but fit to look after the particular children available. For example, there are many middle-class white couples who want to adopt but many more children from lower-class, non-white backgrounds available for adoption. The agencies' aim is to expand the number of lower-class applicants of different ethnic backgrounds rather than to satisfy the needs of the childless middle-classes. If they are unable to do this, then a child may be matched on other criteria, given the available applicants. From the perspective of the would-be parents this process can seem unfair, since it is based on many assumptions which cannot be tested.

The process by which Form F is completed is as important as the criteria observed. For example, it is implicit that the very gathering of such detailed information is a safeguard in itself; the time-scale is recognised as needing to be a matter of months rather than weeks to allow adjustments and reflection to take place on the part of the applicants and the social worker. It is also important to note that the form is designed not just to weed out unsuitable adoptive parents but to provide the information that can be used between agencies to match available children with the most suitable applicants.

Although most agencies use some version of Form F to carry out the assessment of applicants, there is a very wide variety of procedures and skills brought to bear in each case. Some agencies offer preparation to all applicants, some offer nothing. Some involve applicants in the assessment process, others carry it out as a private investigation by the agency.

Prevailing criticisms of the assessment process

The assessment process is the subject of ongoing debate within the field of adoption and has been criticised from both within and without.

Social workers' own attitudes

While the Form F checklist criteria seem sensible, it depends on the sensitivity and perceptiveness of the social worker as to what weight she gives to positive and negative feedback she picks up. The values that each social worker holds are a combination of her own personal experiences of family life, her range of professional experience and the prevailing values of the agency for whom she works and of society as a whole.

It is thus hardly surprising that the selection process is not consistent even within one agency. There are some rules about fair play that are expected by all applicants and by society at large for the selection procedure. For example, Rowe quotes Dorothy Hutchinson:

> the social worker engaged in homefinding should have released her childhood parents from her professional life. She must be emotionally free to make judgments that are neither coloured by a need to appease her own parents nor always to find replicas of them.

(Rowe 1966)

Social workers may fall into the trap of seeking applicants who conform to an ideal, who do not reflect diversity of real family life. Caine describes the preponderance of social workers age 30–50 who have been brought up in the traditional family households of the 1950s. The ideal of a traditional family where husband was provider and wife was homemaker and childcarer was more widespread in the 1950s than it is today, when only 7 per cent of households resemble this model. As time goes by more and more social workers will have personally experienced a greater diversity of family lives themselves and this will inevitably affect the insights they bring to bear on adoption work.

The professional training a social worker receives should alert her to a self-awareness of her prejudices, but there appears to be little systematic acknowledgement of this. For example, Macaskill (1992) describes the unfamiliarity of most social workers with mental handicap and the resulting limitations this places on them when trying to find homes for mentally handicapped children.

The other vital area which is slowly being addressed is the difference between background (particularly class and ethnicity) of social worker and that of applicant. The description of family life-style could be very skewed by a white English person looking at an Asian family, for example. This has been recognised, but it is difficult to change until more mixed backgrounds are reflected in the social work profession.

The social worker's role has changed profoundly from being that of a voluntary and amateur 'do-gooder' to a trained professional who is required to take a very high degree of responsibility in increasingly complex circumstances. The number of factors she has to consider has escalated at great speed, requiring a much higher level of information and training than ever before – all at a time of shrinking resources. It would be very easy to be frozen by fear of failure of placements into not attempting 'risky' ones at all.

Checking police records

One of the areas which poses concern is the checking of criminal records. Since the 1950s adoption agencies have had the legal obligation to make enquiries of the police to check whether the applicant has been convicted of any offence which would render it 'undesirable' that the child should associate with him and this has been extended to include checking the records of all other adult members of the applicant's household.

> As the police make no judgments on the records they send through to the local authority, all offenses however serious or trivial are included. Apart from the clearly serious Schedule 1 offenses of assault on children, the scope for subjectivity on the relevance of offenses immediately comes into play. Do you rule out applicants with offenses relating to dishonesty, fraud, drugs, theft etc? Are such people going to provide good role models for the children in their care, even if they can provide safe and sound childcare?
>
> (Hebenton and Thomas 1990)

As police and social workers increasingly collaborate in child protection work, so the informal channels for communicating are increasing. In the absence of clear guidance as to which offences are deemed acceptable and which are deemed unacceptable, there is a fear that criminal records can be misused:

The problem is one of ensuring the welfare of a child, as well as having an eye to the freedoms and civil liberties of adults. The decisions made every day are ones made largely without the benefits of training or any deep consideration, beyond the immediate and cautious imperative to 'take no chances'. Approval decisions on households are not solely determined by criminal checks, but they are an important element of the process that deserves wider airing than they have received in the past.

(Hebenton and Thomas 1990)

Lack of standardisation and accountability

The variety of procedures means that prospective parents are vulnerable to the whims of the individual agency and of the prejudices of the individual social worker.

A researcher, Julie Selwyn, recently carried out interviews with a number of couples who had been rejected by a local authority adoption panel during the 1980s. Apart from highlighting how deeply these people were hurt, her survey illuminates the gap in understanding between applicants and adoption agency workers about how selection takes place.

They did not know what to expect from an adoption assessment. They expressed worries – would previous marriages or difficult childhoods count against them? Would sterilisation be viewed as their own fault and make them unworthy of a child? One wife thought that the purpose of the assessment was to 'find flaws in my character'. However in spite of fears of prejudice and a general mistrust of social services departments, there was a belief that initial impressions (if unfavourable) would be ignored by the adoption officers, as their training would enable them to encourage an applicant's true personality to shine through.

(Selwyn 1991)

Each family's experience of assessment was distinct, as each had a different adoption officer. One particularly poignant story is that of a family with three children who had applied to adopt and who had been enthused and encouraged by the assessment process. The adoption officer was respected and liked – she showed them their Form F and told them they had a 99.9 per cent chance of approval. The children and parents excitedly awaited the panel date. It came and went with no call from the social worker. Eventually they received a letter stating they had been rejected. The social worker did make one further home visit to try and explain the reasons for rejection but did not include the children in this meeting. The reason they were given made no sense to the couple:

They were told that the panel thought they were a family of achievers and that, therefore, an adopted child would have difficulty fitting in. The husband felt that a reverse form of snobbery seemed to be in operation – 'If we'd lived in a council house on benefits, we'd be ok. We'd done too well and were being penalised.'

(Selwyn 1991)

The experience of rejection has continued to reverberate and affect the relationships within that particular family.

> Ten years on the panel letter had been kept and shown . . . with the same feelings of hurt, injustice and incomprehension . . . [the couple] found advertising campaigns for adoptive parents upsetting: 'if they're so desperate we must have been awful.'
>
> (Selwyn 1991)

In another of her case studies, Julie Selwyn describes a couple who felt instantly disliked by their adoption officer.

> They described the home visits as 'edgy and tense, like we were being interrogated'. . . . The questions asked were not always understood and were described as 'too psychological and academic . . . like she was quoting the last text book she'd read.' They felt their adoption officer had not got to know them at all and they knew little about her: 'one, she hated Christmas; two, she was single.' They did not have the opportunity to attend any group training sessions.
>
> (Selwyn 1991)

The home visits became increasingly distressing and near the end of the couple's assessment the adoption officer told them that 'there was no point putting our Form F in, as it would be thrown out but she would any way to give us a chance.' They were not allowed to read their Form F and were told not to bother asking for a reason if they were rejected as 'no one will tell you the reason'. The couple retained a sense of optimism, believing that the panel would see positives in their Form F and ignore the adoption officer's view. On the day of the panel decision they had a telephone call from their adoption officer informing them they had not been approved but giving no further details. They had no further contact with her. They were left imagining their own reasons:

> Mr B thought he had answered the questions wrongly and expressed himself badly. Mrs B thought it was her fault for being overweight or for something in her family background. She said 'I felt as though they'd thrown me in a dustbin'.
>
> (Selwyn 1991)

Over the past two years I have also spoken to people who have been assessed and rejected by adoption agency workers. Many have had more positive experiences than those described by Julie Selwyn, but even they have focused on the feeling of vulnerability that is brought about by the process. One woman described the social worker as being 'visibly hostile to our middle-class lifestyle. She wanted proof that we had stopped all fertility treatment and that I would give up work if approved for adoption'. Another man spoke of 'the long uncomfortable silences during the adoption worker's home visits – as if she wanted to break down our defences'. One woman who uses a wheelchair described the agency worker's intrusiveness: 'she wanted to see how I managed in the bathroom, how I got dressed – it was as if she couldn't believe me and my husband when we told her that I had coped perfectly well for thirty years'.

Other critics of the prevailing assessment methods have suggested that there is a bias in favour of articulate, well-educated people, as there is much emphasis on 'verbalising' one's feelings and taking a particularly intellectual approach to assessing one's life. This may be seen as merely unfair – or positively dangerous, in that it may exclude exactly the sort of applicants who are desperately needed for certain types of children. For example, Catherine Macaskill has very cogently described how children with mental handicaps often thrive with just such parents who are not particularly articulate or apparently very intelligent but who have the requisite practical skills and acceptance of the child's limitations (Macaskill 1982).

Professionals need to listen to what parents want

Julie Selwyn describes the criticisms voiced by her interviewees.

> Couples would have preferred assessments where they could have been active participants, and based on their present lives. Lengthy theoretical discussions were disliked, with many not understanding the connection between the questions asked and the purpose of the assessment. . . . Couples suggested involving those who were already adoptive parents in the assessment and having the opinion of more than one assessment officer. Several suggested that assessment should concentrate on lifestyle and networks (meeting friends and family, sharing activities).
>
> The role of the panel also came in for much criticism. They were felt to be distant and unaccountable for their actions.
>
> (Selwyn 1991)

There is much dislike of the methods employed to inform applicants of their rejection, and most feel they have a right to an explanation in a face-to-face meeting. The loss of control while decisions were taken and the manner in which the agency treats its applicants can seriously undermine future confidence. The parallels with being rejected for a job are apparent here. In fact one social worker highlights this after her own experience of the selection process:

> I know of no other jobs where interviews take place without the candidate being present. For a group of professionals to spend an hour discussing an applicant whom only one of them has ever met can not only be described as inefficient, if not to say ludicrous but bears a striking resemblance to those occasions when natural parents were/are not invited to case reviews on their children in care.
>
> (Blunden 1988)

In many cases, the likelihood of rejection as baby adopters leads would-be adopters to seek children abroad. Claire Anderson of the support network Stork argues that while social workers are understandably concerned with placing older and handicapped children on their lists, people who want to rear young children also have rights; she believes that prospective parents need to have an equal rating if adoption is to succeed: 'You can't just talk about the needs of a child in adoption. The parents have to have as great a need for the child as the child has for them' (*Social Work Today* 15/2/90).

This brings us back to the issue of children versus parents. The agencies have been quick to point out that their first duty is to the best interests of the child – but should that necessarily imply that the rights of the would-be parents are negligible? The basic rights that Julie Selwyn's interviewees wanted were: 'The right to read Form F in private; the right to know the reason for rejection; the right to appeal to an independent body; but most of all to be treated with respect.'

NEW APPROACHES TO FINDING ADOPTIVE PARENTS

The guidelines accompanying the new Form F go some way to recognising these rights and encourage a more collaborative and wide-ranging approach to assessment. Murray Ryburn in particular has been influential in promoting a new approach to assessment – one which acknowledges that social workers have no superior knowledge base nor any proven methods to objectively assess fitness to be a parent. The picture he presents is one of applicants trying to second-guess the social workers and the social workers trying to second-guess the panel as to what is required to appear to be a fit parent. In a wide-ranging critique of the prevailing methods of selection he presents the argument

> that the observer is always part of and inseparable from what they observe. This view would hold that there is no point of detachment from which we as social workers or panel members can reach an objective decision about the best interests of children, or the suitability of some, and not others, to adopt. Our conclusions will not be a reflection of any objective truth or reality. They will reflect only at one particular time the individually and collectively held idiosyncratic views of assessing social workers and panel members about what the truth is about the suitability of prospective adopters. At another time, with different or even the same assessors, the assessment could have shown quite a different view of objective reality.
>
> (Ryburn 1991)

The consequence of admitting that there is no objective method of assessing parents is that different approaches to finding parents need to be explored – ones which protect the interests of the children but share the responsibility for them more evenly with those people who are likely to have to live with the decisions in the long term – i.e. the would-be adoptive parents and the birth parents. Murray Ryburn describes how this approach was put into practice in his native New Zealand:

> We were committed to the idea that today's not-good-enough adopters by some formal assessment process could become so with the right help and support. We were convinced that like the rest of us different would-be adopters have different learning styles . . . we focused therefore on different

forms of group work to create opportunities for participants to learn in the same group processes from the shared wisdom of others.

(Ryburn 1991)

Medical examinations and statutory enquiries were carried out but beyond that it was agreed that if the applicants completed the agency programme they would be available to be chosen, not by social workers, but by birth families as adopters. Other changes he proposed were to allow prospective adopters to participate fully in the panel process and to involve the extended family of the birth parents in reaching a decision on the child's future.

These ideas have yet to be taken up on a significant scale in Britain but they are none the less moving the process in the same direction as the 'discovery' of the importance of openness in adoption. The actual content of assessment programmes that are preparatory and educative as opposed to investigative remains in the realm of individual agencies to determine. What sort of techniques could they use and do these tell us anything about how to prepare people to be fit parents?

Anne Hartman, another proponent of a more participatory approach to assessment of adoptive parents, in her book, *Finding Families – An Ecological Approach to Assessment* (1979), presents a number of exercises that can be used with would-be adoptive parents and families to help them and the agency worker to understand their situation and expectations in a manner that is of benefit to all, whether or not a placement is the outcome. There are devices that she suggests to explore the family in its environment, the family over time and the dynamics within a family. For many families such an assessment process may be the first time they have actively and jointly explored their own situation and their desire to adopt. It can provide an opportunity for them to understand and resolve their differences as well as to see more clearly the resources they have to offer an adopted child. For the agency worker too it provides a demonstration of what the applicants have to offer so she can see more clearly what sort of child would match their particular situation.

The hope is that for the majority of applicants they will come to understand better their own suitability as adoptive parents and withdraw if they no longer feel adoption would be right for them in their current situation. In a few cases, the agency worker and the applicants may disagree:

> When this differing view of the appropriate decision emerges through the joint assessment process the worker's opinion is based on his or her knowledge of the family, its needs expectations and style. The worker can say with conviction and honesty, 'it just won't work'. The judgement is not based on the view of a family as 'good' or 'bad', as 'functional' and 'dysfunctional', but simply on a prediction that for this family adoption would not work.

(Hartman 1979)

Ann Hartman's work has had a major influence on the new Form F (as can be seen from new sections I have marked with an asterisk) and her approach to assessment of adoption applicants has captured the prevailing mood amongst those who wish to see the adoption process shift away from selection based on 'gatekeeping'.

Such participatory approaches to assessment require greater skills from the agency workers to be effective and this has implications for training and costs. However, they also offer much in the way of increased job satisfaction as pointed out by many social workers who have been involved in new collaborative methods (e.g. Stevenson 1991).

Some agencies have been more ready to adopt new methods than others. Voluntary agencies such as Barnardo's have spearheaded innovative approaches to selecting adoptive parents and there seems to be a general shift towards a greater flexibility and the notion that 'for a whole range of children, a whole range of parents may be suitable' and that it would be foolish to exclude anyone arbitrarily. The BAAF position is that no one has a right to a child but everyone, regardless of age, sex, marital status, race, etc., has a right to apply and be treated sensitively and fairly. In practice, the shift within individual agencies is happening slowly and haphazardly. How much these changes affect practice remains to be seen but what is clear is that, for some time yet, there will continue to be a wide variety of approaches to selection with little regard for 'standardisation, equity and quality assurance' (Selwyn 1991). There is without doubt a need for more information from long-term studies of children who have been adopted to see which factors seem to be most crucial in successful placements.

For my purposes, adoption highlights perhaps the most important aspect of what is required to be a good parent, and that is the ability to create a nurturing relationship with a particular child, not children in general. It is the job of adoption agencies to place children in a manner where their individual needs are best met – not just to find them adults who seem caring. This is particularly true because of the history of displacement, loss and, perhaps, abuse that the child has already experienced – the demands on substitute parents are often greater than on people who bring up their own children, so the issue of fitness to parent a *particular* child becomes crucial. It is this desire to find the most suitable parents for particular children rather than parents who might be good enough that can create a sense of injustice to the people being assessed. In natural parents the biological bond with their children is seen as so important that the latitudes of acceptable parenting are drawn very wide. But for children who are separated from their birth parents there is an onus on those charged with finding new parents who will be better than average for the particular child.

What is slowly being recognised is that the ideal parent for certain children may be from a group that was traditionally regarded as a last resort or totally unsuitable parenting material. Talking to social workers and BAAF, there seems to be no doubt that such applicants are still regarded as lesser parents than the traditional couple and will go through more rigorous assessment. Whether they get a child will depend on the number of choices an agency has for a particular child. One who has plenty of choice will still go to the most 'normal' type of family available.

A disabled, abused or otherwise less desirable child with fewer choices may be placed with a non-traditional applicant. A hierarchy of desirable parents and desirable children still exists and a paradox thus seems to arise that those children who are in need of the most skilled parenting are increasingly allocated to those people who are otherwise regarded as second-class parents. There is a lot of muddled thinking in this area which needs to come out into the open and be debated in the wider public arena, not just between childcare experts. In Part II of this book I will be looking at some of the traditionally ill-favoured groups and examining whether they are justifiably excluded from 'first-tier' parenthood.

WHAT DOES THE ASSESSMENT OF ADOPTIVE PARENTS TELL US ABOUT WHAT IS REQUIRED OF FIT PARENTS?

While there are many issues that are very specific to the particular circumstances of adoptive parents and the children available for adoption, there are a number of general observations that can be usefully drawn from looking at the selection of substitute parents.

Ideal

- Parents should conform as closely as possible to society's perceived norm, i.e. the traditional married couple, and they should avoid eccentric behaviour.
- A child should have two parental figures at most.
- Those with a blood bond to the children are the fittest to be their parents.
- All children need parents for healthy development.
- All parents have an obligation to provide as secure and happy a home for their children as possible.
- Parents should be under 35 when they start a family.
- Parents should not want to have children as accessories or to fulfil their own unmet needs (e.g. for affection or to replace a dead child); they should not place an emotional burden on their own children.
- Parents need self-awareness to understand the influence of their past histories and current circumstances on their parenting potential.
- Parents' mutual support is important to how well they rear the children.
- Educated middle-class parents provide the best upbringing for children.
- Parents should have a wide range of support networks in the community so as to minimise the vulnerability of their families.
- Children's needs are of paramount importance and should be placed above those of parents.

Actual

- Children can benefit from several parental figures.
- A blood bond is neither necessary for fit parenting nor does it automatically result in fit parenting.

- A person may be more fit to be a parent to one child than another. The success of the relationship is dependent on the particular people it involves and their particular histories and external circumstances – in particular their available sources of support within and outside the household.
- Perfection in parenthood is an unrealistic goal – all parents and all children have some weaknesses and some strengths. Some adults may have more strengths than others which may make them more suitable for a wider range of children. Others may have a lot of weaknesses but just the right strengths for their particular children.
- All parent–child relationships are something of a gamble – no one can predict the future, only work with imprecise calculations of relative risks.
- Those whom professionals and lay people regard as fit to be parents are determined by the prevailing cultural attitudes – they are not cast in stone but shift with time.
- Parents' needs are as important to consider as children's needs in order to meet the children's best interests.

3   Parents apart

Who keeps the children?

LESBIAN CUSTODY CASE TESTS PARENTS' RIGHTS

It was a homosexual marriage made in heaven. After 11 years together, Nancy and Michele decided to have children. They found an anonymous sperm donor and in 1980, Nancy had a daughter and four years later a son.

Michele was present at each birth and was registered as the 'father' of the children. But six months after the delivery of their second child, the couple parted and now meet on opposite sides of a courtroom battle that gay activists say could redefine the American notion of parenthood.

(Sam Kiley, *Sunday Times* 8/7/90)

Nancy obtained a court order forbidding Michele from seeing or communicating with the children. Michele was fighting for access but was told that since lesbian marriages are not recognised she had no claim to the children. The San Francisco National Centre for Legal Studies had taken up her case, arguing that such cases should be resolved in the best interests of the child – that if a bond has developed then the relationship should be allowed to grow. Michele argued that though she is not related biologically,

There is more to being a father or mother than donating sperm or giving up an egg. We tried to show our children that parents can do all kinds of things. I was and am part of my daughter's life.

(Sam Kiley, *Sunday Times* 8/7/90)

When film director Woody Allen recently lost his custody battle with Mia Farrow, newspapers all over the world reported the judge's list of his deficiencies as a parent:

NOT FIT TO BE A FATHER

'The film-maker never bathed his children, rarely dressed them and didn't even know the names of their pets', said Judge Elliott Wilk in his ruling in New York yesterday. 'His financial contributions to the children's support, his willingness to read to them, to tell them stories, to buy them presents, to oversee their breakfasts, do not compensate for his absence as a meaningful source of guidance and caring in their lives'.

(Jane Holtham, *Today* 8/6/93)

The case of a lesbian couple or a filmstar duo fighting over their children may seem far removed from the situation of most separating parents but in many ways they graphically highlight the factors which are now considered relevant – without the superimposition of the traditional gender expectations which are being increasingly questioned in all custody disputes. They demonstrate that when parents split up the nature of their relationship with their children comes under scrutiny, by themselves, by their friends and families and by the state. They also demonstrate that the question of who is fit to be a parent looks in two directions. First, it looks back to the parents' past 'performance', the relationship they have built (or failed to build) with the children and the responsibilities they have met. Second, it looks ahead to their potential as separated parents, as single parents or parents in new relationships.

In custody disputes, the issue becomes one not just of parents' rights versus children's rights but between individual parent's rights. The result of two parents separating has always been the question of who 'gets' the children. If both want to continue as parents many questions arise: with whom should the children live? Should either parent be denied contact? How are the children's interests balanced against those of the parents? In the majority of cases the arrangements for the children are agreed without recourse to the courts, but for a significant proportion there is no agreement and the courts are seen as the places to decide on the fitness to parent.

More than either child protection or adoption, the issue of divorce and parental separation is something that touches the lives of vast numbers of people of all classes and backgrounds – royalty, lawyers, doctors, politicians, social workers and media professionals as much as anyone else. The sheer number of people who do divorce now means that it has achieved a certain prominence in the public eye. It has become an area that has been discussed endlessly in the media and been the subject of much academic research. That is not to say that practitioners have necessarily discovered the best way to deal with the welfare of children and separating parents, nor that the level of informed debate between lay people and professionals has been greater.

The history of divorce and custody legislation highlights the shifting definitions of motherhood and fatherhood. In heterosexual relationships, the mother is no longer necessarily the obvious choice to care for the children. As the roles between men and women become more blurred, men are increasingly asking for, and 'getting', the care of their children. So how does the state guide the resolution of such disputes? Who intervenes to assess a parent's fitness to remain involved with their own children? What are the underlying beliefs about how parents should behave and how effective is the state in promoting these beliefs through its intervention? Again, what does this tell us about the expectations and needs of all parents?

A BRIEF HISTORY OF DIVORCE LAW AND PRACTICE

The legislation on divorce was fairly scanty prior to the twentieth century. In many ways the necessity for legislation only became apparent with the recognition of the rights of women in marriage, and, later, with the rights of children. Previously, men's exclusive right to do as they wished with their families, to carry out their obligation to support them or not, was rarely questioned by the state. As illustrated by Thomas Hardy in *The Mayor of Casterbridge*, in certain sections of the population wife sales were once seen as an acceptable way for a husband to end a marriage and to end his responsibilities to support her.

In the rare instances of divorce, children remained the property of their fathers. Men were seen as the heads of households as well as the economic providers, and this enabled family units to remain self-reliant and gave the children not only their name but their status in the community. Therefore by making children the responsibility of men it was thought that they would be supported and not become a burden on society at large in the event of a divorce. The emotional needs of the children were not seen as being the priority – the material needs came first.

A double sexual standard has existed throughout the centuries. Wealthy men have had the legal right since 1753 to divorce their wives on the grounds of adultery but women only earned that right in 1923. The law traditionally always sided with men. Women and children have been dependent on the income that primarily only men could earn, and the state always endorsed that dependency. The absence of legal aid or state support for abandoned women or women who did not wish to suffer at the hands of their husbands made it unrealistic for them to seek divorce, as they would have had no legal rights to any property, to any maintenance afterwards, or to the children.

In many cultures around the world this notion of paternal ownership of children still dominates divorce and custody decisions. It is also true that in most of the cultures where paternal ownership still prevails, the isolated nuclear family has not been the norm. Therefore the child is likely to remain part of an extended family network after divorce rather than become a part of a single-parent family. That obviously has implications for how those cultures interpret whether a child's needs are being adequately met after the loss of his mother.

In Britain, interestingly, the media played a part in creating the need for legislation in divorce.

Titillating accounts of the evidence presented in such cases (of wealthy men taking action for criminal conversation against their wife's lover by a husband) became soft core pornography in the early 19th century. The invention of stenography allowed reporters to write things down verbatim for the first time and cheap broadsheets on the new fast iron presses were hungry for copy. Upper class embarrassment at this publicity as well as weariness with the obvious collusion and connivance involved, and an awareness of the manifest unfairness to women of the existing legal situation led to Palmerston's Divorce Bill in 1857.

(Stone 1990)

The growth of feminism was a driving factor in the progress of divorce legislation, and arguably in asserting the rights of women, helped set the stage for divorce to become a battle between the sexes which all too often included a battle over children.

> For example in the campaign against wife torture at the end of the 19th century, feminists were able to demand reforms such that wives who had taken criminal proceedings against violent spouses were empowered to live apart from their husbands and to take children up to the age of 7 years with them (Matrimonial Causes Act 1878). Here we see the beginnings of a tender years doctrine in which it was assumed that babies and young children would normally thrive best in the care of a maternal figure. The tender years doctrine became a powerful counterbalance to claims based on fathers' rights.
>
> (Smart and Sevenhuijsen 1989)

The legal polarisation of fathers and mothers had begun.

The recognition of the rights of women happened in a piecemeal way throughout the nineteenth century, and the social work element of the courts began as a response to the needs of poor women who could not afford divorce.

> Court social work in magistrates courts developed under the impetus of evangelical and philanthropic philosophies current at the time. The courts' primary objective was to enforce the working man's obligation to maintain his wife and children so that they should not become a burden on the state. Under the provisions of the Summary Jurisdiction (Married Women) Act of 1895 the courts turned to the police court missionary or probation officer to encourage reconciliation. 'Moral rectitude and community self interest went hand in glove.'
>
> (Murch 1980)

This reconciliation role was designed to save the marriage – it was only half a century later that 'child' saving through conciliation became an objective of the court welfare service. In the mid-1920s, for the first time there was a shift away from paternal ownership of children to the principle of the child's welfare being the paramount consideration, but this was interpreted differently to today. Since most divorce was seen to be provoked by adultery, the 'guilty' party was also seen to need penalising by the divorce process. The legal and cultural history of divorce in Christian countries has been rooted in guilt: guilt for sinning against the teachings of the Church, for letting the children down as failed ideal parents, and for letting society down in not preserving the ideal of lifelong marriage union and self-contained family unit. Thus there was period when the welfare of the children was seen as tied inextricably with the innocent party (i.e. the non-adulterous one) while the guilty party was expelled from the family unit, never to return. State intervention remained minimal and there was no investigation into the child's needs.

The growing influence of psychiatry and psychoanalysis in the 1940s and 1950s increasingly examined parenting practices and looked to the causes of adult problems in the parenting they had received as children. This turned the focus of attention to the importance of the mother–child bond, and as the second half of the twentieth century progressed mothers tended to get custody of children unless they were shown to be grossly unfit (e.g. mentally unstable).

At the end of the 1960s there was a move to take away the public shaming aspect of divorce by abolishing the concept of the guilty party. It became widely accepted that children are just as likely to suffer long-term damage in a household where there is prolonged conflict or where one or both parents is deeply unhappy as by the process of divorce. It was thus no longer the state's duty to force couples to stay together when they felt their relationship was over.

The last two decades have seen a phenomenal increase in the rate of break-up of relationships. Since the Divorce Reform Act entered the statute books in 1971, the divorce rate has escalated at an unprecedented rate to the point that one in five children are now predicted to experience divorce in the course of their childhoods. However, divorce statistics do not paint the whole picture. The last twenty years have also seen a steady increase in the number of children born out of wedlock; some are born outside any stable relationship but others are born into stable cohabitational partnerships which may subsequently break up. The means to measure these are non-existent. Thus the full scale of family break-ups is as yet unknown.

What became increasingly apparent was that as parents' parting often led to acrimonious custody battles, the state through its legal procedures became more and more involved in making decisions about who should get custody and who should be allowed access. As neither gender preferences nor allocation of blame were any longer deemed suitable criteria for ascertaining where the best interests of the children lay, courts became increasingly dependent on the welfare officer's investigation of a parting couple's circumstances and their relative fitness as parents. Separating couples themselves became increasingly ensnared by the legal process and dependent on it for resolutions.

The usual outcome for couples who parted was for the mother to gain custody and the father to be granted 'reasonable' access. How this was interpreted varied from one household to the next – the custodial parent could obstruct access by the other parent with virtual impunity. Prevailing views rooted in psychoanalytic understanding of children influenced custody decisions: Goldstein, Freud and Solnit were very influential in the early 1970s, pointing to the necessity of removing ambiguity and acting with speed to resolve children's futures, and that once the 'psychological' parent had been awarded custody this parent should be allowed full responsibility to make all decisions concerning the child without interference from the other parent. Some argue that this encouraged the non-custodial parent to be forced off the scene.

As the number of single parents dependent on the state grew, so did concern about the 'absent' parents. Research into the effects of divorce on children alerted people to the inadequacy of the prevailing procedures. In particular, the discovery that half of all non-custodial fathers lose contact with their children within a matter of months and that many do not continue their maintenance payments made it apparent that, to minimise the cost to the state and the cost to the children, the state had to find ways to encourage parents to take lifelong responsibility for their children. It was recognised that the law needed to be changed to achieve this.

The Children Act 1989 stresses that parental responsibilities are for ever and can only be terminated by adoption. The intention is to encourage separating parents to consider their ongoing role as parents in a manner which promotes the welfare of the children, and it is not for the parents' own convenience or a vent for their own animosity. When a man and woman are married in the eyes of the law they both have parental responsibility for their children. If they are unmarried, parental responsibility is conferred to the mother alone unless the parents have jointly registered their agreement that the father should also have parental responsibility or unless he has made a successful application to the courts to acquire parental rights. This is a recognition of the fact that more children are born outside marriage but into stable cohabitational partnerships. The Children Act 1989 is an indication that the state is recognising that the parent–child relationship is independent of the marriage union and should be encouraged whatever the marital status of parents: married, unmarried or divorced.

So now there is greater significance attached to continuity of relationships with both parents. This is partly pragmatic – to encourage fathers to continue to feel responsible for their children's financial support. It is partly a concession to the growing body of men who are voicing their concerns about being marginalised by the legal and social processes into losing their relationships with their children. As the self-help group Families Need Fathers put it:

> Our main concern is that no parent should have to get divorced from the children just because the marriage has broken up. It has been assumed too long that only mothers care about children.

> (Liz Hodgkinson, *The Times* 9/5/88)

If the mother does not wish to let the father see the child and the child is too young to understand who his father is, there is more ambiguity about whether a father's contact is necessarily in the best interests of the child.

THE TIES THAT BIND?

Last week Irene Parow lost her final appeal in the High Court. The father of her child, a man she has never lived with, has won his battle to gain access to his son. The little boy, now two and a half years old, does not know him and has not seen him since he was eight months old. The court is supposed to regard the child's interests as paramount. In some cases now it seems that judges regard children seeing their unknown biological fathers a self evident good whatever the circumstances.

(Polly Toynbee, *Guardian* 28/4/88)

In many cases mothers with custody of their children have been banned by the courts from moving away from the area where their ex-husbands live so as not to jeopardise the children's continuing relationship with their fathers. For example, a divorced mother who wanted to emigrate with her two young sons (of whom she had custody) to Australia to be near her own mother was told by the Court of Appeal in 1989 that the boys could not be torn away from their father or their roots on the farm in Lincolnshire where they had grown up. The judge said that boys needed a father. The mother had not formed any other stable relationship since divorcing her husband on the grounds of his adultery three years previously. To take them away from their father was not in their best interests – 'the mother would soon get over her bitterness and frustration and survive' (Terence Shaw, 21/2/89 © The Telegraph plc, London).

The case highlights the conflicting interests of parents and children in a poignant way. The mother's hopes to begin a new life with her sons were crushed, her own desires were seen as expendable. One presumes that if she had remarried herself and been able to supply a father figure, the judges might have taken a different line. In any event the children's present needs together with those of the father took precedence. (I have not been able to find any cases of fathers being obliged by the courts to remain living near their children – again it seems that only some courts favour maintaining the bond between children and both their parents.)

The process of divorce, dealing as it does with the untangling of the practical and emotional ties that have bound a couple in marriage, is usually painful, and the current legal system encourages the two parties to engage in mudslinging. There is often an inbuilt need for either one or both parties to prove the other's guilt in the face of the officials of the state machinery. Many unhappy couples tangle with the question of 'can any parent who decides to divorce be deemed a fit parent?'

The stigma of divorce has faded fast, but the notions of guilt and blame are still very much present for most divorcing couples and are fuelled by the adversarial nature of the present legal system. As Judge Joyce Bracewell, a leading figure in the implementation of the new Children Act, points out:

> The situation at present is untenable. If a marriage has broken down, it is counterproductive to make allegations about conduct save in so far as it impinges on a persons ability to care for a child. But while irretrievable breakdown of marriage is supposed to be the sole ground for divorce couples are still having to prove unreasonable behaviour or adultery, or separate for at least two years. It seems bound to create animosity between parents. It very much raises the temperature.

(Patricia Wynn Davies, *Independent* 30/8/89)

There is much pressure to introduce reforms which would place more emphasis on what is called mediation or conciliation (reaching agreement) and less on conflict, but as yet these have not taken place as fully as is necessary.

In presenting a historical overview it is clear that the criteria used by courts to resolve child custody disputes are informed by the changes happening in society at large. In particular, divorce today throws into sharp relief the confusion over the roles that mothers and fathers are 'normally' expected to play. In western countries the role that many men play as parents has been shifting over the past two decades. There are more men seeking custody of their children after divorce or break-up of a cohabiting relationship, there are more lone fathers bringing up children, and there is generally thought to be more involvement by men in the parenting role. But we have not yet reached the stage where men and women in most families are genuinely sharing childcare and domestic duties. The change in attitudes and employment structures that would enable this has yet to happen – as long as women are able to earn only a lesser salary, it will always be they, rather than the men, who look after the children.

The rise of the father has been accompanied, perhaps even pushed up, by the fall of the mother relative to their respective traditional roles. As more and more women go out and seek satisfaction and financial reward in the world of work, their role as rulers of the domestic hearth counts for less. The art of running a home has simultaneously been turned into a series of mechanically aided and unrewarding chores that no longer require a mastery or special training. Likewise, as more and more mothers make use of alternative childcare arrangements (using childminders, nurseries or nannies) the perceived importance of mothers as central to children's needs is being diluted. Clearly others can fulfil a significant proportion of a mother's role. If the mother's two traditional areas of expertise are no longer seen as so expert, the way is open for others to colonise them.

To a lesser extent a similar change in men's traditional areas of expertise has been taking place. With women working, men are no longer seen as the exclusive economic providers. High rates of unemployment have rendered many men unable to fulfil their traditional role for long periods of time, and often this has meant a greater awareness of and involvement in domestic and child-rearing tasks.

At present, in the event of parental separation with or without a dispute, it is the mothers who continue with the daily care of children in the vast majority of cases. The 1989 OPCS (Office of Population Censuses and Surveys) estimates suggest that after divorce, more than one-third of children live with the lone mother, half live with the remarried mother, one in fifteen lives with the mother and her cohabiting partner, and only one in thirty lives with the father.

The shift we are witnessing towards men wanting the right to greater parental involvement is not a shift towards men wanting a greater part in daily childcare. The number of men who want to take on the traditional mothering role remains a tiny but well-publicised minority. The Children Act 1989 is not heralding a new approach to gender neutrality in parenthood as much as endorsing traditional roles of parenthood that require a child to have two parents who, between themselves, take responsibility for his financial, physical and emotional welfare.

THE PROCESS

Under the current system divorce proceedings usually begin by one party approaching a solicitor to serve a petition for divorce on the other party. The latter then hires another solicitor and from then on most communication is done through the respective solicitors. Each party prepares an affidavit presenting his or her case, outlining the reasons for the break-up, and the views they have about childcare and domestic arrangements. Since the purpose of the affidavit is seen as one of making one's own case appear more strong and worthy in the eyes of the courts, there is undoubtedly a temptation to use it to paint a negative picture of the other party. As the solicitor is professionally motivated to do the best for his own client, he may also tacitly or openly encourage this.

The next step is the court – this may be a county court or a magistrates' court. The magistrate or district judge then meets both parties. How much their decisions about future childcare arrangements comes under official scrutiny varies a great deal. If the parents are unmarried and there is no official dispute over who looks after the children, the state is unlikely to become involved. Even if a married couple seek a divorce, as long as they come to a mutual agreement the state does little more than rubber-stamp it. Since the 1950s there has been a requirement that the court establish that the arrangements put forward were satisfactory or the best that could be devised under the circumstances before granting a full divorce, and this has sometimes involved judges ordering investigations even when the parents had agreed a solution. The satisfaction requirement however became a mere formality, and the court rarely took any steps to investigate. The Children Act 1989 has abolished the satisfaction hearing and does not require the court to evaluate the childcare arrangements at all, and it can only delay making the divorce final if there are exceptional circumstances which make this desirable in the child's interests.

However, if there is any dispute over the child's future or firm evidence that the child is in danger, the state becomes involved with an expressed aim of resolving the situation in the best interests of that child. The notions of custody and access have been dropped. The emphasis now is on parents making as many decisions for themselves and the courts only intervening if they absolutely need to – and then only to make orders on those issues that a couple cannot agree themselves. Parting couples can now apply for 'residence' orders if they want the child to live with them and 'contact' orders if they cannot agree on what contact each parent should have.

So if there is a dispute both parties meet the court conciliator, who is a welfare officer. Their discussion is confidential and if they reach an agreement that appears workable in the eyes of the conciliator, they present it to the judge who is likely to rubber-stamp it. If they cannot agree, then the judge decides on how to proceed and gives directions on what information the court requires and over what time-scale. He orders a court welfare report and perhaps other professional reports he deems necessary, e.g. a psychiatrist's report. At this point he also sets a date for the court hearing so that the matter does not drift on indefinitely.

Another welfare officer (separate from the conciliator) sets about making his report. There is no form that welfare officers have to complete. Any information this welfare officer discovers in the course of his investigation, including everything he discovers through the interviews with each parent, is available to the court. Under the Children Act 1989 the emphasis on 'any delay is prejudicial to the child' has meant that court reports should be completed more swiftly: three months, rather than six months as often used to be the case. Some people have argued that the delays in the past (due to shortages of welfare officers or in seeking outside expertise) were no bad thing, in that they often gave the warring parents time to calm down and reflect more soberly on why they really wanted their children to live with them, but it is unlikely that most parents or children experienced delay as a positive thing. Most want a resolution, an end to uncertainty.

The welfare officer makes her report and files it at the court prior to the date of the court hearing. Usually she makes a recommendation to the court but she is not under an obligation to do so. At any time up to and including the hearing an agreement between the parents can take place, but if this has not occurred then the judge or magistrate has to make an order as he or she sees fit. This order is based on the welfare report and on any other information presented to the court. Sometimes the welfare officer may be interrogated on the content of her report, and lawyers for either party may try to discredit that which does not favour them. With older children (usually over 9 years) the judge might also ask to see them.

The order the judge makes may be the end of the matter for the courts – or either party may appeal to a higher court to have the decision overturned, or either party may return to make an application to the court in the future to ask for a new order concerning some aspect of parental dispute over the children. Whoever the child lives with, both parents will continue to have shared parental responsibility and will be expected to deal with day-to-day decisions themselves. If there are irresolvable disputes over specific issues, either party can approach the court to make a Specific Issue Order.

WHO DECIDES?

Once married parents start divorce proceedings or unmarried couples bring a dispute over children to the courts, the professional machinery often appears to take over. A number of professionals become involved, each supposedly concerned only with 'the best interests of the child' – the social work and medical frameworks are far less important than the legal framework in determining outcomes in childcare disputes. All the professionals will be experts in the procedure of the particular courts with which they work, whereas the subjects (i. e. the parents and children) will not. They are thus dependent on the individual professionals to represent them and to represent the law and legal procedures accurately to them.

Solicitors

The solicitor is usually the first representative of the legal system a separating parent meets and is likely to stay in contact with throughout the legal process of divorce and any disputes over children or property. He or she is thus likely to have considerable influence on how the parent perceives the legal process. Each solicitor will be expected to advise his or her own client on how to get the best out of the situation. Past research has shown (Murch 1980) that parents wanted their solicitors to be partisan, to be fighting for them, and were disappointed if the solicitor seemed to be neutral or showed sympathy for the other partner's predicament.

Solicitors are paid by their clients and therefore there is an expectation to achieve what the client wants. The client is the parent, not the child. The extent to which a solicitor encourages the parent to put the children's needs first and take a conciliatory approach to the demands of the other parent varies a lot. Many solicitors now belong to the Solicitors Family Law Association which emphasises a conciliatory, not mud-slinging approach. There are still many solicitors who appear unfamiliar with conciliation procedures and thus do not adequately prepare their clients for the court process by which they could find agreement.

However careful and concerned solicitors are, the process of divorce inevitably encourages a partisan approach even to matters concerning the children. Forty per cent of welfare officers in James and Wilson's survey (1984) thought that solicitors did not give sufficient weight to the interests of the children in divorce proceedings, a view endorsed by Murch's study (1980) which revealed that the vast majority of solicitors did not even see their clients' children, but tended to see the child's interests in the light of the parent they were representing.

Solicitors are not given any training to deal with the complex social and emotional problems that accompany the legal problems of divorce. How good they are at doing so depends on the individual solicitors' own ideas about their role and their experience.

Judges and magistrates

Judges are seen as the final arbiters, the most powerful voice of the state in endorsing who is fit to continue parenting and who is not. It is the judge, not the court welfare officer who decides when to commission a report on a family. There appears to be much discrepancy in what circumstances lead a judge to order a report. Enquiries may be made to police and social services to establish whether the parents have any criminal record or history of welfare involvement. As Murch points out, this leads to one obvious consequence:

> Families chosen for welfare reports will be drawn predominantly from poor working class families because the clientele of the local authority social services and the probation service come predominantly from these social groups. Middle class families not previously known to them will largely avoid being scrutinised.

> (Murch 1980)

One recent survey (Collins and Macleod 1991) found that reports are more often requested when the disputing parents are not married and are usual in cases of unmarried fathers applying for custody. Thus, as with other areas of parental assessment, there are certain groups which are more likely to come under state investigation than others.

Various studies have suggested how little the judges actually get involved in most cases of child welfare after the parents split. The vast majority of children whose parents separate and decide for themselves what to do never have their childcare arrangements examined by the judge. The judges who order welfare reports very rarely go against the recommendations of the welfare officer. So it is actually in a very small proportion of cases that the judge alone is independently coming to a decision involving the child's welfare. The idea that the judges and magistrates are deciding each case on its merits by examining the information and individual circumstances does not appear to be backed up by research. Their greatest significance is to rubber-stamp the decisions of others: of parents, of welfare officers and, sometimes, of children.

There is much criticism of how conservative or out of touch judges sometimes appear to be, but there are undoubtedly also many enlightened ones who recognise the responsibility they carry and also the limitations of the law as an instrument of promoting good parenting. One court welfare officer likens a judge making an order to a car being given an MOT – it is only a certificate pronouncing on the state of the car at the time it was tested, not a predictor of how it will run in the future: that is up to the drivers. So it is for parents: they should not see the courts as being their enduring decision makers.

Court welfare officers

The court welfare officer plays a key role in the resolution of childcare disputes when a couple part. Welfare officers are part of the probation service, though they will have started with a basic qualification which is the same as social workers before going on to work with offenders. Their role over the past two decades has been to report to the courts on various issues regarding the custody of children. Few people are likely to have heard of or met a court welfare officer until the court orders a welfare report on their circumstances. They will have no choice over whether or not a welfare officer is assigned to report on them, nor will they have any choice of officers.

There is much variation in the role that welfare officers think they should play. Their official role is to report and investigate, to be 'the eyes and ears of the judge' – a representative of the court machinery that is concerned with evaluating the child's best interests. However, as with some of the other areas I have looked at in previous chapters, for many professionals, the traditional investigative role has also evolved into a facilitating role. Even prior to the Children Act 1989, many welfare officers recognised that the process of scrutinising and comparing parents encouraged them to see the outcome as winning or losing the 'fitness to parent' test – which was not conducive to ongoing relationships with each other or with the children. In the days when it was expected that the non-custodial parent would withdraw from the family scene, this was not deemed too worrying but with the change in belief about the ongoing necessity for two parents, this mode of investigation was seen to be outdated and conciliation came to be seen as the best way forward.

The adversarial process of resolving disputes . . . is at odds with one of the implicit assumptions of conciliation – that decisions relating to children are the responsibility of their parents. The legal process can allow those involved to collude in making various counter assertions; that after separation, one parent needs to be identified as better than the other; that outside experts are capable of seeking out the correct decisions; and that divorce and separation somehow confer an automatic right on society to put one's abilities as parents under the microscope.

(Francis *et al.* quoted in Murch 1980)

Increasingly, conciliation has become a central aspect of the work of many court welfare officers – encouraging agreement to be reached by the parents themselves. One of the central issues is: who is their 'client'? – the court, the parents or the children? The courts themselves appear to view the role of the welfare officer in different ways (Kingsley 1990). According to one judge, 'The job of the court welfare officer is to look for agreement. . . . He should be after negotiated settlements. ' Another view was: 'The court welfare officer is a sort of arbitrator. He can put forward his own solutions.'

Yet another view was:

We do not want the court welfare officer to resolve the dispute for us. That's for conciliation. We're looking for the court welfare officer to read affidavits, understand the case, confirming the truth of what is said and making recommendations. the court welfare officer is the *court* welfare officer not the family welfare officer.

(Kingsley 1990)

So there are now two prevailing ideologies amongst court welfare officers: 'the courts know best' and 'the parents know best'. The first is the traditional overtly investigative one in which the welfare officers are serving the courts by providing them with information and recommendations based on assessments. One officer who uses this approach described it thus:

Whenever the court asks for a report, even where the parents are agreed the children's responses and attitude should be considered because the welfare of the child is paramount. He also felt that standards of parenting actually differ and that the welfare service should assess that as well. He explained that some parents simply did not look after children as well as others and that it was the welfare service's job to assess that and that parents are not necessarily the best people to decide upon what should happen.

(James and Dingwall 1989)

The second approach focuses on the parents' subjective view of the dispute and aims to facilitate their reaching an agreement without any routine investigation of criminal or social services records or of their home background.

They would present their task as being there to understand why the parents are unable to agree in that they agreed for many years before and they are there to report as helpfully as they can to the court . . . ultimately decisions about the welfare of the child were up to the parents to make. He commented that playing the super-parent was likely to be based on false premises and to undermine the long term potential of those parents to recover their ability to parent and to accept their responsibility as parents.

(James and Dingwall 1989)

These two views represent perhaps the two extremes of what is probably a spectrum of current practice approaches. The varying ideologies mean that methods vary from one service to another and from one welfare officer to another. Most expect to see both parents separately and, if at all possible, together. Practitioners of the 'parents know best' approach are likely to limit their interviews to their own offices and through a process of interviewing, seek to establish the nature of the dispute about the children and attempt to understand the motives of the parents and circumstances of each. Their intention and conduct is designed to be impartial and neutral – so if they spend an hour with one parent they would spend an hour with the other; if they met one parent with the children they would do the same with the other parent. This neutrality is deemed an important aspect of promoting conciliation.

With the greater emphasis on parents making decisions, unless there is a dispute over residence and one party is suggesting that the other's home circumstances are inadequate, the welfare officer is less likely to investigate the home. This is despite the feelings of the High Court and Court of Appeal that reports should include home visits as part of the investigation with attention paid to relationships in the home (Fricker and Coates 1989).

Those who favour the conciliation approach are more likely to co-work on a report with another officer. There is also much opportunity to discuss a particular case with colleagues. All this peer support is a conscious attempt to recognise and share the great responsibility that welfare officers carry and to help the report-making to be as objective as possible.

In the 'courts know best' approach, whom they see and the information they seek out will depend on the individual welfare officer and on the circumstances of the particular family. A detailed survey of welfare officers around England found much variation in whom they interviewed in the process of preparing a report. While parents were always interviewed, children were not, particularly if they were under 5. For those carrying out the investigative approach, other close relatives may be interviewed. Professionals may be approached – most frequently these are the social services, the NSPCC, doctor, health visitor, and police. If the children are of school age the welfare officers would contact their schools. In addition, other people might be approached, e.g. 'clergymen, youth club personnel, play group leaders, child-minders, housing department officials, DSS officials and employers, hospitals, child guidance clinics, friends and neighbours'.

A more recent survey also highlighted the variations in practice, but more interestingly the discrepancy which exists between what welfare officers deem important to do and what they actually do. For example, 'a large majority of welfare officers believed it was desirable to see parents together, but this aim was achieved in less than half of all cases.'

> They also rated child protection as one of their main roles, but each welfare officer interprets a duty to protect children from harm in a different way. No systematic procedure exists for checking records. No consistent approach to attendance of case conferences exists. Court welfare officers show considerable variation in their practice with regard to visiting homes and consulting specialists on a child and family.
>
> (Kingsley 1990)

The picture that emerges is one of welfare officers operating in many different ways with differing views of their roles and of how these should be carried out. They have considerable influence on the outcome of the courts' decisions both in their report recommendations and also in their knowledge of the court system. An illustration of this is found in a description of a court welfare officer described by Dingwall and James:

> Sally was clearly a familiar figure to clerks, ushers, lawyers and judges. This gave her considerable influence over the passage of cases through the system. In one instance for example, her unhappiness with the outcome of an interim hearing led her to negotiate with the relevant court administrator for an early relisting before a judge whom she expected to take a line more in accord with her own.
>
> (James and Dingwall 1989)

Such influence is not surprising, but it does highlight the arbitrariness of the process by which parents may be judged.

Psychiatrists

Psychiatrists may be consulted in a custody or access dispute by one parent, a solicitor or the court or by a divorce court welfare officer. If the nature of their expertise of child–parent relationships is accepted as valid then they clearly have an important role to play, as they can present a view of the child's best interests in which the child is actually the focus of their assessments. In the USA the role of the mental health professional has become increasingly influential in custody and access disputes. In the UK their use is more haphazard and their influence more variable.

Social workers

In some cases social workers may be involved in court cases involving families already on their caselists. If the children have been on their child protection registers, the contribution of the social worker's evidence may be particularly significant to the court's decision making.

WHAT CRITERIA DO THE PROFESSIONALS USE?

The Children Act 1989 features a welfare checklist for professionals to consider in reaching decisions about children.

(a) The ascertainable wishes and feelings of the child concerned (considered in the light of his age and understanding).
(b) His physical, emotional and educational needs.
(c) The likely effect on him of any change in his circumstances.
(d) His age, sex, background and any characteristics which the court considers relevant.
(e) Any harm which he has suffered or is at risk of suffering.
(f) How capable each of his parents, and any other person in relation to whom the court considers the question to be relevant, is of meeting his needs.
(g) The range of powers available to the court under this Act in the proceedings in question.

The Act does not make clear the relative importance a practitioner should ascribe to each of these criteria, nor does it exclude the possibility of putting these issues completely to one side. Their purpose (as with the new assessment procedures described in other chapters) is to encourage a systematic decision-making process. The Act is still relatively new and its full impact has yet to unfold. What follows is therefore an overview of what criteria still prevail at present.

As with the previous areas I have examined, the criteria by which courts reach decisions are not openly available. Prior to the Children Act 1989, a number of rules of thumb seemed to operate which solicitors, court welfare officers and judges were aware of but which were not fixed and varied from one court to the next. Thus solicitors and court welfare officers could influence the outcome of proceedings by selecting a court or judge who was known to favour particular criteria. In custody disputes for example, a man stood a better chance of winning if he had organised good childcare arrangements and could offer a more stable and prosperous home than the mother. Other criteria could be used to score parental fitness:

> For example, a mother might lose points for having a long string of boyfriends and a father gain points if he was going to remarry and provide a more stable upbringing. Similarly I wouldn't be too surprised if a judge was put off a mother who lived in a one bedroom flat. And some judges would be more sympathetic to a religious father than an agnostic mother.
> (Solicitor at The Children's Legal Centre, quoted by Jane Bidder, *The Times* 12/2/88)

The parent who left the family home was seen to be jeopardising his or her chances of getting custody. This led to solicitors encouraging their clients to do everything to make their partners leave the home. Women with lesbian relationships were also regarded with suspicion by the courts, so might be forced to conceal the fact that they could offer their children another stable relationship.

These sorts of rules of thumb form the backdrop to the work of the court welfare officer. The criteria he uses will encompass the following: he will be looking for a sense of the bonds the children have with each parent, the practical arrangements the parents have made, the extent to which they are able to put the children's needs first, the domestic circumstances and provision for continuity of school, other friendships, what their motives are in seeking contact/residence, whether there are any danger signs. If there are accusations of unfitness of one parent by the other he might say, 'Your partner has suggested that you have a drink problem, what do you say?', and if necessary, seek opinions of others as he chooses. Welfare officers often ask parents disputing residence to run through a day in their life with their children, describing in detail the daily routine and how they would deal with each aspect of it. If both parents appear equally competent and loving but neither wants to be seen to be the one who had 'lost' the children, the welfare officer might try and establish which of them is likely to be more compliant about enabling the non-residential partner contact. (One court welfare officer mentioned the 'bus test' might be applied: each partner is asked 'if you were run over by a bus how would your ex-spouse cope with the children?' The answer is often a reluctant acknowledgement that the other is not so unfit after all.)

In the eyes of most practitioners there are some prevailing principles in operation at the moment:

1 Parents are the best people to bring up their own children.
2 Better for the parents to make decisions as they are more likely to make them work.
3 Better for children to maintain contact with both parents after they have split up.
4 Paramountcy of the status quo – welfare officers and courts tend to rubber-stamp the status quo on the basis that any further disruption to children's lives should be avoided.

The status quo principle is also justified in that the parents must be good enough to be coping already, so why change the situation to one which is not tested?

5 Children to be kept together – unless they are actually old enough to express a preference.
6 Boys need the presence of a father to learn discipline and to a lesser extent girls need the presence of mothers.
7 In general there can be no assumption that men are any less capable as parents than women, particularly for school-age children.

All these various criteria are based on a mixture of research, instinct and fashion. When they clash it is for the court to establish which should get priority. In April 1991, for example, a judge awarded the custody of a 6 year old girl to her mother while awarding custody of her three brothers to the father, despite the fact that the girl had continued to live with him and her brothers after her mother moved out. He had rejected the argument in favour of the status quo and concluded that it was natural for the mother to have the care of her 6 year old daughter. The father appealed and Lord Butler Sloss concluded that it was in the best interests of the child to remain with the father rather than be uprooted:

> In custody cases where the child has remained throughout with the mother and is young, particularly when a baby or toddler, the unbroken relationship between mother and child is one which would be very difficult to displace, unless the mother was unsuitable to care for the child. But where the mother and child have been separated and the mother seeks the return of the child, other considerations apply and there is no starting point that the mother should be preferred to the father and only displaced by a preponderance of evidence to the contrary. There is no presumption which requires the mother as mother to be considered as the primary caretaker in preference to the father. (Re A (a minor) Court of Appeal 19 April 1991.)
>
> (*Independent* 29/4/91)

In another interesting case a 7 year old girl who had lived continuously with her mother after her parents had separated but had regular access to her father, was the subject of a dispute. Her mother had formed a lesbian relationship and the father felt that he should be granted care and control of the girl. The court welfare officer's report made no recommendation and the judge granted care and control to the mother, arguing that the girl had a strong bond with her and would in any case find out about the relationship during access visits. The father appealed and the case was submitted for reconsideration with the following justification:

> Despite the vast changes over the last 30 years or so in the attitudes of society generally to the institution of marriage, to sexual morality and to homosexual relationships, it was to be regarded as axiomatic that the ideal environment for the upbringing of a child is a home of loving, caring and sensible parents, mother and father. When a marriage is at an end a choice has to be made for whatever alternative is closest to that ideal. The judge had disregarded the effect on L of her schoolfriends learning of her mother's relationship which would lead to questions likely to cause her distress or embarrassment. This did not mean that the fact that a mother is living in a lesbian relationship should be conclusive or disqualify her from ever having care and control of her child. The court could well decide that a sensitive and loving lesbian relationship provides a more satisfactory environment than a less sensitive or loving alternative. But the nature of the relationship must be an important factor to be put into the balance. It was important that a judge should not reach decisions by relying on his or her own subjective standards but he should start on the basis that moral standards which are generally accepted in the society in which the child lives are more likely than not to promote his or her welfare. These standards may differ between different communities, and in appropriate cases the judge could be invited to receive evidence as to the standards accepted in a particular community. In default of this, a judge was entitled, and indeed bound, to apply his or her own experience in determining what are the accepted standards. (Re L Court of Appeal 24 August 1990.)
>
> (*Adoption and Fostering*, Vol. 5, No. 1, 1991)

This reveals some interesting aspects of the decision-making process. One is that there exists a hierarchy in what is regarded as the best family set-up for a particular child: at the top is the ideal family of loving mother and father, and every other family configuration is, by definition it seems, inferior. Another aspect is that parental deviancy from society's norm goes against a child's welfare. The other important point is that judges are supposed to make their decisions on the basis of those moral standards that are generally accepted in the society where the child is to live. That implies they should be familiar with these. When we look at the social and economic background of most judges, perhaps we should ask how able they are to be familiar with the moral standards of a wide range of communities.

Contact

If the parting parents cannot resolve the contact that the non-residential parent should have, the courts need to do this. So what do they base their decisions on? A knowledge of child development as well as the particular children's wishes and needs are clearly crucial. The court welfare officer needs to look at the child's existing relationship with the non-residential parent. Child psychiatrists may be consulted. Collins and Macleod's survey of reports on unmarried parents' disputes (1991) highlighted the following as important criteria:

1 General backing for the principle of children's access to absent, non-marital parents.
2 No differences in attitudes towards previously cohabiting fathers and fathers who had not lived with their child, although whether the child knew, remembered or had formed an attachment to the father was considered relevant.
3 A break in access was seen as a contra-indication but not a conclusive argument against access – if there had been a break and the mother opposed it, access was usually not recommended.
4 Violence against the mother was not necessarily accepted as an argument against access when supervisory or other arrangements could be made to avoid inter-parental contact.
5 Relevance of race: the racial identity of non-white parents was presented as a key argument in favour of access and custody in those cases where the child was of mixed race.

The courts can lay down the access arrangements but it is for the parents to make them work. It has often been pointed out that the courts do little to enforce access rulings if the custodial parent is obstructive or makes allegations of sexual abuse by the other parent. In a recent ruling, Lord Butler Sloss warned parents awarded custody not to alienate the children from the other parent. In a case involving a woman who had prevented her ex-husband's gifts from reaching their children and had been threatened with imprisonment for so doing, Lord Justice Butler Sloss said:

It is the children's right, not the right of the parent, to have a continuing relationship with the non-custodial parent. This mother might bear very well in mind that she may be storing up for herself the most appalling relationship if the children grow up into teenagers and then find they have a father they should have been seeing and it was their mother's fault they were unable to have a relationship with him.

(Guardian 20/9/90)

In the past there has been an equation in the minds of many parting parents that the father's payment of maintenance 'buys' the right to contact with the child. Many mothers felt that by forgoing maintenance they could be free of the interference of an undesirable former partner. The Child Support Act 1991 is an attempt to force fathers to pay maintenance whether they see their children or not, and has caused some bitterness amongst fathers who have felt forced out of their children's lives and are now to be expected to take financial responsibility without the automatic 'reward' of a relationship with their children.

In trying to discover the criteria that the courts use I have looked for official guidelines, spoken to practitioners, studied the small number of published surveys and looked at some recent judgments. However, looking at previous judgments is only an indicator, not a predictor, of future decisions. As I have shown, the individual circumstances of each case are also affected by the wide variety in professional practice and exercising of discretionary judgement, so in any new case it is extremely difficult to know exactly what criteria will be used and what weight these will be given.

What is the research basis for decision making?

In 1984 James and Wilson wrote that the variation in practice amongst court welfare officers was due to the fact that 'There is no commonly accepted body of theory or knowledge which might help guide practitioners'.

There are theories in abundance but their common acceptance is scant. Goldstein *et al.*, for example, advocated giving sole custody to the psychological parent (the one who has formed a stable and ongoing relationship with the child and may or may not be a biological parent) who, as well as caring for the child, should have the right to deny access to any non-psychological parent because:

Children have difficulty in relating positively to, profiting from and main-taining contact with two psychological parents who are not in positive contact with each other. Loyalty conflicts are common and normal under such condi-tions and may have devastating consequences by destroying the child's positive relationship to both parents.

(Goldstein *et al.* 1973/1980)

This is a psychoanalytic interpretation apparently based on clinical observation of children who have appeared to suffer in such circumstances, but one presumes the authors have not studied children who have not been brought to their attention because no such harm occurred. As Murch says,

We need to know much more about the realities of access provision in the divorcing population as a whole. In particular, we need to study more carefully those families where access works well as well as those where it may be disturbing children.

(Murch 1980)

Again, we see the problematic nature of basing practice on incomplete research. Unfortunately the nature of research into this area is laborious, time-consuming and retrospective. At present the predominating research findings influencing practice are as follows (based on Schaffer (1990) and Richards (1989)):

1 Stability and close affectionate relationships are important to children's well-being.
2 Parental conflict rather than divorce is harmful to children.
3 Boys and girls do slightly better living with the same-gender parent after a divorce.
4 There is no evidence that men are any less capable than women in childcare.
5 Children generally do better when they are able to maintain relationships with each parent.
6 A cooperative and conflict-free approach by parents over the children leads to better adjustment by children after divorce.

Wallerstein and Blakeslee's research in California (1989) and the MRC study in Britain (Douglas *et al.* 1968) have both shown that the repercussions of parental break-up can continue into adulthood. In Britain the MRC study, begun in 1946, interviewed 5,000 men and women about their responses to their parents' divorce or death and found a marked correlation between parental separation in childhood and adult ill-health and lack of academic, economic and emotional achievement. So many children of divorced parents are known to suffer in adulthood in all sorts of ways. What is not known is which aspects affect whether they suffer – is it the negative financial consequences of divorce, is it loss of contact with one parent, or is it a sense of distrust that a loved parent no longer cares?

Wallerstein and Blakeslee (1989) say, 'Children get angry with their parents for violating the unwritten rules of parenthood. Parents are supposed to make sacrifices for their children, not the other way around.'

Her own research and that of others (e.g. Mitchell 1988) shows that children overwhelmingly state they would prefer their parents to stay together rather than divorce, and to get back together if they have already divorced. If it were children's wishes alone that the courts considered paramount, parents would not be allowed to divorce.

She also points out that one cannot predict the long-term outcome of divorce on children from how they react at the outset. What counts most is that children perceive that their parents are committed to them and give them priority. In the context of separation, parental fitness is to do with how parents manage the process to minimise damage to children. It has often been argued that any form of conflict over children is a form of child abuse and the more prolonged it is the more harmful it is to the child.

As with other areas I examine in this book, there is a need for more sophisticated long-term research. As Schaffer (1990) points out, divorce is not a single event but a long process with many different elements:

A whole configuration of factors influences the process of adjustment: the child's age, the child's sex, the nature of previous relationships with each of the parents, the arrangements made for custody and access, the quality of life in the single parent family, the parents' remarriage and so on.

CRITICISMS OF EXISTING ASSESSMENT METHODS

Legal versus social work frameworks

In dealing with parents separating, the professional intervention has largely been determined within the legal framework set by the courts but, as we have seen, the court welfare service has been prominent in operating a social work element to intervention in the investigations it traditionally carried out for the courts. More recently it has been promoting a new area of expertise under the banner of conciliation. The adversarial nature of the legal process is often at odds with the conciliation principle of court welfare work. It also colours the way in which the social work approach operates. For example, the concept of 'fairness' to both parents is a recurring theme in court welfare officers' descriptions of their approach to conciliation, but this has been criticised:

We suggest that any attempt to ensure such fairness represents, in fact an attempt by the conciliator to impose his own views and values on the situation. More than this, it represents a (perhaps legalistic?) distortion of the way in which relationships actually work. Life is not fair; relationships are not fair or unfair, they are what they are. When a married couple are together, no one intervenes to complain that one or other of them has a greater influence in the decisionmaking relating to the children. It is difficult to see therefore why this should change when the couple cease to live together. The way they negotiate will obviously be coloured by the way in which parties relate to each other, and will continue to be so.

(Howard and Shepherd 1987)

Parents' trust in, and recourse to, the legal system is based on the belief that it will be fair to each parent, even if life is not. Effective conciliation however is rooted in the reality of the parents' relationships. It is now realised by those working in conciliation that dealing with parental need to resolve their own emotional confusion is crucial to reaching agreement over the children, so the idea of children being the sole consideration is falling from favour. As in child protection and adoption, it is being recognised that the parent–child relationship cannot be treated in isolation from the other aspects of family life, namely the parents' relationship, property and financial matters. This entails the skills more traditionally associated with the social work approach being the controlling professional framework. Some projects such as the Cambridge Family and Divorce Centre have already started putting this into practice.

The increasing importance of conciliation does however raise issues about confidentiality. A court welfare officer who is also involved in conciliation in the process of preparing a report is bound to make everything disclosed to him available to the court. Other conciliation services depend on offering confidentiality to both parties. There may be a conflict for the welfare officer over how to investigate as well as offer conciliation without offering confidentiality.

The legal procedures emphasise parents getting an agreement, whereas conciliation is more concerned with the process by which parents are enabled to communicate and negotiate mutually acceptable decisions – the difference is crucial, though the end may appear the same to a court. The move away from a short-term legalistic solution to a long-term family solution through more therapeutic intervention by professionals is similar to trends noted in other areas in Part I of this book. However, for this approach to become more widespread entails a huge increase in conciliation service provision for parents which the state has yet to see its way to funding.

Preserving the status quo

This principle of welfare officers recommending the status quo has been criticised:

> It is arguable that such recommendations show an evaluation of factual and theoretical considerations which coincides with the view of the court. However, it may also be a reflection of the fact that welfare officers are aware that their recommendations are unlikely to persuade the court to alter the existing arrangements, and therefore present their reports in such a way as to anticipate the court decisions rather than determining them. If, as it has been argued, solicitors also gear their advice to what they think will be accepted by the courts, then the high level of concordance between welfare officers' recommendations and court decisions is not to be wondered at.
>
> (James and Wilson 1984)

The status quo may make sense to the courts but it does not always seem fair to parents. If, for example, a woman has chosen, in the best interests of her children, to leave the family home rather than disrupt their lives further by uprooting them, it may seem cruelly unjust to the children as well as to her that she should lose the possibility of having them live with her when she has been their main care-giver all their lives. This leads on to the next criticism.

Current criteria ignore parents' interests

In looking at the criteria that are currently used, it is clear that the prevailing belief in the best interests of the child means that parents' interests are put aside.

The emphasis is now on the continuity of children's emotional relationships. Past efforts in caretaking, relative financial benefits of being with different parents and so on are given less priority than making an order that will maximise the possibility of the child maintaining contact with both parents. The court cannot determine the quality of that contact, nor predict its impact on the family dynamics of which the child is only one element.

Many critics argue that the interests of parents should be considered on their own account as long as they do not disadvantage the child. They also suggest that new legislation has given fathers a stronger position in disputed cases than their past efforts in caretaking 'should fairly allow' and poses a possible threat to the custodial parent.

One solution they propose is to solve custody disputes on the basis of the primary caretaker principle. In West Virginia, USA, this principle has been put into practice. The primary caretaker is defined as the parent who:

1 Prepares meals.
2 Changes nappies and dresses and bathes the child.
3 Chauffeurs the child to school, church, friends' homes, and the like.
4 Provides medical attention, monitors the child's health and is responsible for taking the child to the doctor.
5 Interacts with the child's friends, school authorities and other parents engaged in activities that involve the child.

In West Virginia, the Chief Justice recommends the advantages of the primary caretaker rule over the best interest of the child principle thus: a drastic reduction of the need for a protracted, damaging investigation into family life and the fitness of the parents, and the limited possibility of using the children as bargaining factors in the economic settlement – child support, alimony and division of property. He is concerned with protecting women from having to accept anything in order to keep the children. At the same time the rule is gender-neutral and does not exclude the father from the possibility of getting custody. The views of children between the ages of 6 and 14 may be sought and given discretionary weight. Proponents of this model suggest that it stands a better chance of working in the best interests of the child while allowing the parent who has invested most in primary caretaking to continue to do so (Smart and Sevenhuijsen 1989). It also has the interesting effect of minimising professional judgements of what it is to be a fit parent.

Another aspect of this neglect of parents' interests emerges with the 1989 Children Act's combination of stressing that both parents are for life and minimising the state's involvement in their parenting after divorce. (The 1989 Children Act tells the court not to make an order with respect to a child unless it considers that doing so would be better for the child than no order at all.)

The paradox of the Act is that at the same time as there is nothing to fight over (you always remain a parent) there is everything to fight for, because you always have a right to have a say in the upbringing of your child. When there is agreement, problems will be minimised. Where there is routine conflict, imposing a duty to consult . . . might exacerbate the situation. Many women experience emotional and physical violence and harassment in their marriage; to expect them to view with equanimity the potential leverage that the deeper messages of the Act carries is to ignore the physical and psychological realities of their lives. If the courts do not assist in redefining the parental and spousal relationships on divorce, the post divorce situation may be riddled with uncertainty, and thus be a recipe for conflict: none of this will benefit the child.

(Roche 1991)

In the best interests of the child?

Paradoxically, while parents' interests are deemed less important than children's, what is clear is that until now the wishes of children have not been a major criterion that has been represented with any consistency or priority. The 1987 DHSS guidelines emphasise that court welfare reports are not social enquiry reports and should not focus on the misdeeds of parents unless these endanger the child. The moral, mental or physical fitness of competing parents is only supposed to be considered if they affect their capacity to parent. But surveys such as Collins and Macleod's have shown that the most frequent references in reports were to parents' actions and relationships, not to child–parent relationships.

The overriding emphasis on conciliation means that the professionals con-centrate on the parent, not the children. Few solicitors or welfare officers spend any significant time with the children; it is quite possible for the entire dispute to be dealt with without the children being seen by any professional at all or the home being investigated. The welfare checklist is headed by 'the ascertainable wishes of the child', but the notion appears to come second to the notion that decisions relating to children should properly remain the responsibility of their parents. As one solicitor is quoted as saying:

There is an enormous administrative pressure to reach agreement. The case is listed, all parties attend, the court allocates say half a day to hear the thing but puts other matters in the list in case it settles. Everyone is scrambling for court time so it is no wonder people feel pressured.

(Kingsley 1990)

There is a distinct feeling that the tail is wagging the dog, the tail being the overriding need to reach an agreement for the benefit of the court machinery, not the children or their parents.

Court welfare officers provide a largely idiosyncratic and inconsistent service which claims to meet the needs of families and to protect the best interests of the children. In reality this service appears to meet the needs of the courts to achieve agreement between disputing parents, and for this reason is highly valued by the courts.

(Kingsley 1990)

The lack of consultation of children is worrying.

> The implication of this practice, when taken with the low priority given by all court welfare officers to the aims of advising the court as to the wishes and best interests of the children and high priority given to seeking parental agreement, is that many children remain unseen and unheard and waiting on the sidelines for a decision to be made about their future.
>
> (Kingsley 1990)

Many who have studied the new Children Act are similarly cautious about the extent to which it will actually protect a child's best interests.

> The new restriction of the judge's power to take an overall view of the quality of the parents' decisions about what is to happen to the children is significant. . . . It does seem to give the parents a freer hand than they, at least theoretically, had previously but it is debatable whether this is encouraging responsibility or irresponsibility.
>
> (Eekelar and Dingwall 1990)

The challenge is for practitioners to improve their communication with children and their knowledge of child development to enable the voice of the child to be heard on all reports.

Inconsistency is a bar to fairness

I have already described the challenge posed by the different approaches employed by welfare officers in preparing court reports. But there is another aspect which adds to this inconsistency. As with social workers involved in assessing parents for adoption or for the purposes of child protection, there is also the concern over court welfare officers' scope for imposition of personal moral and social standards on those whom they are reporting.

> Perhaps the most worrying is the subtle and probably largely unconscious imposition by litigants of the welfare officers' personal values during the time when the investigation is taking place when many parents feel particularly vulnerable emotionally. Then, implied or other criticism of their values or behaviour may serve only to weaken their morale and render them less able to adapt more realistically to what may be a rapidly changing and emotionally fraught situation, or may even alienate them from the system of law which is trying to find solutions to their problems. At the very point when they may need encouragement and a degree of personal validation they may face disapproval the harder to deal with if not acknowledged by the officer concerned. Welfare officers may need to remember that we are not talking about people who have broken the law, but about citizens whose private morality may merely differ from their own. Yet the problem is that the welfare officer may consider quite seriously that the parents are behaving in ways which

cause unnecessary suffering to their children. The welfare officer may take the view that is worse than minor crime.

(Murch 1980)

Whether parents actually are subjected to such disapproval or merely feel so is difficult to measure – divorcing brings parents under the scrutiny of their families and friends, perhaps their employers, their children's teachers and others. Thus the sense of disapproval may be a general one which the parents experience and is ascribed to the particular welfare officer or professional. The impact on the parents will in itself risk changing what it is the welfare officers are assessing. It may also affect what they choose to note and what they choose to ignore.

The picture that emerges is one of widespread variation in the beliefs and practices by which an influential document is prepared – so can anything be done to make the process more systematic? There seems to be some anxiety about addressing this issue:

> The possible implications of such variations in practice in terms of the information made available to the court are clear although a move to standardise practice would create practical and ideological difficulties including the question of how far state intervention in family life in the children's interests can be justified.

(James and Wilson 1984)

One approach to more standardisation is:

Explicit criteria

As we have already seen the criteria that are used by professionals are far from consistent or explicit. It has been argued that this impedes both the possibility of child-centred decision making and parental agreement. For example Murch's survey (1980) found that 'some welfare officers forget that parents do not always understand or share their belief that early childhood experience determines later behaviour.'

This professional view of what children's needs are and how to assess them is one that is rarely shared with parents who are the subject of assessment. It has been suggested that

> the value of explicit criteria would help mark out the boundaries for courtroom discussion about the child developmental needs. Secondly these criteria would facilitate a greater understanding by parents of the information base used by welfare officers in their reports. Thirdly the criteria would improve the level of communication between the report writer and the adjudicator.

(Gibbons 1989)

The following criteria, he suggests, should be agreed and made explicit:

- Child's view.
- Existing care arrangements: living conditions, time spent each day with child; work/school; what kind of daily routine the child experiences.

- Previous parenting experience: who put the child to bed? Who did the child go to at times of distress? Who did the day-to-day caring?
- Personality and character of parent: what would the child experience in terms of discipline, play and meeting developmental needs? What is the degree of affinity/bonding between parent and child?
- Future role of non-custodial parent: overnight parenting experience; help with child's interests and activities; caretaker role; sharing parental concerns about the children.
- Personal support network: proximity of grandparents; relatives; schoolfriends, other significant relationships; distance from school and progress in school; general practitioner/medical concerns; clubs; guides, scouts; playgroup.
- Cohabitees (if applicable): attitude of new partner to non-custodial parent; relationship with child concerned; permanence of relationship; interaction between cohabitee's children and those of natural parent.
- Access: child's rights to see both parents as frequently as possible; future arrangements; value of access in meeting child's developmental needs; parenting role for non-custodial parent.

This list is more comprehensive than the welfare checklist in the new Children Act which only covers some of these areas and still leaves a lot open to individual professional discretion. Explicit and agreed criteria could make a big contribution to the way parents approach settling childcare disputes and to their perception of the fairness of professional intervention.

Empowering parents

There seems to be a professional view of parents who are in a dispute which tends towards paternalism. For example, there is no consistency about showing welfare reports to parents, and although the new law emphasises parental responsibility there is often a sense of parents not behaving responsibly and needing to be dealt with firmly: 'Of course, some parents at a supervised handover behave well, especially when there have been clear statements by the supervisor as to what is acceptable or unacceptable behaviour' (Johnson 1991).

Since welfare officers' professional experiences of parents are limited to those who have a dispute of some sort, they are undoubtedly seeing the more 'troublesome' ones and this will colour their views of parental behaviour. While the processes of the legal system itself encourages an adversarial view of divorce, if parents rise to the challenge this presents they are criticised by the professionals:

> Parents need advice and education. Sometimes determined parents will shop around to get the professional advice that suits them. It is sad that some parents will put their children through medical examinations, or psychiatric assessments, in order to sustain their belief about the unsuitability of their former partners.
>
> (Johnson 1991)

It is sad that parents feel driven to seek this sort of professional expertise in order to play the same game as the courts. It is precisely because they know that courts think that 'individual parents' perceptions can be unreliable' that they seek professional evidence that will stand up in court when their own opinions will not. It is often at the suggestion of solicitors that parents do so.

The new laws emphasising parental responsibility are an encouragement for professionals such as court welfare officers to help parents reach their own agreements and not impose their own solutions. But this is not necessarily straightforward if, as we have seen, the pressure is for the obtaining of an agreement. James and Dingwall, for example, quote the following from case records: 'It is time you both began to put the interests of your children before your own feelings or one or both of you may lose your children' (1989).

Another report records that 'In the end they were unable to agree so . . . we concocted our own arrangements and said that we would insist upon these arrangements being followed out.'

This is an important reflection of the discrepancy between professed ideology and the realities of putting it into practice. However, for parents to behave responsibly it needs more than laws, it needs an approach which empowers and prepares parents for the new experiences they are facing. As Clulow suggests:

> How difficult it can be for a couple in the throes of separation and divorce to make and sustain the distinction between parent and partner when the two roles converge on one and the same person. Information, including an understanding of how loss can affect behaviour and the capacity to be an effective parent, can be an invaluable asset for parents and professionals alike when the familiar world seems to be falling apart.
>
> (Clulow 1989)

As far as empowering parents to continue to take responsibility for their children there appears to be a great need for parents to have a full understanding of the consequences of divorce for themselves and for their children. Here there is an analogy with pregnancy and birth. Like the beginning of parenthood,

> the ending of marriage not only brings with it many practical problems about such matters as housing, employment and money, but it also disturbs the basic structure of daily life, calling into question most of what has been taken for granted in terms of domestic routines, patterns of friendship and social support, and the social identity that will usually have been built around the marriage.
>
> (Richards 1989)

At present, the information and experience that comes from seeing large numbers of others going through separation lies with the professionals – more effort needs to be made to pass this on to parents. One attempt is through divorce experience courses being run in a few centres around Britain, often set up by practitioners involved in conciliation. These courses cover the different aspects of divorce (legal, emotional, financial) in a way which allows people to learn in the company of other people at similar stages to themselves (much like antenatal classes preparing parents for birth). They encourage parents to see that (just as childbirth) divorce is only a beginning, not an end in itself.

Withdrawal of state and professional responsibility only makes sense in terms of children's interests if it goes hand-in-hand with empowering parents to understand the influences on their parenting abilities.

THE POST-DIVORCE PARENT – WHO IS FIT?

When parents part, the question of who is fit to be a parent leads to many further questions – who is fit to be a single parent, who is fit to be a step-parent, how can a parent not living with his children be a fit parent? Again, most parents who find themselves in these roles have no preparation for them and often no one to turn to to help them adjust (De'Ath 1992). It has been suggested that

> greater deprivation and disturbance to children can come after the marriage break up rather than before. Custodial parents have less time and affection to offer, non-custodial parents are less involved, over-indulgent. Emotional scars aside, economic consequences can be considerable.
>
> (Dr Martin Richards quoted by Anne Woodham, *Guardian* 13/5/85)

The non-residential parent

As far as the state is concerned, the non-residential parent remains a fit parent by remaining involved with the child, providing financial maintenance, and a safety net should anything happen to the parent with whom the child lives. But as far as the children are concerned how does the absent parent remain a fit parent? According to the current philosophies:

- He/she remains involved on a regular basis (this includes writing and telephone calls as well as personal contact).
- He/she has a cooperative relationship with the other parent.
- He/she maintains a loving relationship with the children.
- He/she recognises their need to know their origins and their need to maintain contact with both parents for a sense of identity and belonging.
- His/her continued involvement counters the suspicion that they might have done something to drive the parent away.
- He/she turns up as arranged or ensures that plenty of notice is given if an appointment cannot be kept.

(Johnson 1991)

The handover from one parent to another can be extremely stressful to a child who is likely to already have some divided loyalties and confusion about how to behave. The fitness of both parents in such situations is also measured in terms of how they manage these handovers to minimise distress to the child.

Parents not living with their children have a particularly ambiguous role in relation to their children and this highlights the extent to which the parenting role is rooted in daily domestic routine as much as in a culturally constructed ideal of a blood bond. Demonstrations of affection and support are much more difficult to engineer in constrained circumstances of environment and time. Since it is most often men who fall into this role, many will not have previously had much daily involvement with their children and so have an even more scanty base on which to build. In Britain, one senior court welfare officer I spoke to commented on the need to educate fathers on how to get more involved with their children rather than just taking them to playgrounds, zoos or McDonald's. Somehow it is accepted that contact is important, but how the relationship is to flourish in the constrained circumstances of limited contact is for each father to discover for himself.

As Judith Wallerstein put it, 'Should he be a pal, an uncle, Santa Claus, or a playground attendant?' In California her team has set up groups for divorced parents (former partners attending different sessions) to come and discuss such practical aspects as where children should sleep, what they could do, what they could talk about. This type of work has led to a sharp decrease in the number of fathers losing contact with their children after divorce – thereby proving the importance of preparation for this variation on 'standard' parenting.

Step-parents

There are a large number of routes by which step-families are formed; many divorced and separated parents will go on to form another relationship which results in their children acquiring step-parents. Research following up divorced and lone parents suggests that within two years over half the non-resident parents (usually fathers) have remarried and within five years about half the resident parents (usually mothers) have remarried (De'Ath 1992). For parents this represents a new opportunity to find personal happiness, but for children the situation is often more ambiguous.

Despite the huge number of children who find themselves in this situation there has been little recognition of the specific challenges that such families face. While childcare arrangements may be scrutinised when couples separate, there is no such corresponding interest in children's welfare when their parents form new adult relationships. Yet there is much evidence that an equal amount of concern and support is required. At the end of 1991 the Family Policy Studies Centre produced evidence that where a divorced parent, usually a mother, has remarried the children come off worse compared with those in two-parent families and single-parent families. They are more likely to leave school without qualifications, more likely to leave home by the age of 18 (some to join the homeless on city streets); girls are more likely to leave school before 16, more likely to marry before the age of 20, and more likely to become pregnant in their teens.

These findings emerged from analysing the lives of a group of children born in 1958 whose parents divorced in the 1960s. If the results can be extrapolated for children whose parents are divorcing and remarrying now, there are serious implications. Not least is one of the common assumptions in custody disputes favouring the partner who is in a new stable relationship and that a new two-parent family is socially superior to a single-parent family. While the single parent may be free to concentrate on her children, any new relationship she forms brings competition and many difficult new relationships which are not of the children's choosing and are perhaps rarely embraced wholeheartedly by the step-parent.

When two people jointly choose to become parents it usually results in reciprocal relationships with the child, but when the parent–child relationship has been chosen neither by the child nor by one parent, there can be no assumption of such mutual bonds and many step-parents feel they should grow to love the other partner's children. This puts the step-parent in a difficult situation – what role should he or she play? The pressures to become replacement parents are great – but children do not readily accept this if they already know their natural parents. Step-parents may also mean new step brothers and step sisters, or new children born of the new adult partnership – all these produce additional possibilities for conflict and resentment, but also for support and friendship. For the children, new partners often mean new households with new rules, new networks of extra-familiar contacts at the expense of previous ones. The new partner's presence may affect the amount of contact the children have with their non-residential parent.

Parents in such situations can feel pulled in every direction in their attempt to be perfect and yet they may end up feeling failures. Their own new relationship may become threatened by the stresses of parenting in such unfamiliar circumstances. Breakdown rates for second marriages are notoriously high. The research on children of single parents and those who acquire step-parents is not encouraging and, whenever it is reported, paints a very bleak picture – which in itself places a huge burden of guilt on many such parents. Again there seems to be little emphasis in researching what specific aspects of being in a single-parent or step-family are potentially damaging and what measures can minimise the effects on children and their parents. In the absence of such data, prejudices born of ignorance can serve to penalise such families further.

WHAT THE ASSESSMENT OF SEPARATED PARENTS TELLS US ABOUT FIT PARENTS

Ideal

- Parents are for ever – children need continuity of relationships with both their parents.
- A man and woman living together in a loving and supportive relationship are most likely to provide good parenting.
- The parent–child relationships are inextricably embedded in the parental relationship.
- However poor the parental relationship, children's needs are best met if the parents stay together.

- Successful parenting is very closely tied up with the continuity and stability of the domestic and daily routines a child experiences.
- A woman is the fittest person to nurture her children.
- A man is the prime economic provider for his children.
- A boy needs his father as a gender role model.
- A girl needs her mother as a gender role model.
- Parents have rights and duties to their children which are inseparable.
- It is the parents' duty – and not that of the state – to ensure their children's welfare.
- Decisions relating to children are the responsibility of their parents.

Actual

- Parents' individual involvement with their children may fluctuate over the course of their lives.
- The parent–child role changes and evolves with time; in particular the closeness with either parent may vary.
- Successful parent–child relationships can exist independent of the parents' relationship.
- The parenting role is directly affected by the quality of relationships, in particular that between parents.
- A relationship full of conflict may do more damage to children than a divorce.
- Parents need to do their best to ensure as short a period of conflict/uncertainty as possible in the event of a breakdown of parental relationship.
- Parents need to seek out appropriate support to help their family through crises.
- Men and women can be equally fit as lone parents.
- Parents can continue to be good enough parents even when not living with their children, but this requires adjustment and some relearning of the parental role and creating new routines.
- Parents try to provide stability and reassurance for their children even when under stress.
- Parents have responsibilities and privileges with regard to their children, not rights.

4   Playing God

The medical gift of children

In 1987 a woman who had entered a US$10,000 contract to be a surrogate mother for the child of an infertile couple came to the attention of the American courts. Having received the sperm of the man by artificial insemination she became pregnant and gave birth to a daughter. However, instead of handing over the child to the couple she decided she wanted to keep her, and refused payment. There followed a bitter court wrangle in which the relative merits of all four would-be parents were openly debated.

> It came down to a classic custody case: who was the best parent? Judge Harvey Sorkow was vehemently critical of her character. Throughout the three month trial experts portrayed her as something of a diabolical person – an ill-educated former nightclub dancer who was unstable and, by implication, unfit to be Baby M's mother. And yet she and her husband, a refuse collector with an alcohol problem, have two school-aged children of their own both living at home. Nobody has ever suggested removing them because of unfit parents, the court heard.
>
> (Christopher Thomas, *The Times* 2/4/87)

It soon became inevitable that the child would go to the middle-class home of the professional couple who could provide a materially better life-style (including music lessons) and, it seemed from the Judge's appraisal, better social values. His decision was based solely on what he called 'the best interests of the child'. He felt the father would be a better parent than the surrogate mother's husband.

This story and others involving the human consequences of the new reproductive technologies highlight an important historic shift that has taken place in the last decade. For the first time in history the biological bond of gene transfer between adult and child is no longer the fundamental basis for parenthood. Our very definitions of mother and father are no longer clear: providing semen to create a child does not entitle a man to be called the father of that child. Becoming inseminated, carrying a foetus through pregnancy and even giving birth to a child no longer automatically means the bearer can call herself the mother.

This is contributing to an overall shift in attitudes to who is fit to be a parent – it is no longer assumed that a genetic relationship can define parental rights or responsibilities. The relative merits of those responsible for creating a child as fit are called into question, but there remains a difficulty in considering the future welfare of a child who is not only not yet in existence but whose existence remains the gift of doctors.

A BRIEF HISTORY OF MEDICALLY ASSISTED PARENTHOOD

Over the course of this century the medical profession's involvement with the process of becoming a parent has become more and more profound. Medical intervention has gone further and further into the reproduction process removing more and more of parents' authority over their own reproductive lives: from advising on nutrition and child-health, to managing women's labours in increasingly technological ways, to supervising pregnancy which includes a growing number of tests and medical procedures, and to controlling fertility itself. The development of chemical contraceptives such as The Pill and the media attention it received heralded the first public acknowledgement of the separation of sex from reproduction. The full range of medical family planning techniques came to be widely promoted, so endorsing the idea that every child should be a wanted child and a healthy child and all fit parents should therefore plan their children's births and do all they can to ensure they develop healthily. The only way they could do this effectively was through seeking medical help and accepting the expertise of the medical professionals.

Thus the private biological process that lay in the natural powers of most men and women has increasingly become a medical and technological process that takes place in clinics and hospitals, arenas of professional power. It has now reached the stage where the very process of conception can be controlled by doctors, with the would-be parents only playing a very subsidiary role. The advent of techniques and drugs that can influence who can have children has given them new God-like powers and in the last two decades has brought about a phenomenal revolution in what medical science can do for fertility and childbirth.

The apparent motivation to intervene has been to ensure healthier mothers and babies, to minimise the risks of childbirth and multiple pregnancies which caused so much death and misery in centuries past. The intention of assisted reproduction was to treat those with 'medical' problems that prevented them from the 'normal' process of conception and pregnancy. The 'goodness' of such motives was almost indisputable and the headlines focused on the happiness of the proud new parents and on the patrician benefactor figure of the doctor who had made their parenthood possible.

The earliest form of medically assisted reproduction, donor insemination, has been on record for nearly a century, but its wider availability on the NHS was a matter for considerable debate – a commission led by the Archbishop of Canterbury in 1950 concluded that it should be made a criminal offence, such was the danger it posed to family life. The advice was not accepted and its use continued in a limited fashion, drawing criticism and concern but not active discouragement. There seems to have been a feeling that, since such a small number of people were availing themselves of it, there was little reason for the state to intervene.

The growing demand for assisted reproduction has been influenced by trends in the other areas considered in this book so far, in particular adoption and divorce. The difficulty of adopting a baby, combined with the desire to have something created especially for oneself, has increased the number of people seeking medical treatment to become parents. The preference that infertile couples are increasingly showing for medically assisted reproduction rather than adoption reflects in part at least a desire to have as much of a normal experience of family life from as early as possible. The increase in divorce and subsequent remarriage has led to an increase in desire for children at a later age when natural fertility is lower, or when the male may have previously had a vasectomy. There is also evidence that fertility has been dropping over the century, possibly due to environmental pollution.

The possibilities of medical assistance in reproduction caught the imagination of many and have quickly taken it to the stage where perfectly healthy, fertile women are demanding donor insemination purely because they have not found suitable men to impregnate them or do not want to involve a man. Grandmothers are gestating their infertile daughters' children, couples are adopting the fertilised eggs of others and having them implanted in the adoptive mother who will then give birth to a child that is genetically not her own and so on. Who is fit to be a parent now comes with a corollary – how many fit people does it take to parent a child? The man providing sperm, the woman providing the egg, the woman whose womb will carry the baby, the woman and/or the man who will care for the child? And if the custody of the child comes into dispute, how will it be resolved in line 'with the best interests of the child' when those best interests include the possible need to have contact with his biological parents? And what effect does the existence of such artificially created families have on society? Can any future child trust his parents to be who he thinks they are? Will we see a backlash from the children as they approach adulthood and discover their true genetic parentage?

Throughout the developed world, the law is having to engage with family situations never before contemplated and regulatory authorities are having to acknowledge that they may not be able to control all the new methods of parenting. Opponents argue that it is a Pandora's box – that assisted reproduction techniques should not have been made available until other social and moral and practical issues have been resolved. They fear that just as high-tech hospital births have come to be regarded as normal, so high-tech conception will be too, and just as problems are being recognised with the technologies and drugs used in pregnancy and labour so may other problems emerge with assisted reproduction. They also express concern that the huge funds required to provide such treatments divert attention and resources from dealing with the consequences of infertility and underline the social pressures on people to have children.

As more and more people are now seeking help in *making* and *having* babies, feminists and right-wing traditionalists alike are accusing the medical profession of having turned parenthood into a consumer-led manufacturing process, whereby designer babies can be made to order on the production lines of laboratories and clinics for those who can afford them. The consumers are thus encouraged to see medical intervention as ensuring quality control of their products. Doctors argue that they are providing services for which there is a huge demand and point to the happiness of the parents who have succeeded in getting what they wanted.

In Britain it is no longer an option to discontinue these services, merely a matter of how to regulate them effectively (Morgan and Lee 1991). Such is the demand that they are here to stay and it is for society to come to terms with the new notions of family that they bring (Glover *et al.* 1989).

THE PRINCIPAL TECHNIQUES AND THE ISSUES THEY RAISE

Artificial insemination by donor (AID)

For donor insemination all a woman needs is a syringe and some fresh semen obtained from a willing man. Private arrangements rarely come to light unless there is a dispute over custody of the child. (For example, in America a lesbian couple who had received sperm from a homosexual friend split up and all three were awarded visiting rights to the child.) But the recent spread in sexually transmitted diseases and in the HIV virus, as well as the growing concern to avoid genetically inheritable conditions, has increased the number of women seeking medically supervised AID. The expectation is to get sperm which has been obtained from a healthy donor of good genetic stock. With adoption becoming so difficult, AID is often the only answer for a couple where the woman is fertile but whose partner is infertile or a carrier of some genetically transmittable disease. The success rate for donor insemination is high.

AID is now available from any willing gynaecologist on the National Health Service in Britain as well as from private infertility clinics. The selection criteria vary – some refuse treatment to single women, some to lesbians, some to women deemed unsuitable mothers for other reasons, e.g. health, age, job. Some state policies such as not inseminating anyone whose partner is not in agreement. However, few investigate the background of the couple. In 1989 the newspapers reported the case of a British husband who successfully divorced his wife on the grounds of unreasonable behaviour after she received AID without his knowledge or consent and subsequently gave birth to a daughter.

MP Ivan Lawrence QC, chairman of the Tory backbench legal committee, was among those who questioned the vetting procedures of sperm bank clinics. He warned: 'If we are not careful, we will take a giant step towards the destruction of family life by making too freely available to single parents the opportunity to have children this way' (Justin Davenport, *Daily Mail* 16/10/1989).

Egg donation

For women who cannot produce their own eggs, receiving the eggs of another woman can often enable conception. Egg donors are not as numerous as sperm donors, partly because more intervention is required to remove the eggs. Frequently it is a sister or friend who provides the eggs, and often women who come to a clinic for other forms of treatment are also asked to donate eggs. Whether such women are the most suitable to provide eggs is questionable, since they are usually older and therefore considered more likely to increase chances of foetal abnormalities which lead to a higher risk of miscarriage and of babies with handicaps.

Surrogacy

This is the process by which a woman agrees to bear a child for someone else to rear. It is most commonly used by couples where the woman is infertile and who 'commissions' another woman (often a relative) to receive the husband's sperm and carry the baby in her womb until birth before handing the baby over to the commissioning couple.

Surrogacy exists in different forms, official and unofficial. It can be effected by a man having sexual intercourse with the surrogate mother. It can be done by artificial insemination of the host mother with the man's sperm (e.g. the recently reported case of the Boston lawyer who sent frozen sperm by air courier to California where a nurse successfully inseminated herself. The resulting baby was then handed over to the Boston couple). Avoiding expensive fertility clinic fees is obviously a motivating factor in such cases. None the less, the commissioning parents still have to make their own judgements about who they want to carry their child through pregnancy – someone who is healthy, not a drug user, smoker or alcoholic, and someone who is likely to behave in such a way as she would if the child were hers for ever – and yet be prepared to hand over the baby.

Modern surrogacy uses egg and sperm from the commissioning couple, fertilises them in the laboratory and transfers the fertilised embryo to the host mother who then carries the baby and gives birth to it. The baby is thus genetically unrelated to the host mother but the commissioning couple none the less have to adopt the child and 'to prove themselves to be fit parents'.

There are potentially many dilemmas over who has legal ownership of a child born in this way. The commissioning couple cannot be sure that the surrogate mother will hand over the child after birth. In Britain she retains the right to change her mind and no financial contract is legal (but in many states in America commercial surrogacy is legal and contracts enforceable). And what if a couple split after surrogacy has been embarked upon? It resulted in three adults claiming custody of a baby in the widely reported Moschetta case in California.

In Britain the only test case was that of Kim Cotton in 1985, whose surrogate pregnancy had received widespread coverage in the media, generally painting a black picture of the woman who could deliberately create a baby only to give it up in return for money. Her situation was caricatured by many media professionals as that of a greedy and heartless attention-seeking woman who was prepared to put her own selfish needs before her family's – there was almost gleeful reporting of the rifts in her family that had resulted from her decision to become a surrogate mother and from the subsequent intense media scrutiny.

In a dramatic and eventful evening at the hospital in the full glare of publicity, the fate of Baby Cotton was taken out of her mother's hands. The local social services arrived while Kim Cotton was in the throes of labour to check rumours that she did not intend to keep her baby. As soon as the baby was born she was made a ward of court and neither Kim Cotton nor the commissioning parents were allowed to take her home. Eight days later, the High Court

> deemed the father and his wife to be a warm, caring sensible couple who would give the baby a good home. They were a professional couple, well able to meet the baby's emotional needs and to handle the complex questions of her birth when they arose. . . . The couple who lived abroad . . . had both a town house and a country home . . . flew out of Britain with Baby Cotton at the weekend.
>
> (Cotton and Winn 1985)

The case of Baby Cotton, coming as it did at the time that the Warnock Commission was in the process of publishing its findings, received a huge amount of publicity and is said to have accelerated the steps to make commercial surrogacy illegal in Britain. It was another interesting example of the media not just reflecting public opinion or reporting events but actually setting the agenda for the state's actions. In fact the media had been responsible for introducing the idea of surrogacy to Kim Cotton in the first place, and in defining many of her attitudes to going ahead. She felt no desire to hold on to the baby as it was 'not born from love' within her own marriage. It was an act that she says she did not regret but her story is a vivid illustration of how much social as well as biological events, pregnancy and childbirth are. Her belief that it would just be a personal business was dashed by the wide-ranging effects it had on a large number of other people in her family and social network. Surrogacy is clearly not a job to be undertaken lightly.

The director of Bourn Hall Clinic in Britain, announcing the start of their surrogacy programme, acknowledged the many dilemmas:

> Professor Robert Edwards, the test tube baby pioneer, predicted the technique [surrogacy] could one day be used by career women who did not wish to give birth themselves. . . . The concern is that it could lead to exploitation: 'there could be pressures to make this into a trade'. He went on to say that the clinic would not offer the technique for convenience – 'this is something that has to be done in love. It is one of the greatest gifts that one woman can give to another woman'.
>
> (Aileen Ballantyne, *Sunday Times* 19/8/90)

It seems probable that if the surrogate mother is a relative or close friend of the mother, she is more likely to be motivated by love, but also more likely to find it difficult to give up her relationship with the baby afterwards. For strangers, the motives are more difficult to ascertain. Kim Cotton says she was motivated by the idea of doing something worthwhile and getting paid for it, but also by the challenge of doing something unusual. In the USA Phyllis Chesler reports that many of the women offering themselves as surrogate mothers are poorly educated, leading lack-lustre lives, who have low self-esteem and who see surrogacy as a way of becoming important to others as well as making money. Others have been sexually abused as children and see the use of another man's sperm to produce a child as a way of cleansing themselves of their past. Most see themselves as fairy godmothers to whom infertile couples will be forever indebted but all too often find that, as soon as the child has been handed over, the couple want to break off all communication. More information is clearly needed about why women become surrogate mothers and the long-term effects on them (for example, do some experience the debilitating sense of loss that has been identified in women who have given up children for adoption?).

In Britain, for official surrogacy taking place under the aegis of a fertility clinic, the surrogate mother has to be in a stable relationship and have a child of her own. Bourn Hall has drawn up guidelines (with its local ethics committee) on who will be given surrogacy treatment. They are likely to be women who do not have wombs or have had over ten unsuccessful attempts at IVF, and women who have medical conditions that would be made worse by pregnancy such as heart disease or high blood pressure. In the USA some states have tried to introduce legislation that would limit surrogate arrangements to married couples who have undergone detailed psychological assessment.

Opponents to surrogacy include organisations such as LIFE, who are against all artificial methods of reproduction. A LIFE spokesman believes that surrogacy poses risks of psychological damage to all involved: 'We are opposed to any technique which treats human beings almost like consumer products for the convenience and benefit of other people. We don't believe it is in the best interests of the child' (Aileen Ballantyne, *Sunday Times* 19/8/90).

Many feminists oppose surrogacy on the basis that it deliberately sets out to deny a child the continuity of a relationship that began at conception, that it trivialises women's role as mothers by separating pregnancy from motherhood, and that it promotes the possibility of wealthy women exploiting poor women. (There was a well-publicised case in the USA relating to a Hispanic woman who alleged she had been forced to enter a surrogacy agreement by her family to make money from her rich childless employers.) It has also been pointed out that women seeking to become surrogates are subjected to more scrutiny than men seeking to become donors; thus the implication is that carrying a baby is a more significant act than insemination (Lasker and Borg 1987).

In vitro fertilisation (IVF)

This is the process pioneered by Patrick Steptoe and Robert Edwards in the 1970s by which eggs are taken from a woman and fertilised outside by the sperm of her partner under closely controlled laboratory conditions. A small number of selected embryos are then transferred back into the woman's womb and the woman then hopes for a successful pregnancy. The success of this treatment varies with the age and individual circumstances of the woman and from clinic to clinic. Few women get a baby with just one course of treatment, and most of the women undertaking such a programme go through several cycles before they are successful or before they give up. The most successful clinics rarely have a 'take-home' rate of more than 25 per cent. The price for such treatment can be high – emotionally, financially and physically. Those who succeed in becoming parents may feel the cost is justified but there are many who will be disappointed.

The rigorous selection of parents is even more important because of the difficult circumstances they will have to cope with, both in the treatment and in the associated risks of, for example, multiple births and neonatal problems, and not all couples can cope with this. Counselling, which includes why the couple want children, can help by considering alternatives to medical treatment. It has been suggested (Hanmer 1991) that many infertile women will pursue every available medical channel to conceive as a way of resolving the ambiguity of their childless status to those around them ('Look, I've tried everything, and there is no way I can have children'), and many women describe the enormous sense of relief when they finally stop having treatment.

'Off-the-shelf babies' – frozen embryos

Fertilised eggs can be frozen and stored for future use for up to five years. The question of who exercises rights over how these are used has created another angle on 'who is fit to be a parent?'. Already in the USA there has been a 'custody' battle over such embryos after a divorced wife chose to have further children from the stored embryos created during her marriage. The husband's lawyer argued that fatherhood should not be imposed on his client – particularly as he would be legally liable for child support.

The development of embryo freezing also has implications for parenthood. Women are at least risk of producing chromosomal abnormalities between the ages of 20 and 30 but may be too busy with a career to have children then, so perhaps they should have the choice of storing fertilised embryos for a later stage in their lives. At first sign this may seem unacceptably selfish and with no obvious medical grounds for treatment. However, as with the argument for providing treatment to single and lesbian women, some have argued that this service would be a pre-emptive medical measure, reducing the possibility of handicapped children and the 'burden' they might become to their parents and to society.

Bourn Hall has recently announced that it will make frozen embryos available for adoption by infertile couples, should the donors be willing for them to be used in this way. The embryos, frozen at two days old, could be implanted in the womb of the infertile mother, who could then give birth to the child who would bear no genetic relationship either to herself or to her partner.

Mary Warnock has discounted opposition to using embryos in this way by stating: 'These embryos exist, so why not have someone look after them. It's a better way of adopting' (Aileen Ballantyre, *Sunday Times* 15/12/91).

The appeal to infertile couples will be understandably great. For £850 they can go through the socially acceptable way of becoming parents – pregnancy and birth. No one need know how the woman came to be pregnant. It is likely to be the only way a childless couple can adopt a baby since baby adoptions through agencies are so rare nowadays. It seems a perfect solution for the genetic parents who do not want their unwanted embryos to die.

TACKLING THE DILEMMAS

In contrast to the other areas I have thus far considered in this book, the speed with which the new technologies have been developed and fear of the mind-boggling consequences of their unregulated use have alerted everyone to the need to face up to the ethical dilemmas. This has created an unprecedented burst of concentrated activity to discuss the issues in a public and systematic way. The Warnock Commission brought together leading medical specialists, philosophers, church representatives and lay people to investigate and report on the moral dilemmas and how these could be tackled. The Commission's report and the media coverage it received did much to bring the issues into the public arena and it has become the one area so far examined that seems to be most open to the public. Anyone may contact the Licensing Authority that was set up to regulate clinics and get information about the guidelines that are issued to them and how the Human Fertility and Embryology Authority (HFEA) inspects them. Anyone may contact a particular clinic and get details of their overall policies regarding who they will treat. This apparent openness in the face of public concerns has probably been a significant factor in the acceptance of the new techniques. However, it should be noted that there was a long period during which the embryologists were first developing their techniques when everything was shrouded in secrecy, and it was only with the birth of the first test tube baby that the matter was presented to the public, as a wonderful breakthrough in the treatment of infertility – by then it was a *fait accompli* and the medical lobby had set the agenda for the ensuing public debate. Critics suggest that the present guise of openness is a small concession by the medical establishment in return for being allowed to get on with their self-serving, high-tech experiments.

The Warnock Commission drew attention to the following:

- that the moral and ethical dilemmas are significant;
- that they cannot be resolved by professionals alone;
- that the work of the clinics needs to be monitored carefully to ensure good practice and to avoid exploitation of a vulnerable group.

The current consensus seems to be 'yes, there are concerns, but at the present time there appears to be no conclusive reason why clinics should not provide help to those who want children, that we should continue as a society to be vigilant to the consequences of such treatment and take reasonable steps to minimise its negative outcomes'.

From the start it was inevitable that this would produce the dilemma of *who* should be permitted to become a parent through medical assistance and *how* this selection would be carried out. As a result of the Warnock Commission's deliberations on the ethical questions raised by the new technologies, in 1991 a permanent supervisory body, the HFEA, came into being to license clinics and regulate their work. HFEA inspectors visit every clinic before granting a licence, meet the staff, and ask questions about selection criteria that are to be employed by that clinic. The aim is also to inspect each clinic annually thereafter to review all aspects of their work, including the sort of clients they have treated and those they have refused. The aim of the inspecting team is to be constructive, so they argue there is no reason why the clinic staff would want to lie or to deceive them. The Authority is made up of twenty-one professionals (e.g. research scientists, professors in obstetrics, child psychiatry, sociology, genetics, lawyers, a bishop, a social worker, education and nursing lecturers) and lay people who can be seen as representing the public interest as well as understanding the scientific and ethical issues. There is no doubt that much thought has gone into considering how best to regulate the treatments that enable parenting by artificial means.

So does all this openness and monitoring mean that 'who is fit to be a parent?' has a straightforward and consistent answer as far as medically assisted parenthood is concerned?

THE CURRENT OFFICIAL BASIS FOR SELECTION OF WOULD-BE PARENTS

Scientists argue that, if the techniques are available, they should be available to all who want them. Those alarmed by the implications of their widespread take-up argue that their use should be tempered by the consideration of the future of children born by such methods. Rather as the opponents to divorce argued that one had to think of the outcome for the children before allowing their parents to choose to split up, opponents to open access to assisted reproduction are arguing for the future welfare of such children, in particular the stigma and possible sense of loss of biological identity they might experience. However, as with divorce, there is no doubt that as there are more and more children born by such methods, any stigma will give way to a degree of social acceptance. (Unlike divorce, the children need not know of their unusual beginnings until they are 18 and choose to check their records.)

The HFEA has produced a voluntary Code of Practice which presents guidelines on selection in accordance with the HFE Act 1990. The Act states that a woman 'shall not be provided with treatment services unless account has been taken of the welfare of any child born as a result of the treatment (including the need of that child for a father)'.

One of the general obligations of those offering treatment is:

In deciding whether or not to offer treatment, centres should take account both of the wishes and needs of the people seeking treatment and of the needs too of any children who may be involved. Neither consideration is paramount above the other, and the subject should be approached with great care and sensitivity. Centres should avoid adopting any policy or criteria which may appear arbitrary or discriminatory.

The Code of Practice avoids laying down precise guidelines as to who might be considered undesirable but urges a systematic approach to gathering and recording information before taking a decision.

Where people seek licensed treatment, centres should bear in mind the following factors:

1 their commitment and that of their husband or partner (if any) to having and bringing up a child or children;
2 their ages and medical histories and the medical histories of their families;
3 the needs of any child or children that may be born as a result of treatment, including the implications of any possible multiple births, and the ability of the prospective parents (or parent) to meet those needs;
4 any risk of harm to the child or children who may be born as a result of treatment, including the implications of any possible multiple births, and the ability of the prospective parents to meet those needs;
5 the effect of a new baby or babies upon any existing child of the family.

Where people seeking treatment are using donated gametes, centres should also take the following factors into account:

1 a child's potential need to know about his or her origins and whether or not the prospective parents are prepared for the questions which may arise while the child is growing up;
2 the possible attitudes of other members of the family towards the child and towards his or her status in the family;
3 implications for the welfare of the child if the donor is personally known within the child's family and social circle; and
4 any possibility known to the centre of a dispute about the legal fatherhood of the child.

Paragraph 3.16 heightens further factors which will require consideration in the following cases.

1 Where it is the intention that the child will not be brought up by the carrying mother. In this case, centres should bear in mind that either the carrying mother, and in certain circumstances her husband or partner, or the commissioning parents may become the child's legal parents. Centres should also take into account the effect of the proposed arrangement on any child of the carrying mother's family as well as its effect on any child of the commissioning parents' family.
2 Where the child will have no legal father. Centres are required to have regard to the child's need for a father and should pay particular attention to the prospective mother's ability to meet the child's needs throughout his or her childhood, and where appropriate whether there is anyone else within the prospective mother's family and social circle who is willing and able to share the responsibility for meeting those needs and for bringing up, maintaining and caring for the child.

As far as the actual gathering of relevant information is concerned the Code of Practice says that this should be done by taking a medical and family history from each of the prospective parents and that they should be seen together and separately. It also requires the centre to satisfy itself that the client's GP knows of no reason why the 'client may not be suitable to be offered treatment, including anything which might adversely affect the welfare of any resulting child'.

It goes on to say:

> If any of these particulars or inquiries give cause for concern, e.g. evidence that the prospective parents have had children removed from their care, or evidence of a previous relevant conviction, the centre should make such further inquiries of any relevant individual, authority or agency as it can.

Other people can be approached only with the consent of the client – the HFE Act does not confer any legal powers on centres to get such information otherwise. If the consent is withheld, that also has to be taken into account. It does not specify what would be considered a relevant conviction (child abuse? drug misuse? prostitution?).

> (3.25) The decision to provide treatment should be taken in the light of all the available information. Treatment may be refused on clinical grounds. Treatment should also be refused if the centre believes that it would not be in the interests of any resulting child, or any child already existing, to provide treatment, or is unable to obtain sufficient information or advice in order to reach a proper conclusion.

> (3.26) If treatment is refused for any reason, the centre should explain to the woman and, where appropriate, her husband or partner, the reasons for this, and the factors, if any, which might persuade the centre to reverse its decision. It should also explain the options which remain open, and tell clients where they can obtain counselling.

> (3.27) Centres should record in detail the information which has been taken into account when considering the welfare of the child or children. The record should reflect the views of all those who were consulted in reaching a decision, including those of potential parents.

The Code of Practice also includes a conscientious objection clause which entitles any member of staff not to become involved in anything to which they have an ethical objection.

The wording of the guidelines seems to emphasise that the client is the would-be parent and that the clinic should act in a manner answerable to the client. Thus, unlike with adoption, the child is not seen as the client and his future well-being is dealt with in a fairly superficial manner. Whereas selection for adoption is concerned with whether an applicant will be a fit parent and every effort is made to discover this, for medically assisted reproduction the effort is fairly minimal and is designed only to exclude those who might seem grossly unfit. Thus a criminal record or a physical disability would not of itself exclude fertility treatment whereas for adoption it would be a very significant negative factor. The procedures and record keeping are clearly designed to protect the centre from criticism – 'We did all that we could reasonably be expected to do' – rather than to protect the best interests of the resulting child; e.g. there is no attempt to investigate the home or family of clients, and no obligation to check criminal records.

THE ACTUAL CRITERIA AFFECTING SELECTION OF WOULD-BE PARENTS

Current practice interprets the guidelines in different ways. The NHS centres, under acute pressure of long waiting lists, apply more demanding criteria than private centres. But even amongst the NHS centres the criteria are not uniform. Some only provide treatment to married couples, while others will provide treatment to a cohabiting couple. A couple who had been living together for six years were barred from treatment recently because they were not married. The consultant, while believing that marriage gave a child a more stable home, was clearly concerned by more than just the future welfare of the child: 'This treatment is in the public eye. We've got to be purer than the driven snow' (Tom Merrin, *Daily Mirror* 25/7/91).

For fertility treatment doctors the question of who is fit to receive treatment has two parts – the clinical and the moral. The clinical aspect is of far more interest than the moral, and more time is spent taking the medical history of the patients and evaluating whether their infertility is amenable to medical correction. The doctor's skill and training to do this is beyond doubt. However, they cannot be said to have the same training to address the second question, namely who is likely to be an unfit parent, and this undoubtedly receives less attention.

Most clinics emphasise that their role is to provide a service, not to play God. Most shy away from the idea that they have any responsibility to vet future parents. They argue that NHS treatment is only restricted by virtue of finite resources – to those with a good chance of success and the most deserving (i.e. to people who do not already have a child). Private clinics may claim they do not screen at all – anyone who can pay will get treatment. But in practice the local ethics committees advise on general suitability and it is at the discretion of the consultant as to who gets treatment.

Should fertile people get infertility treatment?

The medical framework is all-pervasive in the selection process. Becoming a parent is seen almost entirely as a medical process. The doctors are carrying out their professional obligation to cure illness – in the only way they are empowered to do. They cannot give infertile patients other people's children to adopt, they cannot remove the social pressures to reproduce or the inbuilt desire so many people powerfully experience to nurture – but they can in many cases cure the illness by helping the infertile produce children.

But if the adult seeking treatment is not ill – i.e. does not have any medical condition preventing reproduction but lacks the social conditions to enable parenthood (namely, a willing partner of the opposite sex) – should doctors get involved at all? In some countries fertility treatment is restricted to those who are medically infertile as opposed to socially incapable of reproduction. In Britain the official view is that no group should arbitrarily be excluded and recognition is given to the fact that the single and the gay can become parents in non-medically assisted ways which pose more potential risks to them and their future children. In their case the provision of medically assisted reproduction is a way of minimising the risks of future medical problems. Not all gynaecologists will provide treatment to fertile people.

In Britain the media recently featured the row over the costs and morality of fertility treatment to a single mother who gave birth to sextuplets. The media uncovered the fact that she already had a child, was not married to or living with the father and that the father already had three children from a previous marriage. The usual celebration of multiple births quickly turned sour:

> MPs have criticised the doctors who selected them for fertility treatment from hundreds of other desperate couples. The cost of the treatment and the hospital care of the babies may total tens of thousands of pounds.
>
> *(Sunday Times* 22/5/93)

The implication is that couples are more deserving than single people.

Peter Brinsden, Medical Director of Bourn Hall, says that they do not offer treatment to single women.

> I know this upsets women's rights organisations but I do not plan any changes. We have a clinical ethical committee which has lay people including a lawyer, a scientist and a gynaecologist. It decided that the prime concern is for the baby – not the women – and that it was not right to deliberately create children, in addition to those produced accidentally, in an environment that might not be ideal.
>
> (Christine Doyle 12/3/91 © The Telegraph plc, London)

However, he is then quoted as saying that he receives two or three requests from single women a month and 'sends as nice a refusal letter as possible and will very occasionally suggest a clinic where they may be helped'.

It is clear that there is some ambiguity as to whether single women are inherently less good potential parents or whether most gynaecologists simply do not want to be seen to be enabling them to become mothers. The BMA's position is that while doctors should observe the law and 'must consider the type of environment into which the child will be placed, it is up to society as a whole, not doctors, to decide if single women should be denied artificial insemination' (© The Telegraph plc, London 12/3/91).

Other countries such as the USA and Denmark have clearly stated that being single does not exclude a woman from treatment. Sweden has clearly forbidden it. Britain has left the position legally ambiguous and thus it is at the discretion of individual consultants, guided by their local ethics committees.

Evaluating potential parents

That discretion is based on a fairly limited investigation of a person's background and personal judgement about that person's parenting potential. The conscientious objection clause can be invoked whenever there is doubt in the consultant's mind about someone's suitability. What is discovered about a person's suitability as a parent is largely discovered in the course of the clinical interview. If the referring GP has provided any evidence suggesting marital violence or substance abuse, the fertility consultant would raise it as a subject for discussion. The GP is seen as the person who knows the patient in the community and therefore would disclose any adverse information or not refer the person for treatment. The infertility consultant might read between the lines of the GP's referral; e.g. a GP might hint that his patient has had problems handling stress in the past or is in a stormy relationship. If he had any cause to believe that the adult's problems had not been resolved he might decide to withhold treatment. Again the medical model prevails in selection – only children who are at obvious risk of physical harm at their parents hands (i.e. if the would-be parents have a known history of physical violence, AIDS or drug abuse) are likely to be prevented from coming into this world. As far as many doctors are concerned if people ask for treatment, they should get it.

In an interesting parallel with adoption, for NHS patients the long waiting lists (two to four years is common) mean that doctors believe that only people who are seriously committed to becoming parents are likely to get treatment. This in itself is seen as evidence of their fitness to be parents. But what about those who (because they can pay) can get 'quickie' treatment at private clinics? Will their commitment have been adequately tested? The other argument used against vetting potential parents is that people able to have children normally are not vetted, so why should those that need assistance? As Brian Leiberman at St Mary's in Manchester put it, 'we believe that all adults should have an equal opportunity to get to the starting line (i.e. become parents) and thereafter they should be under the same public scrutiny as any other parent – no more, no less.'

Sceptics have argued that this is a form of passing the buck on to social workers at a later stage.

The local ethics committees determine some overall principles about whom a particular clinic should exclude. For St Mary's private IVF programme, the ethics committee permits treatment for single women but a different ethics committee attached to the NHS centre is more conservative and has laid down guidelines excluding single and lesbian women. Back in 1984 when they were first considering guidelines it was felt that all the research suggested children were best served in a stable heterosexual cohabitational set-up and they have not seen any reason to shift from this position.

St Mary's Hospital in Manchester is the longest-running NHS centre in Britain (it has been operating since 1983) and in many ways has set standards for other clinics. It was the first to involve an ethics committee and to draw up its own criteria for who should get treatment.

The stated criteria are as follows:

- Woman less than 36.
- Man less than 46.
- Couples living together for at least three years.
- No children living with couple.
- Living within geographic catchment area of north-west Manchester.
- Female must be close to ideal body weight for height.
- Must not have had more than two complete IVF courses of treatment before applying.
- In general, must fulfil adoption criteria.

Since 1987 these criteria have been made public so the large bulk of referrals are for people who fulfil these criteria and are likely to be accepted on to the waiting list. Once accepted they face a long wait. When their turn finally comes, and if they still fulfil the criteria, a medical history is taken and treatment discussed. No detailed psychosocial history is taken. Dr Lieberman acknowledges that the screening is quite superficial but cannot see a practical alternative.

In 1987 St Mary's Hospital was taken to court by a woman who, having initially been accepted, was then refused treatment by the clinic. The Press reported the fact that she had a past conviction for operating a brothel and thought that this was why she was being refused treatment. The consultant argues that this was not the reason but that it had become apparent in the course of interviews that the couple had a history of domestic violence and 'didn't seem to have a clue about what having a child involved'. The court upheld the hospital's decision, saying that unless the doctor had applied his discretion in a manner in which no reasonable consultant would have done his decision to reject the woman could stand. It effectively endorsed the right of the medical establishment to determine parental suitability. For those with a physical disability the prevailing approach appears to be not to exclude arbitrarily but to look at each individual and the threat, if any, to their own personal health. For those who risk passing on a condition (e.g. muscular dystrophy or cystic fibrosis) Dr Lieberman said he would offer genetic counselling and, having ensured they had the full information, leave the decision to them. Although Dr Lieberman states that there are certain adults to whom he would refuse treatment (e.g. drug addicts and people who are HIV positive) not many such people come looking for treatment. In June 1991 the *British Medical Journal* reported the dilemma of doctors at St Mary's Hospital in London where a couple who were both HIV positive sought fertility treatment. After serious consideration the doctors decided not to provide treatment because of the risk not only of the child getting AIDS but also of becoming orphaned at some stage in his childhood.

The doctors, however, admitted that the obverse viewpoint could also be argued, i.e. that 'aware, consenting patients have the right to determine the course of their childbearing in much the same fashion as HIV-infected women can elect to continue their pregnancy' (*British Medical Journal* 10/6/91).

Their decision appeared to receive the support of other fertility specialists and experts in law ethics. What was not reported was how much the couple had already considered the risks and decided they were worth taking. The vertical transmission rate (i.e. the risk of passing on the virus to an infant) is thought to be between 13 per cent and 30 per cent – recent figures suggesting a lower rate than previously. And of course, even if the infant were born with HIV, would it develop AIDS? If other inherited traits can be passed on subject to the parents' choice, why not HIV? This is a subject to which I will return later but it has much to do with the way society perceives risk in terms of what it finds most frightening. AIDS is a topical and alarming disease; there is therefore perhaps more readiness to intervene to prevent the possibility of it being passed on. The doctors are also aware of developments across the Atlantic: 'It might be interesting to consider whether the child could bring an action against the gynaecologist for "wrongful life"'.

What is clear is that whether we as individuals agree or disagree, it is the fertility specialists who hold the balance of power in deciding who is fit to become a parent, and the state endorses their authority to do so. The precedents that are being set are unlikely to be upturned in the short term.

Other factors undoubtedly affect the selection of would-be parents. There is a considerable degree of competitiveness between fertility clinics, and as all clinics want to improve their take-home baby rate they will tend to select those who have the greatest chance of success. This is particularly true of NHS clinics. Private clinics are prepared to offer treatment more readily to those with less chance of success – they stand to gain financially and can argue that they are providing hope to those who would otherwise have none. Thus a 50 year old woman recently gave birth to a baby as a result of treatment at a private clinic – she would have been refused treatment by any NHS clinic.

Counselling versus assessment

More strongly than any of the previous three areas I have looked at, the need for the assessment process to be therapeutic has been recognised as central to those seeking artificial means of creating children.

The HFEA Code of Practice states preconception counselling should be made available to all and distinguishes between the different forms it should take. There is an acute shortage of trained infertility counsellors and the HFEA makes no provisions for funding more training. At St Mary's Hospital in Manchester, the take-up rate for counselling is low. The official explanation is that all who are accepted have had a long period of time to adjust to the idea and also receive ongoing support from the clinic's nurses during treatment so they do not need it. There is however a concern that many people do not accept counselling because they fear that admitting a need for it might be seen as a sign of weakness and undermine their chances of treatment. Some clinics are more rigorous in their provision of counselling prior to treatment being agreed. There is the possibility however that information which emerges during counselling might be used against the would-be parent. A leading infertility counsellor in London spoke of the pressure on people seeking treatment for infertility to hide their ambivalence towards technological intervention for fear that if it is their only option then they do not want to compromise their chances to get it.

And the need for counselling and support may not end with treatment. Such are the social pressures to found families in as normal a manner as possible that many people seeking artificially assisted parenthood are forced to conceal the fact. Combined with the demands of the treatment itself, it has been suggested that this secrecy can place undue strains on the family, particularly on its relations with the extended family and friend networks. According to some, this secrecy about the origins of the child may continue beyond the child's birth and have profound repercussions on the parents and their experience of parenthood (Snowden and Mitchell 1981). There does not appear to be much support for such after-effects of assisted reproduction – the doctor's role ends with the successful conception, and the patients are expected to go off and play their longed-for roles as ordinary parents. The HFEA Code of Practice does suggest that counselling services should be made available at any time after that, but few people are likely to take this up.

SELECTING PARENTS: THE MEDICAL FRAMEWORK VERSUS THE SOCIAL FRAMEWORK

Many people who seek medically assisted pregnancy or use surrogacy would be deemed unsuitable material for adoptive parenting. This may be simply because of their age, but it may be because of their home circumstances, a past criminal record or other factors which social workers would deem less than ideal for children. A recently reported case illustrates the potential for dual standards. It involves a couple becoming parents through surrogacy, using the husband's sperm and the wife's sister as the host mother. The couple had been rejected for adoption because 'The woman suffered deep depression over her childlessness. Such was her mental condition that adoption agencies decided she would not be a suitable parent' (Annabel Ferriman, *Observer* 11/1/87).

Social workers tried to influence the HFE Act to permit them to play a greater role not just in counselling but in the assessment process for fertility treatment. This was not heeded. The medical lobby had defined their natural authority many years before. A report issued by the Royal College of Obstetricians and Gynaecologists in 1983, for example, stated that as physicians

> are taking part in the formation of the embryo . . . that role brings a special sense of responsibility for the welfare of the child thus conceived. . . . Therefore most practitioners will intuitively feel that IVF and embryo replacement should be performed in the most natural of family environments.
>
> (Hubbard, in Arditti, Klein and Minden 1984)

They appear to be comparing themselves to mothers who intuitively feel responsible for the children they create. This point further emphasises how professionals making assessments see themselves as parental figures themselves towards those whom they assess.

The exclusion of social workers was at least partly a result of professional rivalry. Social workers' hopes that more provisions for information access be included, namely, discretionary powers to get medical or criminal records without the consent of the applicant, were similarly rejected. Unlike adoption, the rights of would-be parents to privacy seem to have prevailed over the rights of the future child. Or perhaps more accurately, the rights of doctors to retain absolute discretion in selecting *patients* prevailed over the rights of parents or their children.

As we have seen, the HFE Act, unlike the Children Act, promotes the notion that the welfare both of the parents and of the children is important but neither is paramount. As a spokesperson for the HFEA said:

> the sheer number of people coming to clinics means that they cannot be expected to investigate them beyond taking a medical and family history and perhaps contacting the GP. There is a limit to how much a clinic can delve into the life of a particular client. Yes the welfare of the child is important but this has to be weighed up against the welfare of the parents.

So it is primarily a pragmatic decision – if there were unlimited resources Dr Lieberman at St Mary's says he would undoubtedly want to see more in-depth counselling of applicants and more investigation of their backgrounds. On the whole there is a feeling that few people who currently receive treatment are likely to be grossly unfit. After all, the argument goes, the child is a longed-for and wanted child and that is seen as evidence that the parents are no less suitable than any fertile person who wants a child and can have it unassisted. Other children cannot choose their parents so why should those who would otherwise remain unborn be given more choice?

An ongoing internal study (D'Souza *et al.* 1990) of children born through the St Mary's IVF programme since 1983 has suggested no cause for concern – the parents appear to be 'good' parents despite the stresses surrounding their children's conception. It seems to have been a helpful factor in their closeness. The cases where extra stress is noticeable is in families with multiple births – since IVF poses an increased risk of twins and triplets. However, there has been little independent long-term research into those children born by artificial means. For example,

> If our prime concern should be for the child, it might be thought that there would be a follow-up of the AID family but usually interest ceases with the achievement of conception. Many AI practitioners do not even inquire about the outcome of pregnancy, preferring to remove themselves from the scene as soon as conception using donated semen has taken place. Others continue to have an interest but such a follow-up is not usually undertaken in a systematic

way. Indeed it is difficult to obtain unbiased information from such observations which would enable us to reach some valid conclusion about the effect of AID on the developing child.

(Snowden and Mitchell 1981)

It seems that until a child is born, the welfare of the would-be parents (including their desire to have children) is given more importance. Once the child is born – and only if there is some dispute or evidence that the child is in danger – then the state will intervene in the usual way to consider his welfare and rule in his best interests.

The state is thus permitting doctors to decide whether or not to bring a new child into this world for the benefit of would-be parents. Doctors have neither the skills nor the resources to carry out detailed screening of all would-be parents. The state has in effect decided that detailed screening is not necessary and that the rights of people to become parents are on the whole greater than the rights of the unborn child. The social framework has been virtually ignored and the medical one has ruled supreme.

So far I have laid out how the HFEA Code of Practice seeks to influence clinics in their decisions regarding selection of would-be parents. However, the Code of Practice only covers licensed activities – not all medical treatments are licensed: for example, artificial insemination using the husband's sperm.

It remains entirely in the hands of the individual gynaecologist whether or not to provide such treatment. One prominent consultant gynaecologist graphically illustrated this with a story of her own experience with a couple who had been unable to consummate their marriage but wanted children. The woman could not bear the idea of penetration but begged for artificial insemination. The gynaecologist had grave reservations about the psychosexual problems in the couple's relationship but reluctantly agreed to make six attempts – the number which usually produces a pregnancy. The woman put up a great deal of resistance to attempts at inseminating her with the husband's semen, screaming loudly throughout. After the agreed six attempts, no pregnancy happened and the gynaecologist was relieved to be rid of the dilemma as well as the unpleasant experience.

Individual gynaecologists are faced with many such dilemmas about parental suitability (e.g. couples where there is evidence of mental instability, promiscuity, or 'mere' poverty) and act according to what they feel they can justify to themselves. What has not happened hitherto is a debate to share that responsibility.

WHAT THE ASSESSMENT FOR MEDICALLY ASSISTED PREGNANCY TELLS US ABOUT FIT PARENTS

Ideal

- A man and a woman need to have sexual intercourse to produce a child.
- This act leads to a pooling of genetic material to create a baby which gives those two people rights and responsibilities to that child as well as a natural blood tie.

- Parenthood is a biologically and socially constructed activity that begins with the marriage of a man and a woman and results from sexual intercourse between them. The baby is carried in the mother's womb until birth and is thereafter nurtured by her with the support of her husband.
- The role of parents begins during pregnancy and lasts for a lifetime.
- The family unit is based on shared genetic material.
- People need to be young when they embark on parenthood.
- Children are a blessing, not consumer goods to which all parents are entitled.

Actual

- Sex is not essential to procreation.
- Becoming a parent is a socially created role more than a biological one.
- Pregnancy and birth are desirable but not essential experiences of parenthood, nor are they necessary for a full bond with the child.
- While blood ties between a child and his extended family are desirable they are not essential to successful family life.
- Parenthood may begin at any time: pregnancy, birth, or after birth.
- Who is fit to be a parent changes over time in response to changes in technology and science. Social attitudes follow.
- A wanted child is more likely to be well looked after by the parents.
- Merely being a genetic parent does not confer any responsibility towards rearing a child.
- No one is too old to become a parent.

5 Key themes from Part I

In examining these four facets of the assessment 'pyramid' some key themes have emerged about their common base.

The professionalisation of parenthood

The role of defining fit parenting appears to have been hijacked by a relatively narrow band of professionals over the last forty years. The very appearance of the word *parenting* signifies its transformation into a category for study and expertise, no longer just one aspect of daily living but something that requires particular skills, behaviours and knowledge – which only professionals can know. Professionals have unwittingly created closed systems largely impenetrable to an outsider not versed in their professional rules. Their language and processes have built up a whole new way of looking at parent–child relationships which is often alien to the experience of most ordinary people. This growing gulf between professionals and those ordinary people who are subject to their procedures has made the possibility of fair assessment more difficult.

The importance of research

During the whole course of this century, but particularly over the past twenty years, a growing body of research into child development has given professionals a sense of knowing more about children than do parents. Thus professionals confidently tell new mothers that their babies' smiles are only wind or that they are born virtually blind even when mothers suspect otherwise from observing their own children. The information that comes from studying large numbers of children can be valuable and the desire many parents have to learn about their children's development is shown by the popularity of books and magazines which translate and update the findings of research for a popular audience. However, the professionalisation of child expertise can also be a disempowering process that makes all parents feel inadequate and unconfident in their own judgements.

In the assessment processes and criteria in most of the areas there appears to exist a professional consensus that parents should have a knowledge of child development and a quality of interaction which enables them to understand what is regarded as 'appropriate' for fit parents. Such expectations are not made explicit and raise the question of to what extent can the state 'nanny' parents who do not have such knowledge and skills. Again and again the use of research to justify and help decision making is mentioned, but in very different ways. As Schaffer (1990) points out, the quality of the research itself is a matter of great significance. What he does not make explicit, but which his clearly and simply written book *Making Decisions About Children* could itself encourage, is more widespread dissemination of the professionals' research base to the general public. If the existing research together with its limitations were common knowledge, it would be easier for a wider range of people to contribute to the debate on how parenting should be assessed. What all areas have in common is a need for more longitudinal and sophisticated research to show the impact of professional intervention into family life. Until that is available, one person's opinion is not necessarily any less valid than another's. And professional opinion is not necessarily any more accurate than that of parents or would-be parents.

Conflicting professional frameworks

I introduced the idea of three different professional frameworks in the first chapter of this book. It is clear that the three models overlap in each of the four areas to different degrees:

Child protection: legal and social work and medical roughly equivalent.
Adoption: social work predominates.
Divorce: legal predominates.
Assisted reproduction: medical predominates.

There also appears to be a number of conflicts between professionals of different disciplines in each of the areas. Each professional approach represents different value systems which are particular to the history of the profession. Each has a predominating approach to its relationships with clients which are paternalistic but each area is seeing some small shifts towards more partnership with parents and would-be parents.

Quiet revolutions

Each of the four areas has witnessed a major revolution whose origins can be plotted at some point during the 1970s. For child protection, the death of Maria Colwell in 1973 and the subsequent public inquiry led to an unprecedented scrutiny of the role of social workers. That public scrutiny and frequent hostility towards those involved in child protection has been a major theme in their work over the ensuing two decades. For adoption, the revolution also occurred during the course of the 1970s – the work of adoption agencies was transformed from the relatively easy job of placing babies with readily available infertile couples to the more difficult one of finding homes for older and handicapped children. The change in skills and approach that this has required has completely transformed the nature of adoption work. In the case of divorce, the 1971 Divorce Reform Act was followed by a steep increase in the number of people seeking divorces and the associated increase in the involvement of professionals dealing with the public effects of the failure of a private relationship. The role of court welfare officers has similarly been transformed from one of trying to preserve the marriage to one which is concerned with protecting children from the excesses of their separating parents. And finally, fertility treatment; as we have seen, the birth of Louise Brown in 1978 heralded a veritable explosion of new reproductive technologies which had barely existed previously and which have revolutionised the way in which professionals affect how families can be created. Each revolution's origin represents a point of no return as far as the traditional view of family life is concerned.

New demands

The impact of these revolutions on professionals and on individual families has been and continues to be huge, yet there seems to have been a slowness to respond to the need for different types of professional intervention that they have all created. The move has been away from the traditional investigative role to a more therapeutic one but the professional structures have not changed to accommodate this. There is a growing recognition that for good parenting to take place, parents need to feel empowered and confident in their role – this has significant implications for the nature of professional intervention that is most effective.

Who's the client?

One of the recurring themes in examining the four areas is the problem of who various professionals are working to serve. Professionals whether they be legal, social work or medical have different views on who their client is: the child, the parent/would-be parent/the state/professional peers. This ambiguity makes it difficult for clear thinking to take place on whose rights should be considered uppermost and how assessment of a particular situation should be carried out.

Although the term 'client' is used it is not an accurate description of the situation of most parents or children under assessment since they do not have much influence on how and by whom they are assessed. Power is very much with the professional to decide on the course of professional intervention. To an outsider, assessment appears to be a matter of balancing children's interests and parents' interests when there is a conflict – what has become apparent is that assessment procedures are also governed by the need to serve professionals' interests such as the need to achieve results that are required by the state, to retain authority over other professionals, to stay free of criticism from one's peers and from the media.

The impact of the media

The media have played a number of significant roles in the recent history of all four areas of professional intervention. The most significant role of the media has been as an agent for change in what is considered normal. By showing different ways of being, and by enabling people to feel they belong to a wider community than their immediate geographical one, the media have opened up the range of options people are likely to consider for their own lives. Thus the interest in fertility treatment, the destigmatisation of divorce and single parenting, the explosion of interest in international adoption that followed – for example, the 1991 news footage of Romanian orphans – are all attributable to the impact of the media.

There is no doubt that in each of the four areas the professionals' task of assessing parental fitness is greatly influenced by the consideration of what the public, in particular the media, will make of their decisions. At times this borders close on paranoia. The fear of being discovered to have made a 'wrong' or unpalatable decision can encourage a defensive and over-conservative assessment of parents. Whether parents and their children are given the fairest and most helpful support from professionals in this climate is questionable. The influence of the media often appears to be a phantom presence hovering over the professional making assessments.

The media play the role of bringing to light what they deem to be in the public interest to know but also serve to act as society's mirror reflecting its developments, warts and all. Just as with research, the viewpoint and coverage by the media is constrained by two demands: funding and impact. There is an inherent tendency therefore to only present things which will make people sit up and listen or will encourage people to buy a particular newspaper or magazine. Programme makers are more likely to get funding and slots for programmes which have impact and this usually means trying to find controversy. There is a marked tendency to create scapegoats in the coverage of all these areas – where the child was not protected from an abusing parent, or if children are placed with gay foster carers or if judges rule in a surprising way in custody cases or if doctors appear to be tampering with nature by offering fertility treatment to particular groups.

All too often, as I have shown, adverse media coverage (or the fear of it) sets the professionals' agenda. Those involved in public services are always vulnerable to public scrutiny, be they police or social workers. If they have a bad image it is not just the fault of the media, but a reflection of the lack of standardisation or equity in the service they provide.

Lack of standardisation and equity

One of the recurring themes in reading and talking to professionals and parents involved in each of the four areas is the absence of a coherent professional approach to family intervention and support. This is partly a natural reflection of the fact that the subject itself is dynamic, not static; one set of rules might be appropriate for a certain time and place but not for another – again very much like parenting. But there appears to be little attempt to find consensus. This results in a situation where some parents are scrutinised more closely than others and thus are more likely to be found wanting. It also means that different criteria are used by different professionals so that parents are vulnerable to the whims and policies of the particular professionals.

Pooling professional resources

There is little evidence of consistent sharing of expertise across different professional disciplines in any of the four areas. Yet this sharing of expertise can be invaluable (e.g. Adcock and White 1985). Adoption work, for example, has pioneered many new approaches to the assessment of families and has much to offer other areas where practical intervention in the parent–child relationship is required. Adoption has been concerned with looking for what makes good parents, so it has built up a body of practical knowledge of what factors encourage better than good-enough parenting to take place. This knowledge could be more widely shared. For example, the approach of the Form F checklist could be used as the basis for preparing any adult for parenthood, particularly prior to and during pregnancy. The Hartman (1979) ecological approach could also be adapted for use with those counselling people seeking assisted reproduction or custody after divorce. In fact, all prospective parents/step-parents may benefit from being taken through such awareness-raising exercises: to feel supported and to develop a greater understanding of themselves as potential parents. If this were a service available to all prospective parents it would not stigmatise the few parents who are obliged to go through it.

While pooling resources can act as a check against subjectivity of individual professional approaches it can also lead to an uncritical building of the wrong type of consensus which excludes the expertise and input of other significant voices – most notably parents and children themselves. The need to put aside professional territorialism and seek a wider range of inputs is long overdue. Doctor Jonathan Miller once suggested that novelists and playwrights are better observers of human nature than most doctors – his argument could be extended to incorporate others whose expertise in predicting human behaviour may be equally valid. One group I would be interested to involve would be insurance risk assessors, who are particularly skilled at evaluating relative risks of different human behaviours – perhaps their expertise could be harnessed to evaluate the relative risks of different decisions concerning children?

Parents' interests versus children's interests

In saying that the interests of the child are paramount we are in danger of thwarting those very interests if we do not also consider the needs of the parents of those children. It is easy to feel compassion for a neglected two year old but less easy to feel so towards his alcoholic, unemployed father. It is as if it embarrasses society to be confronted with adults who 'fail' as parents, for there are few resources directed towards preparing people for parenthood or rehabilitating those who appear not to be able to cope with the responsibilities. The need for assessment to be therapeutic in its intention rather than to police parents has to be addressed more imaginatively, even if the outcome is still the removal of children into care. All too often failure to do this means that the 'careless' parent continues to produce 'replacement' children who are also at risk.

The way that professionals currently work, and the way that the media reports their work, often polarises the interests of parents and children as being mutually exclusive. Yet the notion of fairness rests on the assumption that parents have natural and legal rights to be supported in caring for their own children and that these rights should be considered whenever professionals intervene. It also rests on the assumption that children have certain rights to minimum care and to remain with their birth families. Thus there is an overlap of interests: both parents and children have a common interest in staying together. Trends in each of the four areas suggest some recognition of this.

Time is of the essence

Time is an essential factor in assessing parents. Adoption agency workers and welfare court officers and solicitors often build in time for reflection to take place; those assessing parents of children at risk need to balance leaving children in a dangerous situation with assessing parents over a period of time. Longer-term observations from teachers, doctors and social workers are necessary supplements to the time-specific assessments by psychiatrists, for example.

One concern is that such an assessment might be too time-specific and give rise to a misleading and possibly unfair appraisal of the parent's overall abilities. There is clearly a danger that a child psychiatrist or court welfare officer seeing parents and children only over a short period of time and at a time of crisis may get an unbalanced picture of the parents' skills for childcaring activities. Most often the period of contact between professionals and families is short, the decisions are made and the contact – particularly with individuals – is ended. There is thus little follow-up to the decisions to see their effectiveness or to give an opportunity for parents to assess their impact.

Who decides what is normal?

In all four areas, the belief that there exists only one ideal version of normality in terms of family life is the danger that professionals have to guard against when assessing fitness of parents. They have to operate within the framework of taboos that society at large propagates: universally accepted ones such as protecting children from sexual interference, excessive physical violence, exposure to criminality, and less clearly held ones such as the status of children in single-parent or homosexual households. But they also have to rise to the challenge of being open to the merits of each situation and not be blinded by the poorly thought-out prejudices of society at large. Rather like parents, professionals will never satisfy everyone all of the time – that goes with the job.

Professionals, by the nature of their experience and expertise, may also be in a clearer position to feed back into the values of society at large about its norms. If, for example, professionals observe that children are just as capable of thriving in non-traditional families, then they can make that message clearer to the lay public. Dora Black, in *Child Psychiatry and the Law*, says:

> In court one is often dealing with value judgements held by other people rather than objective information about a person's ability to be a parent. Thus terms like 'mentally retarded', schizophrenic, drug addict, alcoholic, psychopathic, personality disordered, etc. may be used to suggest that a parent is inevitably incompetent or unsuitable. The child psychiatrist's role often may be to translate these value laden labels into everyday language and to explain how such conditions in parents may affect children's well-being. Diagnostic labels are impressive and may carry powerful stereotyped connotations, which will be used by skilled advocates in an attempt to disqualify a parent or parents.
>
> (Black *et al.* 1989)

The professionals and the media have done much to promote certain concepts of what is to be considered normal. The professions concerned with family intervention first became prominent with the inception of the welfare state of post-war Britain at the time when the traditional family was at its peak. Many of the most fundamental ideas about how the state should intervene and involve itself in family life date from then and it sometimes appears that progressive professionals are struggling to shake off the legacy of those early years which have become anachronisms in current society. One wonders how much the family ideals of those who began working in the 1950s have continued to influence practice and whether, as they retire and leave the professions, the younger intake will reflect a different and more varied set of family norms.

There is growing emphasis in all areas of supporting opinion with fact as a check against the individual assessor's subjectivity but this is only a limited measure. The culture-specific perspective being employed and how sensitive any professional carrying out such an assessment can be to different cultural norms is particularly difficult to envisage when professionals themselves are so rarely from the groups they scrutinise.

When one looks at the composition of government-appointed commissions, ethics committees, adoption panels, those present in case conferences, those involved in courts, etc., one becomes very aware that there is a preponderance of professional white males while those they are assessing are largely females from non-professional classes. There is also a distinct feeling that the people who predominate in such panels and commissions all hold intellectual positions which are more similar to each other than they are to those they judge.

This is a point that recurs again and again, even though professionals themselves often dismiss it. Parting parents in Murch's study talked of their greater trust in court welfare officers who have children, people seeking to adopt questioned the judgements of agency workers who were childless, those who are infertile question the ability of the childless to judge their situation. For example, Kim Cotton recalls her feelings about awaiting the judgment of the Warnock Commission on surrogate pregnancy:

'I was a little frightened of them at that stage. I desperately hoped they were looking into every aspect of surrogate motherhood. I kept thinking, "I bet they all have children. I bet there isn't anyone sterile on the board. Will they really know what infertile couples go through?"'

Because she didn't know much about the committee, she thought of them as bureaucrats removed from real life rather than, as was the case, experienced people professionally concerned with the problems of infertility.

(Cotton and Winn 1985)

The questioning of the qualifications of those who assess others leads to two possible scenarios. The first is to admit the bias in the professionals' judgements and to counter it by involving a wider range of people in the assessment process. One move that might improve the likelihood of more appropriate intervention is (as the Magna Carta suggested a millennium ago) for people to be tried by their peers. This would require the professional to facilitate the involvement of the community to which the family or adult feels they belong. Such a group's values would be more transparent to the family and more likely to expose the issues that matter. An example of this is the involvement of extended families in decisions about adoption as described by Murray Ryburn (1991). The second is to produce evidence that shows professionals are fit to judge others from different walks of life.

Is less state intervention in children's best interests?

In each of these four key areas, there is a slow but perceptible trend away from state intervention unless absolutely necessary which has heightened the tension between whether parents know best or professionals know best as to what is right for children. The trend is least noticeable in child protection and more so in the selection of would-be parents for fertility treatment.

Child protection – less power to social workers, making an order only if it would be better than making no order at all; children remain parents' responsibility for life unless adopted.

Adoption – away from excluding potential adopters to including as many as are willing to take damaged children.

Divorce – away from investigating childcare arrangements or homes, towards encouraging parents to take as many decisions for own children without recourse to the courts.

Fertility treatment – minimal investigation procedures for those seeking assisted reproduction.

What underlies this desire to withdraw from policing family life?

Pragmatism – the sheer numbers of families that would require it (under previous ideological thinking) have been rapidly growing to the point where the resources needed to police them effectively are considered too large. Child surveillance shows up a huge and apparently unending queue of vulnerable children, many of whom may need substitute parents, large numbers of parents splitting up inflates the number whose childcare arrangements would require scrutiny, and the numbers of people seeking fertility treatment is growing fast.

Assessment is a contextual exercise – it has to be linked with the resources actually available. So instead there has been an ideological shift, as embodied in the new Children Act, away from professionals taking decisions over what is best for children to parents taking more responsibility for their own children. However, as has been pointed out (Eekelar 1991), how parents should exercise that responsibility towards their children remains vague; the state appears more concerned that it relieve itself of the burden of being responsible for children.

Do professionals know best? There is increasing doubt, generated by many professionals themselves (e.g. Ryburn 1991), as to whether the knowledge base actually exists for them to be able to judge who is fit to be a parent and who is not. Those in the social work profession at the vanguard of adoption reforms are emphasising the importance of admitting that they cannot be expected to predict who will be a fit parent. And as Ryburn says,

> Nor do I think any other professional group of assessors would do it any better, because traditional assessment processes are based on what in my view is the unattainable search to find objective criteria to measure parenting suitability.

Others in court welfare work have similarly questioned the assumption that conducting extensive investigations with the individuals concerned will somehow lead to a discovery of who is the better parent.

Does investigation help anyway? The process of policing parents is being shown to be notoriously ineffective when combined with the belief that children and parents should stay together. There is little study of the outcomes of professional decisions but, given that such a high number of adoptions fail and children of divorced parents continue to suffer, there is growing doubt over whether investigation is the answer. Traditional investigation procedures are seen to be disempowering and it is now recognised that to enable parents to be fit parents requires an emphasis on empowering parents and would-be parents to make informed choices for themselves.

The overall trend away from policing parents may be a temporary swing. It certainly seems contradictory to the notion of protecting the child's best interests and the promotion of children's rights. There seems to be a widening gap between what have been termed social children and private children – ones that come into the arena of professionals require the best interests principle to be considered, those that do not or can be prevented from doing so are afforded minimal state protection, remaining the responsibility of parents and families.

And as we have seen, when it comes to understanding what is 'in the best interests of the child' the state's involvement through professionals is characterised by inconsistency and idiosyncrasy. The situation all too often resembles the story of the six blind men and the elephant each seeing only one aspect of a situation and believing it is all. The elephant could be seen to be a metaphor for 'the child's best interests', the blind men professionals from medicine, social work and the law and, to some extent, the media.

> It was six men of Indostan
> To learning much inclined
> Who went to see the elephant
> (Though each of them was blind)
> That each by observation
> Might satisfy his mind

The first hits the side of the elephant and concludes it is a wall, the second feels the tusk and concludes it is a spear, the third grabs the squirming trunk and decides it is a snake, the fourth touches a knee and concludes it is a tree, the fifth feels the ear and calls it a fan, the last seizes the tail and declares it is a rope.

> And so these men of Indostan
> Disputed loud and long
> Each in his own opinion
> Exceeding stiff and strong
> Though each was partly in the right
> And all were in the wrong!

> The Moral:
> So, oft in theologic wars
> The disputants, I ween,
> Rail on in utter ignorance
> Of what each other mean,
> And prate about an elephant
> Not one of them has seen!

(Saxe 1980)

My own examination has suggested that most professionals are genuinely concerned to act in children's best interests but are often blind to what those interests are and how they should be assessed. What can make this blindness even more marked is that so many of the professionals concerned with making decisions about children do not even go to 'feel the elephant' first-hand but sit in their offices groping at the replicas made by other blind men.

Accountability and control of discretionary power

Most professionals are aware of the responsibility they carry in assessing parents and determining children's futures. The task is not taken lightly, yet there are few opportunities for professionals to be in any way answerable to the parents or would-be parents they assess. (Children are generally not regarded as being answerable to – it is assumed their best interests are at the heart of all professional decisions.) Professionals sometimes behave as the sort of parents they would disapprove of themselves in assessments: authoritarian and secretive. There is a big gap between what professionals expect of the assessment process and what parents or would-be parents expect. Adoption panels are secret, they do not have to explain their decisions. Social workers assessing parents in child protection cases have been notoriously inconsistent about involving parents in decisions about their children. The Children Act and the HFE Act seem to recognise the need for more accountability as the price for parents shouldering more professional responsibility. Hence there are some trends for more partnership (allowing parents to attend case conferences, see welfare reports, to be told why they were not accepted by fertility clinics, etc.).

What is not addressed is the issue of staff continuity or follow-up. If professionals could take more personal responsibility for their decisions by making face-to-face contact and remaining accessible beyond the decision, it has been argued that this would encourage professionals to take more note of the consequences of their own decisions and the continuity of staff would be of benefit to parents and other professionals (Wolff 1991).

At present there remain extensive areas where professionals can continue to exercise their discretion as to who is fit to be a parent and who is not and can be protected by the professional cloak of secrecy and anonymity. None of the professionals who are involved in the assessment of parents have been elected to do so, nor do they have a clear public identity as to who they are and what level of power they exercise. This, combined with the lack of a commonly accepted and proven knowledge base, makes their expertise questionable – and yet their professional judgement is deemed authoritative.

As I have already shown, this encourages the possibility that the practitioners will impose their own moral standards on people who have come to them seeking support with their family problems, often with little choice or knowledge about the individual professional. It also means that the decision-making system appears arbitrary and the people who are its subjects have no control over the processes.

So how can this professional power be exercised more responsibly? The answer once again is openness:

> The seven instruments that are most useful in the structuring of discretionary power are open plans, open policy statements, open rules, open findings, open reasons, open precedents and fair and informal procedures. The reason for repeating the word open is a powerful one: openness is the natural enemy in the fight against injustice.
>
> (Davis 1969, quoted by Murch 1980)

In the context of assessing who is fit to be a parent this openness means:

1 Open access to the research and professional ideologies with which most parents – who will be subjected to its influence – have no familiarity.
2 More open debate, which includes the views of those people who are the recipients (voluntary or involuntary) of that professional intervention.

3 Assessment criteria that are readily available and whose relative importance is made clear and then consistently observed by professionals.
4 A clear and honest outline of the assessment process, its motives and time-scale that parents and children can expect as well as flexibility to accommodate them on their own terms as far as possible.
5 More direct access by people to the professionals who assess them and a right to appeal against their decisions.

When I started to research this book I expected there would be clear guidelines to professionals which their administrative structures would expect them to follow and which, when requested, would be readily available to the public for scrutiny. I expected these guidelines to reflect a standard approach throughout the country with, of course, some scope for professional discretion but only if it was within a regulated structure that allowed such individuality of response to be assessed by other professionals and, if necessary, independent outsiders. That this was not the case perhaps should not have surprised me. But what was disturbing was the general reluctance and suspicion of professionals to expose themselves to any scrutiny from an outsider. Individual people did talk to me but usually only after consulting their peers and superiors and they were, on the whole, keen to stay off the record and not be identified.

Few ordinary people feel able to question professionals by calling them up or writing to them. Few professional journals are accessible to the lay person or available at local libraries and even if they were, most are unintelligible to the lay person, immersed as they are in technical terms and ideas that presume a professional expertise. The burgeoning number of self-help books shows that parents do feel a need for the information by which they can meet professionals as equals and not as vulnerable subjects of investigation. But books only reach a small number of the public; many people are not accustomed to reading books as a way of addressing the challenges in their lives. They expect to be treated fairly and expect professionals to exercise their power fairly. The onus should thus be on the professionals to communicate their knowledge base in an accessible manner and to be honest and open in their dealings. The media share that responsibility to communicate and to inform debate between professionals and the public they serve.

I started this book with a desire to find out how the state currently defines the current job description for fit parents – to continue the analogy, what appears to be needed is an agreed job description based on openly agreed criteria, fair selection processes with an emphasis on equal opportunities, and plenty of readily available on-the-job training.

Part II

Parents on the edge

In Part I we learned a little more about what criteria for fit parents emerge from the assessment procedures of professionals, but the societal values underlying these criteria appeared confused and conflicting. There seems to be a growing feeling that professionals, and therefore the parents they assess, are being made to dance to a frenzy of different tunes played by a hidden orchestra.

To try and understand the music and who is playing it, it has become clear that we cannot just ask 'what is a fit parent?' and get a complete answer. So I have decided to examine who is considered unfit and attempt to extrapolate from that. I will look in turn at some of those groups that have traditionally been deemed unfit but whose numbers are growing and who are challenging traditional notions of family. What are the underlying social values that they are seen to be contravening and what do these tell us about the value expectations of all parents?

As before, I wanted to begin with a historical perspective – to see what basis there might have been for the labelling of certain groups as unfit for parenthood. I found that in the past there has been no shortage of opinions as to who should be stopped from becoming a parent.

UNFIT TO PARENT – FOR THE SAKE OF THE NATION

The biological basis for selecting who is fit to be a parent has long been promoted in cultures throughout the world. In Plato's *Republic*, the rulers determined who could have children. They were particularly keen that the offspring of the depraved or those imperfect in any way should be removed and allowed to die. Many traditional cultures today discourage the marriage of those who are of questionable moral or physical perfection. The underlying belief has been that undesirable characteristics will be passed on from one generation to the next, 'polluting' the community.

Charles Darwin's *Origin of the Species* is well known for his theory of the biological evolution of plants and animals whereby those best adapted to their contemporaneous environment continued and those least suited died out. What is less well known is how he extrapolated from this to encourage a particular theory of social evolution. In *The Descent of Man* (1871) he argued:

With savages the weak in body and mind are soon eliminated . . . we civilised men, on the other hand, do our utmost to check the process of elimination; we build asylums for the imbecile, the maimed and the sick; we institute poor laws and our medical men exert their utmost skill to save the life of everyone to the last moment. There is reason to believe that vaccination has preserved thousands, who from weak constitution would formerly have succumbed to small pox. Thus the weak members of society propagate their kind . . . excepting in the case of man himself, hardly anyone is so ignorant as to allow his worst animals to breed.

(Darwin 1871)

As Stephen Trombley demonstrates in his brilliantly researched and written book *The Right to Reproduce?* (1988), many prominent writers, doctors and politicians of the late nineteenth century concluded that certain sections of society were unfit to produce children and argued that society should check their capacity to reproduce. They varied in their targets but broadly concurred: 'Persons in any rank of life who are not in good physical and mental health have no moral right to have children' (Arthur Marshall, a leading medical man and embryologist addressing a conference in 1885).

A popular author of Darwin's time, W. R. Greg, was one of the first to suggest eugenic solutions to social problems and to acknowledge the reluctance of the public to accept these. He identified three problems afflicting nineteenth-century society which were promoting the decline of the British race:

We are learning to insist more and more on the freedom of the individual will, the right of everyone to judge and act for himself.

We absolutely refuse to let the poor, the incapable, the lazy and the diseased die. We are lenient with criminals.

(Trombley 1988)

The great mistake of modern social and political thinking, he argued, was to place the rights of the individual above the individual's duty to the state.

The founder of eugenics, Sir Francis Galton, proposed segregation and/or sterilisation of all those deemed unfit. In Britain he never achieved his practical aim, although many prominent politicians were influenced by his thinking well into the twentieth century. Elsewhere in western Europe and the USA, sterilisation of the institutionalised 'feeble-minded' did take place, often on a scandalous scale. The Nazi adoption of eugenics and the resulting atrocities put paid to any idea of an overt eugenics programme in Britain. However, it seems that Churchill shared something of Hitler's views on the causes of national decline. As Home Secretary he once wrote to Prime Minister Asquith: 'the proliferation of the unfit, combined with the low fertility of "all the thrifty, energetic, and superior stocks" was a "very terrible danger to the race"'.

Sir William Beveridge, so-called founder of the welfare state in post-war Britain, had earlier put forward proposals to deal with the unemployed, suggesting that only those who were employable deserved full citizenship rights such as liberty, political power, fatherhood, conduct of one's own life and government of a family. All those deemed by the state as unemployable should, he suggested, be detained in colonies and permanently lose all such rights.

Many of those accredited with progressive thinking on matters of sex and contraception were firm advocates of eugenics. Sexologist Havelock Ellis argued that eugenic certificates ('a patent of natural ability') should be issued on a voluntary basis. These would help people to make a wise choice of marriage partner, and to obtain certain jobs.

In response to criticisms of the 1933 Nazi sterilisation law which legalised wholesale compulsory sterilisation of a wide range of the unfit on social as well as medical grounds, Ellis argued that Hitler's views were based on genuinely scientific work.

Marie Stopes, best known as the pioneering advocate of birth control, was a fanatic supporter of eugenics.

> In a contribution to *The Control of Parenthood* (1920) she wrote 'Utopia could be reached in my life time had I the power to issue inviolable edicts'. She wanted legislation that would enable compulsory sterilisation not only of the insane and feeble minded, but of 'revolutionaries', 'half-castes', the deaf, the dumb, the blind and anyone else who might threaten the vigour of the race.
>
> (Trombley 1988)

She tried to prevent her own son's marriage to a woman who wore glasses on the basis that it would be a crime against his country. Sydney and Beatrice Webb, two of the principal founders of modern socialism, believed that since the consequences of unchecked parenthood would be public problems, it was the duty of individuals to put the state above personal freedom in the matter of fertility.

UNFIT TO PARENT – FOR THE SAKE OF THE CHILDREN

The spectre of Nazi crimes against humanity shifted the debate. The political and social climate no longer put the good of the nation as high as personal freedom. Politicians could no longer talk openly about controlling fertility for the welfare of the nation but for the welfare of children. Over the course of this century politicians from both ends of the political spectrum have voiced opinions on the dangers of uncontrolled parenthood. As recently as 1974, Keith Joseph in a famous speech, said:

> The balance of our population, our human stock is threatened . . . a high and rising proportion of children are being born to mothers least fitted to bring children into the world and bring them up. They are born to mothers who were first pregnant in adolescence in socioeconomic classes 4 and 5. Many of these girls are unmarried, many are deserted or divorced or soon will be. Some are of low intelligence, most of them of low educational attainment. They are unlikely to be able to give the children the stable emotional background, the consistent combination of love and firmness which are more important than riches. They are producing problem

children, the future unmarried mothers, delinquents, denizens of our borstals, subnormal educational establishments, prisons and hostels for drifters. Yet these mothers, the under-20s in many cases, single parents, from classes 4 and 5 are now producing a third of all births. A high proportion of these births are a tragedy for the mother, the child and for us.

Yet what shall we do? If we do nothing the nation moves towards degeneration, however much resources we pour into preventative work and the overburdened educational system. . . . Proposals to extend birth control facilities to these classes of people, particularly the young unmarried mothers, evokes entirely understandable moral opposition. Is it not condoning immorality?

I suppose it is. But which is the lesser evil, until we are able to remoralise whole groups and classes of people, undoing the harm done when already weak restraints on strong instincts are further weakened by permissiveness in television, in film, on bookstalls? . . . In general, research showed that children of fatherless families with adolescent mothers had small chance of satisfying lives.

(Sunday Times 20/10/74)

This speech may have lost Keith Joseph the leadership of the Conservative Party but in truth he was voicing what many in his party believed and what many supporters of the Conservative Party and of 'traditional values' wanted to hear. The situation today as we approach the end of the twentieth century is ripe for a replay of some of the arguments presented by Greg, this time fuelled not so much by a nationalistic concern for the 'British race' as for the well-being and rights of children.

Today, the focus for assessment of parental fitness has shifted away from whether people can produce the right quality of genetic offspring to whether they are up to the actual task of child-rearing. This has been largely a result of the increasing knowledge and concern about the influence of child-rearing practices on adult well-being and the realisation that the environment (in the form of human relationships as well as physical circumstances) played a greater influence than biology, certainly as it has hitherto been understood.

It has been recognised that there is a need for more carefully considered research to inform professional judgements about what parental characteristics serve a child's best interests. In the following chapters, I focus in turn on some of those groups that have been regarded as unfit material for parenting to explore what the objections have been and to examine to what extent these are now being challenged. By examining why those groups have been treated as 'marginal', I hope to learn more about what has been regarded as 'central' to fit parenting. As more and more of these traditionally marginalised groups enter the mainstream, there is the opportunity to study what criteria are actually deemed necessary for fit parenting.

I should like to stress that the group labels are not of my choosing but they are part of the pathologising process that I wish to study, so I have retained them in the form in which they are still commonly used, e.g. terms such as disabled parents, mentally handicapped and so on. The order in which they appear is related loosely to how strongly and openly they are regarded as deficient as potential parents and I begin and end with areas with which I have direct personal experience.

6   Disabled parents

My husband's sister stood up in court and said 'She'll never be fit and able to
look after a child'. The judge, in his infinite wisdom, said 'Well, we don't
know what quality of life you'll have in a wheelchair so your child is better
off with an able bodied parent'. He took away everything I had. I was Fiona's
mother. He told me I could no longer be that person.
                                    (Gwen Reid, BBC's *From the Edge*, October 1992)

Disability and parenthood are words which still seem to come together only
uncomfortably in our society. The choice of parenthood is withheld from many
disabled people through the disapproval of others, through lack of accurate
information and lack of role models. If parenthood is embarked upon it is often
made more problematic and stressful because of the lack of understanding from
professionals. The media reinforce public prejudice, taking little notice of disabled people as parents except to publicise the stories of children being removed
from parents deemed unfit or the plight of young children who are forced into
caring for such parents.

However, several factors have combined to produce a growing number of
parents with disabilities in recent years. Medical advances have enabled many
disabled children to survive into adulthood and medical treatment has also
enabled many people to conduct fuller adult lives, although certain disabling
conditions are on the increase, e.g. AIDS. In Britain, the Chronically Sick and
Disabled Persons Act (1970) set in motion the integration of disabled people into
the community, underlining their right to live independently. The disability
rights movement which developed in the 1960s has resulted in a greater con-
sciousness amongst people with disabilities of their rights to self-determination.
So more disabled people are now living in the community and pursuing ordinary
lives – yet as parents they remain an invisible group. There are several reasons
for this:

- They wish to avoid any attention which focuses on their disability as a
  negative trait.
- Many of the public places where parents and children are normally seen such
  as shopping centres, playgroups, school gates and leisure halls are inaccessible to people with disabilities.

- They have yet to be recognised by the media or advertisers as people who do lead family lives.

  One exception to the almost complete absence of pictures of disabled people as parents is the photographs which accompany the 'Tragic But Oh So Brave' stories about disabled parents which appear from time to time in newspapers and magazines. Text and pictures are used to underline how exceptional these individuals are considered to be. Such pieces reinforce the message that disabled people do not generally become parents, while those few that do are a curiosity on the margins of society.

  (Wates 1993)

Over the past few years, I have spoken to many hundreds of parents with physical disabilities and some specific themes recur constantly. Disabled people are still more likely to be offered abortions and sterilisations and to have more professional supervision of their pregnancies and parenting. Too often the professional (e.g. doctor, health visitor, social worker) who is approached for expert advice is ill-equipped to give it. Particularly where medical evidence is lacking or insufficient, personal opinion may be presented to dissuade a disabled person from contemplating parenthood. Disabled people find it difficult to adopt, and in cases of divorce a disabled person is less likely to be seen favourably by the courts as a prime carer. For many people with disabilities, fear of the negative judgement of professionals is a disincentive to become parents or to seek help from them.

Society still objects to disabled parents. Those with physical disabilities and those with learning disabilities are seen as two categories, the latter being regarded as more seriously deficient as potential parents. So, although all categorisation is artificial I will look at them together and then at attitudes to those with a learning disability separately in Chapter 7.

All disabled people are the same

This assumption appears to underlie many of the objections to disabled people as parents. Yet disabled people do not form a homogeneous group. The label 'disabled' covers such a wide range of medical conditions and social experience that it is virtually impossible to make any general statement other than that it confers on its recipient a second-class status in many areas of daily life which then leads to a number of problems such as isolation, undermining of confidence and lack of access to information and support.

The very definition of disability is fraught with problems because it seeks to make homogeneous a disparate group. Conventional definitions have focused on physical impairment and lack of functioning, e.g. 'Disability is regarded as a problem for those individuals who fail to achieve the standards of functioning prevalent in their society' (Grimshaw 1992). Advocates of the disability rights movement argue that the disability has nothing to do with their physical difference and everything to do with society's intolerance: 'Disability is the disadvantage or restriction in the organisation of a society, which prevents an individual with a functional limitation or impairment from fully participating' (Hurst 1992).

The nature and extent of one person's disability is not something that can be objectively measured. Every observer will interpret it differently according to his or her own expectations of what is normal and desirable. Those who have been born with an impairment or have had it since childhood are likely to have a different experience to those who have become disabled in adulthood. The nature of the onset of the disability, whether progressive or sudden (e.g. through accident or stroke), and the prognosis for the future may all affect the individuals' perception of themselves. Those who have been institutionalised and segregated in their early lives may differ in their sense of identity to those who have remained integrated and also in their experience of family life and domestic practicalities. The acceptance of the impairment by family and friends will significantly affect the person's self-confidence. Furthermore, disability and illness are not synonymous. Many people have disabilities which, because of their static nature (e.g. a missing limb or club foot) or because appropriate measures can be taken (e.g. diabetes or epilepsy), have no impact on their day-to-day health. Others have developed strategies which maximise strengths and minimise weakness (e.g. pacing themselves, building in rest periods, not staying up late, etc.) which enable them to lead as full lives as those without the physical impairment. Yet others do have to deal with being ill and trying to maintain their roles as parents and partners.

Disabled people should not have sex

Childlike, abnormal and therefore unattractive: these are the stereotypical views of people with disabilities which imply that they cannot form normal loving relationships and should therefore be asexual. The enlightened attitude of policy makers in the first half of this century was to put disabled children into institutions regarded as safe havens where they could be with other disabled individuals, but as they grew older they were kept separated as far as possible from members of the opposite sex. Thus the chances of forming stable relationships, setting up home or embarking on parenthood were fairly limited for many disabled people. Although institutionalisation of disabled people is decreasing, the segregation mentality still persists.

If disabled women do become pregnant, that is uncomfortable evidence that sex has taken place. Often there is the assumption that it must have been an accident or rape – which is considered to be no way to start a new life. There is much explicit and implicit discouragement of sex.

> Sadly it's not just medical experts who are guilty of ignoring the sexual rights and needs of people with disabilities. The movements for sexual and reproductive freedom have paid little attention to disability issues. And the abortion rights movement has sometimes crudely exploited fears about defective fetuses as a reason to keep abortion legal. . . . Yet for disabled women, the right to bear and rear children is more at risk.

Yet the disability rights movement has not put sexual rights at the forefront of its agenda. Sexuality is often the source of our deepest oppression; it is also often the source of our deepest pain. It's easier for us to talk about – and formulate strategies for changing – discrimination in employment, education and housing than to talk about our exclusion from sexuality and reproduction.

(Finger 1992)

Apart from the taboos surrounding the sexuality of disabled people there are also practical barriers – lack of information and advice about sexual matters makes it difficult to build the confidence needed to embark on and maintain relationships. Those who do may be undermined by outsiders who express distaste at, or voyeuristic curiosity about, their sexual practices.

Disabled women will have hazardous pregnancies

For a small proportion of women with disabilities, pregnancy may pose a high risk. The lack of familiarity with disabled women in pregnancy and the absence of a comprehensive knowledge base often prevent health professionals from giving correct advice or managing the pregnancy and birth in a non-alarmist way. There is much anecdotal evidence that disabled women are more likely to undergo more medical intervention, often to allay the anxieties of the professionals around them. Labelling a disabled woman may in itself lead to unnecessary complications.

The child will be born handicapped as well and deliberately producing a deformed child is irresponsible

It is a commonly held belief that disability is something that is inherited or can be caught like a cold and it is therefore irresponsible to have a child. In fact very few disabling conditions are inherited and most children with deformities or disabilities are born to able-bodied adults, but many disabled people have been given inaccurate information which has prevented them from making informed decisions. For example, until quite recently it was commonly thought that cerebral palsy would be inherited and so all adults with cerebral palsy were dissuaded from having children.

But some disabling conditions are genetic, with varying probabilities of being passed on. The growing medical concern with antenatal screening and the increasing attitude of prospective parents wanting 'perfect' children prejudices society against those who may not fulfil our expectations of normality – but that may be more society's failing. The logic that says 'If the status quo is that such a child would suffer prejudice and lack of opportunity, so it shouldn't be born' is a sure way of perpetuating that prejudice. A recent vivid illustration of this took place in California, inspired once again by the media.

Is it fair to bring a child into the world that you are pretty sure has a very good chance of having a disfiguring disease? We are talking for the next hour or so about the case of Bree Walker who is pregnant. She has a genetic deformity and there's a 50-50 chance that her baby will in fact have that deformity, so is this an appropriate thing to do? Is it fair to the kid to bring him into the world with one strike against him? We'll be back to the phones.

(KFI Radio host 1991)

Bree Walker, a well-known Los Angeles television news presenter with a condition called ectrodactylism that results in the fusing of fingers and toes, became the subject of a nationwide controversy as a result of this radio phone-in. She and her husband filed a complaint against the radio station for infringing their privacy and many disability rights activists came together to voice their concern.

Phone callers to the radio show had criticised her decision with comments such as:

'I would rather not be alive than have a disease like that when it's a 50-50 chance.'

'If you could prevent someone coming in deformed – you know, I'm not God, but I don't think it's fair to the child.'

Later Bree Walker and her husband appeared on a television show to defend their decision:

Walters: Why bring a child into the world who is going to have so much personal, emotional and perhaps physical pain? Why do this to a child?

Bree Walker's husband: Because we're confident that we can provide the love and support necessary to offer our child as worthwhile, as valuable, as meaningful a life on this planet as his mother has had.

Bree Walker: And here's the problem with saying that it's not right to bring a child into the world who may not have that kind of difficulty to face. That is saying that there is only one set of standards that's acceptable and that devalues all of us. If we have such a narrow-minded look at what's valuable in life or what kind of life is worth living, then how can we ever feel we're in a society where everybody can feel great about trying to contribute.

(From *20/20 Vision*: 'My Baby, My Right', October 1991)

Although Bree Walker grew up with the deformity and the pain herself, her adult life is without significant handicap – she can do most things, leads a full and productive life and does not consider herself disabled. She is a strong role model for her own children and seemingly well-equipped to help them handle the challenges they may face.

Bree Walker: This was just not that big a deal for me and I'm not so presumptuous as to say it won't be a big deal for my children, but I do spend an awful lot of time thinking about the right way to encourage them and to make sure they aren't limited just because other people might say they are.

Walters: What will you say to your daughter if she says 'I've gone through a lot, Mummy, and I'm not sure that I want to bring my own child into the world'?

Bree Walker: I'll tell her to think about it a lot and to make sure she's ready to handle it if it happens. I'll also tell her how much I wanted her. I'll tell her that she couldn't be more loved and that physical perfection is a very empty goal, that it's just a shell. This is just a shell that we're given for short period of time and that what's inside is what's important.

(From 20/20 Vision: 'My Baby, My Right', October 1991)

This optimism and strength of purpose have been echoed by many disabled parents I have spoken to but it is tempered by the realities of living in communities which systematically exclude disabled people. The issue of raising disabled children when the parents are disabled is little studied. Again the problems of inaccessibility of buildings and transport, fear of professional scrutiny and exclusion from support networks can prevent disabled parents from getting the sort of resources (such as they are) that exist for able-bodied parents of disabled children. Micheline Mason, a writer and prominent campaigner for the mainstream integration of disabled children and also a disabled single mother of a disabled daughter, described the process of building everything from scratch:

> The initiative I have had to have in order to manage my life with Lucy has been a never ending necessity because it seems no one can imagine or work out in advance the fact that we will need assistance to do such and such a thing, or that we might be in a state of urgent need, unless I constantly spell it out . . . I have had to learn the art of spreading the load, widening my group of supporters, returning in some other ways the favours, researching and organising paid support, stretching inadequate state benefits, dealing emotionally with the unavailability of certain people, saying goodbye to many temporary helpers, and constantly training new people to take their place . . . there must be better ways in which communities can work together than this.

(Mason 1992)

And these are just the practicalities – dealing with the emotional upheavals can seem just as mountainous. Anne Finger powerfully captures this in describing the ambivalence she felt about wanting her child to survive his traumatic birth, knowing that he might be severely disabled.

> Will I have to relive through him the world of stares and loneliness and shame? Of hospitalisations, cold stethoscopes against a warm chest, waking in the night alone in a metal bed? I wanted something perfect to come out of my body. All my life I've had to fight for everything. Walking across a room is work. I wanted something to just happen. I wanted something not to be hard. Other people have babies and all they have to deal with is diaper rash and sleepless nights.

(Finger 1992)

These practical and emotional challenges caution against too ready an assumption amongst adoption social workers that disabled children should be placed with disabled parents, but they also remind us of the enormous impact of the dominant value systems which promote a narrow view of what sort of humans are to be deemed acceptable. The growth of 'wrongful life' and 'wrongful birth' suits in the USA where parents are suing doctors or children are suing parents for allowing birth to a child with a deformity or handicap are a dangerous trend in underlining the expectations that only the able-bodied and healthy can have lives worth living (Carey 1991).

Disabled people are dependent so cannot have other people dependent on them

Even in families where disabled parents may need a lot of assistance in managing practical tasks, they may still be the source of emotional strength that binds a family together. Disability alone is not an indicator of the ability of an individual to care for and support others. It is interesting that the word 'care' has come to mean solely physical care (as with professional care staff in nursing homes) rather than an emotional commitment to the person being cared for. It is also interesting to note that dependency here is seen as a negative helpless state and independence as positive and desirable. In western societies parents tolerate the dependency of children by thinking of them as totally helpless but, guiltily or not, try to avoid others becoming dependent for fear of limiting their own independence. We thus think of dependency in pathological terms rather than as part of a dynamic, mutually beneficial two-way pattern in all our relationships with others.

Producing a child when you cannot be sure of your own health or long lifespan is irresponsible

Anyone can become ill or disabled. Not all disabled parents were disabled (or as disabled, in the case of progressive and unpredictable conditions such as multiple sclerosis) before having their children. Even those who have a disability prior to becoming parents could legitimately argue that no parent knows how their life will turn out or when they will die. And who can assert that the quality of relationship that parents with a disability develop with their children is not good enough?

Underlying this sort of criticism are the beliefs in the guilt of the ill and disabled. Many religions treat the ill and disabled as sinners, paying for misdeeds in past lives. This parallels the secular, but none the less equally onerous, late twentieth-century belief that we are responsible for our own health – so that if we become ill or disabled it is our own fault and we should therefore suffer the consequences. Both the medicalisation of disability and the growing promotion of the Body Beautiful through exercise, diet and surgical treatment have encouraged this belief to the point that we are becoming more intolerant of those who are unable to meet the standardised requirements.

Children are in danger of neglect because disabled parents won't be able to look after their physical needs

It is difficult to generalise about this when so little is known about the lives of families where one or both parents are disabled. The effect on their caring abilities will depend on the nature of their disability as well as many other factors such as access to information, peer support and role models, all of which are often more difficult for disabled people. It cannot be categorically stated that disability means that a parent will neglect the physical care of her child. What is needed is more awareness of the many families that are functioning well and to learn from them what the significant factors are.

Every well-meaning parent cares for her child in the way that works best for both the child and herself and that applies just as much to parents with disabilities as any others. Those parents who are unable to deal with specific aspects of physical care for their children will tend to find other sources of help from family and friends and perhaps from social services. It could be that a responsible parent is one who ensures the welfare of her child by orchestrating whatever combination of support is required. It is only if that support is lacking, or suddenly disappears (e.g. a spouse leaves or dies) or if the parent is too frightened to ask for help that the danger of neglect may become significant. The fear of professional intervention leading to the removal of the children is an underlying fear amongst many disabled parents who therefore avoid seeking professional help.

Two other relevant facts are worth mentioning here.

1 An important body of videotaped documentary evidence collected by *Through The Looking Glass* in the USA (Kirshbaum 1988) shows very clearly how even tiny babies adapt to their regular care-givers' particular ways of handling them, e.g. curling up so as to be easier to pick up or lying still for a nappy change. So, far from being passive recipients of care, children actively participate in a two-way, dynamic relationship. There is clear evidence that different ways of handling and caring for young children can be readily accommodated by the children themselves as long as they have the regular contact with each care-giver to recognise their individual style.

What this work has highlighted is the need for observers to take care before passing value judgements on the different ways in which disabled parents may undertake babycare. This is well-illustrated by the courtroom scenes in *The Tiffany Callo Story* (Mathews 1992) where Megan Kirshbaum is called to defend a young woman with cerebral palsy whose fitness to care for her baby son is on trial. Step by step, Kirshbaum dismantles the simplistic and ill-informed assessments by psychologists and social workers who have no familiarity or empathy with disabled people as parents. For example, a video tape of Tiffany Callo slowly changing her baby's diaper is used as evidence of her incompetence. Kirshbaum presents a more positive view of the slow pace of disabled people's lives:

> Their diapering is slow. The professionals, non-disabled professionals can get very judgemental about that but it focuses on the slowness of the enterprise,

and indeed there can be incredible slowness in the care. But the fact is that parents and babies can get through that in a very appropriate way. In some ways the slow pacing, which is, in the disabled community, sometimes called 'crip time', in different families seems to be almost a cultural characteristic of a slower-paced life, slower-paced approach to work, more tolerance of slow pacing.

(Mathews 1992)

Kirshbaum goes on to suggest that this could actually be advantageous to babies as it more accurately matches their own pace. It can also be a time for developing communication and playfulness between parent and child which secure the bond between them.

Not all disabled parents instinctively have the adaptive skills or access to appropriate equipment to deal with all aspects of childcare, but these are skills and information which can be passed on by others. At no stage did Kirshbaum take her role as an assessor to be other than therapeutic as well – she worked with the mother to develop strategies which addressed the different problems the latter was having, often with brilliant success. The process by which she assisted the mother to develop adaptive techniques for caring and relating to her baby during his brief visits to her is fascinating and very illuminating. What she brought to the process was her experience of working with many other disabled parents which enabled her to offer a range of ideas in order to develop the one that might work for Tiffany Callo. Kirshbaum's work needs to reach a wider audience, and *Through The Looking Glass* is planning to produce Guidelines for Assessment and Intervention in 1994 which should help other professionals provide better support in the future.

2 The physical needs of a baby are very different to those of a ten year old. It is important to remember that dealing with nappy changing and feeding is a very short-lived stage of a relationship that may last for fifty years and that children do not necessarily focus on parental disability as abnormal. For example, older children usually see their parents' disability equipment such as sticks and wheelchairs as an ordinary part of the environment: 'I think we have much to learn from the children of disabled parents; from their viewpoint the definition of childhood can often include disability in a matter of fact way' (Kirshbaum in Mathews 1992).

While finding a way to deal with physical care and safety are obviously important they should be kept in context of what a parent can do at other times – not necessarily to be seen as compensation but as different and equally valid and valuable to the child. In an important custody case in California some years ago, a supreme court judge awarded custody to a physically disabled parent, noting that 'the essence of parenting lies in the ethical, emotional and intellectual guidance the parent gives to the child throughout the formative years and often beyond' (Carney v. Carney, 24 Cal 2d 725 (1979)).

The child will have to take unreasonable involvement in household chores and caring for disabled parent

> Disabled people with children may be thought to bear a heavier load than most. But it is often the children who really bear the burden.
>
> (Christine Webb, *The Times* 8/5/87)

> On the basis of a survey in Tameside and estimates by the National Carers Association it is thought that there could be 10,000 young people under 18 who are fulfilling the role of primary carer in the household.
>
> For these young people it is reasonable to assume that the possibilities of a conventional parent–child relationship are sharply reduced. With the parent as carer and child-as-dependent, roles are reversed, the young person could face complex psychological problems, with their education and friendships damaged by the stress of caring.
>
> (*Community Care* 22/2/90)

There has been in recent years a spate of publicity about children caring for disabled parents. The justifiable need to draw attention to the hardships faced by some such children has unfortunately reinforced the impression that all disabled parents are a burden on their children. The young carers are invisible – they do not generally identify themselves readily and since under the age of 16 they are not entitled to register for any carer's benefits, there are no official ways of measuring their numbers. So no statistics exist to refute such impressions and it is easy to see why they prevail: most professionals who come into contact with families where there is a disabled parent are likely to do so because the family is in need – those who are coping well are not observed. Yet glimpses of a different reality emerge occasionally:

> Some of the children we saw were perhaps doing a little more housework as a result of their mother's or father's illness. Some were probably doing less, where their mother's illness meant she was at home rather than out at work, or where she was trying to compensate them for what she saw as the terrible burden her illness inflicted upon them.
>
> (Segal and Simkins 1993)

A pattern that has been recognised amongst some families where children become carers is that the mother becomes disabled, the father leaves the family and the mother becomes progressively more dependent on the children for physical care and housework. State services may provide help during the day but are usually absent at night times and weekends, the expectation being that the children can cope: 'Young carers are sacrificing their childhoods to the care of another family member' (Christine Webb, *The Times* 8/5/87).

Housework, caring for the weak, and self-sacrifice are all seen as primarily the role of the parents, in particular of mothers, so any suggestion of role reversal is often interpreted as evidence that the parent is inadequate. Could it not also be seen as part of a fair and reciprocal relationship (Grimshaw 1992)? What degree of helping with the running of the household and caring for parents becomes unacceptable?

In the western world children are not expected to participate in the domestic chores or caring roles – both are undervalued and seen as a burden to be avoided. It is a cultural issue – most societies with only a minimal state welfare system have expected and depended on exactly this sort of relationship between children and parents. The able-bodied (whatever age) help the less able. The crucial difference has been the ready availability of the wider family network which usually prevents this from becoming an unbearable burden on a single child. If in the industrialised world we decide that each child has a right to a childhood unencumbered in this way, the welfare provision should be there to prevent it. But despite the sentimental sympathy for lost childhoods, the practical support is far from evident.

> Young carers tend not to draw official attention to their own needs out of fear that disclosure would mean they are taken into local authority care and the family broken up. Their contributions go largely unrecognised and their problems remain invisible until family problems develop into a crisis.
>
> (Bilsborrow 1992)

All too often the professional interest is focused on either the child or the parent rather than on the family as a unit and the response is to seek to remove the children or to put the disabled parents into residential care. This may be the only solution for a small number of families but is unlikely to be the best. Such situations beg a whole host of other questions – where are the family and community support networks which turn a blind eye to such children's domestic lives? The Merseyside survey highlighted the importance of the extended family as a resource; the young people who had spent time in state care were the only ones with no extended family to call upon. Could earlier supportive intervention from professionals prevent the caring from becoming a burden? In Britain both the Children Act 1989 and the Community Care Act 1992 emphasise the need to keep parents and children together but in practice the resources and will to back this up are not easy to identify.

Finally, caring for a disabled parent may not be a totally negative experience. Many of the respondents in Bilsborrow's study felt they had benefited from a closer relationship with that parent and the maturity and sense of responsibility that had come with being more involved with the household running.

Disabled people cannot support their families financially

One correlation all over the world is that of disability and poverty. Prejudice as much as the practical and medical limitations caused by the disability itself prevent people with disabilities from getting a good education and job opportunities. This then affects their earning power and ability to be self-sufficient. So it is hardly surprising that this notion of burden on the state underlies many of the objections to disabled people becoming parents. If it is the father who is disabled and unable to earn a salary he is seen as inadequate as the traditional hunter-gatherer-provider for the family. This may affect his own self-perception and his quality of parenting.

It is interesting to note here that for fostering and adoption, disability in the father often appears to be seen as less problematic than in the mother, presumably because she is traditionally expected to run the family home and care for the children.

It is also important to note that basic living costs are frequently higher for disabled people because the environment and standard mass-produced goods and services are not designed to accommodate their individual needs. Costs associated with getting usable equipment, accommodation, transport, clothing, as well as personal and domestic assistance, can all make a big dent in already low incomes.

The family cannot be self-sufficient and therefore will become a burden on friends/neighbours and society

Exceptional resources, including a united and supportive family, good personality adaptation of both parents and secure material circumstances are needed to compensate children for the parental disability. We cannot at present rely on community services to make up for what the individual family lacks. Although we tend to assume that there is a safety net of health care, education and welfare support, these services are in fact drastically short of resources.

(Wolff 1991)

This paints a very bleak and unfounded picture of families with disabled parents. If disabled parents had equal access to the same range of resources that other parents have, only a few would need additional community services. So the lack of access to good education, well-paid jobs, appropriate housing, to social situations where friendships and mutual support networks arise – all these would eradicate the perceived over-dependence on the state. At present the combination of ignorance, prejudice and lack of accessibility of information, transport and buildings can handicap disabled people as parents more than does their physical condition.

Furthermore, the exceptional resources which this author suggests that children of disabled parents need (supportive family, secure material circumstances, etc.) are arguably a priori requirements for all children. This notion of all disabled parents as dependent and needy needs to be questioned. Many disabled people are members of communities who care for others, they are not just cared for themselves (Wates 1993). They would be more visible as such if physical and social barriers could be broken down so that they could participate more freely in community activities.

The cost to society also needs to be kept in perspective. Taking a child into care is a far more expensive way of dealing with a family where a disabled parent is thought not to be coping than to provide appropriate services for the periods when they are required. In many areas social workers do precisely this – for example, organising home helps or transport for mothers of young children. But often the help is not tailored to what the family actually needs to get over a crisis (e.g. hospital stays) or a particularly demanding stage of childcare (e.g. a new baby). The constant stress on resources often seems to mean that professional intervention is limited to vetting parents rather than supporting them, and finding reasons to deny equipment or financial support in the short term which would minimise problems in the long term.

Parents can only be normal if they can prove themselves to be totally self-reliant at all times

Can you be a fit parent if the only way you can deal with your children's physical needs is with able-bodied help (either family and friends, paid help or through state support)? This calls into question the general desirability of the isolation of any parents in bringing up their children. The quality of the child-rearing experience for parent and child anywhere is unquestionably enhanced by the availability of support in all its different forms (family, friends, neighbours, self-help groups, professionals). All parents take advantage of this according to their needs if it is available – so why should disabled parents be penalised? Lack of accessible transport and accessible venues can impose more isolation on those who may need social networks most.

A child will suffer because of the parent's disability

> The rights of the disabled for as normal a life as possible are agreed but we should be clear that their children will start life from a position of disadvantage.
>
> (Wolff 1991)

People with disabilities do not form a pathological group whereby such a statement can be made. It begs the question of what picture the author has in mind of 'the disabled'. It suggests that all people with disabilities are incapable of providing a good standard of childcare and that the children will be handicapped by the stigma of having disabled parents. There is no evidence to support these positions.

There has been little useful research into the impact of disability on family life until very recently. Most of the previous research into this has treated parental illness and disability as synonymous and has concentrated on looking for problems that children might have experienced rather than looking at what they might have gained or what positive attributes and achievements the parents might have passed on. Ranjan Roy's review (1990–1) of the relevant research was more illuminating than most of the original research itself. He set out to try and answer:

1 What may be the prevalence of physical, emotional and psychiatric problems in the children of the medically ill compared with the general population?
2 What may be the risk factors that predispose children of medically ill parents to psychological and medical vulnerabilities?

He examined findings of research into children of parents with depression, cancer, spinal injury, myocardial infarctions, dialysis, multiple sclerosis, tuberculosis and Huntingdon's. Most of the original research appears to be seriously flawed in its methodology and limitations of sample size so it is difficult to know whether the findings are worth publicising or not. But in the absence of 'good' research it is tempting to quote the good news (e.g. children of spinal cord-injured fathers interviewed in adulthood showed that parental disability had little long-term effect) and to ignore the questionable negative findings (e.g. regarding the emotional and behavioural problems of children of parents with multiple sclerosis). Roy concludes that it is impossible to answer either of his original questions and suggests that the research raises more questions than it answers.

> First, the samples are inevitably clinical and generally speaking the sample size is small. Secondly, little thought was given to controlling for age, sex, socioeconomic status, duration of illness of the children or parents, degree of disability, and an increasingly important variable, the role of buffers or protective factors that may offset or counteract the risk factors for the children. What kind of measures were used to assess the children's responses to the parental illness? For the most part, information . . . was obtained from the parents themselves and only in exceptional circumstances from the children either by interviews or objective tests or some other independent source was used to verify parental observations such as the family physician or the school.
>
> (Roy 1990–1)

He concludes that in the absence of properly designed and executed long-term research there is really no way of clearly establishing the power of parental illness to cause long-term damage. More enlightening sources of information on how families deal with parental disability are now emerging piecemeal, written by those with direct experience of living in families with disabled parents as well as by those who have worked with them. For example, *My Mum Needs Me* (Segal and Simkins 1993), written by those with experience of counselling a large number of families with parents who have multiple sclerosis, provides a useful insight into how different members of the same family can react to parental disability and how to address the stresses on relationships that might result. Another study, *Children of Parents with Parkinson's Disease* (Grimshaw 1992), also shows the specific issues that concern children and parents. Both these pieces of work are mould-breaking in that they report the views of children directly and show the variety of experience – positive and negative.

Some points are worth noting from such research:

- Parental disability is just one type of stress factor that may affect families and may not be the most central one.
- All members of the family need access to accurate information so that they do not blame themselves unnecessarily for changes in the parent's physical and emotional health.

- Family adjustment appears to be directly related to the level of adjustment of the disabled parent.
- The age of children at the time of onset of the parent's disability may be an important factor in how well they adjust and in particular on how they themselves come to view illness and disability.
- Middle-class families with a stable marriage and good income minimise the negative consequences of parental disability.
- Social support is significant in minimising hardship for all parents.

Having more accurate information about families where parents are disabled and understanding their particular individual circumstances, expectations and aspirations can enable more constructive approaches by professionals.

Only those who are considered physically normal have a right to parenthood

Historically, I have already shown the eugenic arguments that have prevailed in the West and which continue to do so in other parts of the world. But arbitrary discrimination against disabled people still goes on in so-called modern societies.

> After spending about two hours with us, he said that he had enjoyed talking with us but because he did not know of a disabled person becoming approved as an adoptive parent he was not able to help us with our application. He felt that even if we did get approved by the adoption panel we would not get used. . . . It seemed that because we were not a standard family he would have a harder job getting us accepted by other social workers, who would be more likely to choose a standard family to place a child with.
>
> (*PPIAS Newsletter* No. 61 (1992))

It is the common approach of non-disabled observers and researchers to seek out what makes disabled parents different from rather than the same as able-bodied parents and then to ascribe value judgements about those differences – whereas children and parents with disabilities may see it as no more significant then any other aspect of their family life:

> Family life and parenting are not straightforwardly affected by disease and disability. Children showed an awareness of parents' normal activities such as going to work, shopping and cleaning. It can be argued that such visible activities may be important in confirming the children's sense of parents' normality as active household members.
>
> (Grimshaw 1992)

Perhaps much of the discomfort of the able-bodied about disabled people is rooted in our own fear. We label them as abnormal in order to try and reinforce our own ideals of how 'normal' we are. It is something that has been explored by disability rights activists:

With the rise of industrialism, words like normal and defective, words which had once only been used to refer to things, began to be used to refer to people. The shift in language mirrored the shift in belief which mirrored the shift in social reality. In the industrial age, a new degree of uniformity was expected of people. The rhythms and pacing of life could no longer be organic. People became expected to function like things.

(Finger 1992)

Looking at those who are considered non-standard or abnormal teaches us a lot about that which we consider to be normal. Parents with disabilities often talk about the fact that they just lead normal lives like other families, about how having children made them feel that they had achieved something normal, often for the first time in their lives. While becoming disabled is seen as a process of becoming abnormal, having children is seen as becoming a normal member of society. So, while the interests of children are obviously important, perhaps it is time that society recognised the opportunity for fulfilment and 'normal' life that raising children can bring for disabled people.

Many of the barriers in society facing people with disabilities are also those facing most parents of young children. Isolation, juggling limited amounts of time, energy and money, the difficulty of getting around crowded shopping centres with children, getting on and off public transport, through heavy shop doors, up and down endless steps, finding toilets, carrying heavy loads of shopping, the lack of respect and tolerance of needing to do things at a different pace – all these are reasons for uniting and working together to make our environments better for everyone. By focusing on the disability we ignore the commonality of experience as parents and their particular expertise.

Because disabled parents are amongst those most harshly affected by the constraints and under-resourcing of parents in our society, we are also amongst those who are furthest along the road to finding solutions. This is one of the reasons why our experience is worth looking at.

(Wates 1991)

USEFUL POINTS FROM THE EXPERIENCES OF DISABLED PARENTS

Kirshbaum's work noting the synchronicity of the slower pace of many disabled people with a child's pace has already been mentioned but there are other benefits that have often been observed:

- Children are likely to grow up more sensitive and tolerant of difference.
- Children may have stronger role models of parents as resilient and resourceful.
- Many disabled parents can offer more time because they are less likely to be rushing around trying to do too many things. While this time can be valuable to all children it may be a particular extra resource for children who have had very disrupted lives and need that extra attention.

Although my disability has prevented me from going on long walks with her, swimming and other activities, it has given me more time to spend with her. I am always here to play games, to listen and talk, and this has been an advantage.

(*PPIAS Newsletter* No. 61 (1992))

In reference to the ideal father, Roy said he couldn't play football, but one of their daughters would take on all comers. In reality they wondered how many fathers want to play football and cricket. Because of her natural disposition, Doreen does much of the listening to the girls' problems, though she feels her husband also gives them more time than some able-bodied men who are always doing DIY and snooker. 'He is a proper family man.'

(Caine 1990)

Examples like this are confirmation – for those who need it – that disabled people can be as good as most able-bodied parents but even better than others. As parents they cover the same spectrum as other people who do not have a physical disability.

Another advantage of 'abnormality' has been the understanding it has brought about in the way that babies develop. Much is made in childcare manuals of the importance of face-to-face contact with babies, the use of singsong 'motherese' to teach babies language. But by looking at how parents who are blind or deaf communicate and by observing their children, the theories about what is essential to communication have been modified. What becomes clear is that there are different routes to development of skills, such as language, for example (Collis 1991; Sacks 1990), through the use of sign language instead of speech, which are equally successful. Knowing about such variety can enable a greater range of options to help those children (of whatever parentage) who have difficulty acquiring skills through the standard route or to help disabled first-time parents improve their parenting skills.

The research and videotapes by Kirshbaum add to the body of knowledge which shows how babies are actively influencing the care they receive from their guardians. All this type of work shows that parental responsiveness is what babies need but that it can come from whatever combination of touch, sound and movement the care-giver is comfortable with.

In the coming years we should see more of this type of information and experience as more parents with disabilities enter the mainstream – but it is a process of discovery to which the rest of society has to make itself open.

WHAT THE ASSESSMENT OF DISABLED PARENTS TELLS US ABOUT FIT PARENTS

Ideal

- Should only have children if they are physically healthy and if they have no reason to expect a short lifespan.

- Be responsible for doing everything in their power to have healthy, able-bodied children.
- Should be financially self-sufficient,
- Should follow accepted ways of babycare.
- Should not expect children to help with domestic chores or in any physical care of parents.
- Should conform to society's expectations of normal-looking parents.
- Should only expect to care for their own children if they are able continuously to prove that any disability is not a handicap to the children.

Actual

- Parents do their best to ensure that every child, whatever his physical health, achieves his full potential.
- Parents' essential role lies in the moral, intellectual and spiritual guidance they give to their children throughout life.
- Successful parent–child relationships can exist under a variety of conditions.
- There are many ways in which the needs of babies can be satisfied and the only guide to which is best is what the regular care-givers feel comfortable with.
- Children are active contributors to how they are parented.
- Good material circumstances can help families cope with stressful situations.
- Parenting is a lifelong relationship of which babycare is an important but very short-lived stage.
- Parents seek out support networks that are appropriate to their particular circumstances.
- Lifelong health cannot be guaranteed for any parent or child. While it may be desirable, it need not be essential to successful child-rearing.
- The family unit is subject to many external and internal pressures as a result of factors other than and including disability.
- All parenthood requires continuous adjustment to external circumstances and to individual needs. Society more or less hampers certain parents in going about their child-rearing.
- Class (as determined by employment and financial security) is a major factor in how parents cope with stress factors.

7   Mentally handicapped parents

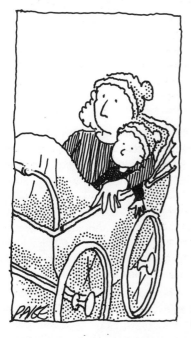

(© *New Statesman and Society*/Solo 1988)

HANDICAPPED COUPLE FIGHT MOVE TO TAKE BABY AWAY

We feel the couple cannot look after the baby. If I can have firm evidence that this is not the case, I will look at it again. The man is genetically handicapped and the woman is as she is because of a severe accident. They are both extremely forgetful. The woman plays with dolls and our fear is that she would treat this child like a doll. There have been chip fires in the house as well.

> (Social Services Committee Chairman quoted by Paul Hoyland,
> *Guardian* 2/7/87)

A case of guilty until proven innocent? This newspaper extract reporting the views of a social services Chairman highlights a random selection of misfortunes and negative traits – childlike, forgetful, dangerous – which any sensible person would immediately agree seem to confirm unfitness to parent. The report does not provide any evidence of rigorous assessment or attempts to support the parents.

Can mentally handicapped people cope with caring for children?

The gut response, given most people's limited direct experience of people with learning disabilities, seems to be no. Yet more and more people traditionally labelled as mentally handicapped are becoming parents, presenting a major challenge to those professionals charged with protecting children and forcing everyone else to examine our assumptions more closely.

All of the assumptions and objections that apply to parents with physical disabilities also stand for those with a learning disability. The objections are however even stronger, and whereas many people would avoid openly suggesting that physically disabled people should not become parents, most seem to have no such inhibitions about those with a learning disability.

Mentally handicapped people are all the same

Most of the objections seem to lump all mentally handicapped people together but there is clearly a wide variety of individuals covered by the label. What does mental handicap or retardation actually mean? What is low intelligence? Despite people's ready use of the terms, surprisingly, there are no clear answers to these questions. In the not so distant past, many people have been labelled mentally retarded and institutionalised without any rigorous assessment of their intelligence. Over the centuries the terminology has changed: within my own lifetime terms such as imbeciles, feeble-minded, half-wits, mentally retarded, gave way to mentally handicapped and, more recently, to developmentally disabled and people with learning difficulties – although most of the academic literature still refers to mental retardation. The terms tells us nothing about what has caused the handicap nor what potential the individual may have to develop. Genetic conditions such as Down's Syndrome are the commonest cause of learning difficulties but the rest have a variety of origins which as yet are poorly understood.

Mental retardation has been defined in terms of IQ (Intelligence Quotient), a system of tests intended to measure intelligence. The scoring methods treat mental retardation to be an IQ of below 70. Thus mild mental retardation is defined as a score between 70 and 55; moderate retardation between 54 and 40, and severe retardation as below 40. IQ has by no means been accepted as an accurate indicator of intellectual potential but, in the absence of any other objective standard measuring techniques, it has been widely adopted by those working with children and adults with perceived learning difficulties.

IQ is not an accurate indicator of how well an individual might function in society given appropriate education and training. Nor does it recognise the inherent role of the social and physical environment in which the individual lives. For example, referring to the situation in Pakistan, it was found that

> Nearly 80 per cent of the individuals identified on the basis of intelligence test results as mentally retarded were not perceived to be so by the community when the norm utilised was one of adequacy in social functioning. In simple rural and agrarian community where stress on education is low and where collective and cooperative living – rather than individual striving and competition – is the general rule, many of the mildly retarded individuals do fulfil the social functions expected of them and hence do not get identified as mentally retarded.
>
> (G. Prabhu 1983 quoted in Miles 1992)

It seems to me that the most accurate definition is not one that measures IQ or tries to ascribe a medical label but is 'people who are perceived by their families or communities as having a noticeable level of deficit from culture-specific norms of learning, behaviour, intelligence and competence' (Miles 1992).

To what extent this deficit has negative connotations depends on what expected norms are unfulfilled.

> 'Mental retardation', understood thus is socially and individually noticed, constructed and felt. If one of the [Pakistani] educated elite has a teenage child who has not learnt to read even after tutoring and who cannot be trusted to serve tea and make polite conversation with parental guests, the child may be deemed 'stubborn'. However, the criterion of 'failure to learn to read' would hardly indicate mental retardation in the general population where less than 30 per cent of adults have learnt to read. 'Unreliable in polite talk and in serving tea respectfully to guests' would equally be misleading as a criterion of mental retardation if applied to English adolescents.
>
> (Miles 1992)

The cultural norms are thus significant in what we label as abnormal. For example, the notion of independence of family is a cultural norm of the West, not of countries like Pakistan. So the failure of a child to develop into an adult independent of his elders is not seen as an immutable objective and need not prevent marriage or childbearing.

It is worth noticing these culture-specific aspects of how we perceive mental retardation because it encourages us to ascribe less of the problem to the individuals we have labelled. It also helps us understand more about the values we have elevated in western society such as literacy, employment, independence, self-sufficiency. It also calls into question the status we attach to high intelligence. It has often been argued that intelligent people can do more damage to society than those of low intelligence. (It is also interesting to consider, as you read this section, how many of the communication problems experienced by mentally handicapped individuals are very similar to those facing immigrants who do not speak the local language – again suggesting a cultural dissonance.)

We clearly need to be wary of generalisations. Some people with learning disabilities have been brought up in institutions, some in families, some have physical disabilities, many do not. Some have been accepted by those close to them while others have been rejected. Some are better equipped than others to handle day-to-day living. Many are poor and living on the margins of society, without the trappings of what is considered normal life. Because of their lack of literacy and status, their own views and experiences remain largely unrecorded.

They should not be having sex

APPEAL COURT RULES THAT RETARDED GIRL BE STERILISED

The retarded girl, referred to only as 'Jeanette', is now becoming sexually aware and the consequences of her becoming pregnant were frightening, Lord Justice Dillon said.

(Independent 17/3/87)

A spate of well-publicised court cases in recent years concerning sterilisation of mentally handicapped young women brought to the public's attention the fact that they do have sex but this is seen as undesirable and problematic – either it is a sign of abuse or of promiscuity. Above all they are childlike and so should not be interested in sex. The latter view is at least partly the result of being cared for into adulthood by parents and institutions, neither of which are comfortable about the sexual maturity of their charges.

It is interesting to note that the focus has been on the sterilisation of young women with little regard for the contraceptive responsibilities of the men who are their sexual partners.

It may be objected that male sterilisation would not solve the problem of the woman's fertility; that she could become pregnant through intercourse with another man. But this argument presumes the woman's promiscuity. In individual cases the premise could be defamatory. Would it be appropriate for a husband to object to a vasectomy on the grounds that his wife might become pregnant by another – without substantial proof of the likelihood? There is no justification for a general assumption that all women with learning difficulties are promiscuous. If individuals are promiscuous they need special services to protect them from the sexual disease that sterilisation does not affect.

(Carson 1989)

Furthermore, there is the danger of imposing one's own prejudices on mentally handicapped women:

We would not, for example, be surprised that a 17 year old woman was not interested in or indeed did not like babies or children. . . . We would ordinarily allow for people's attitudes to children to change in the future. It is a sexual stereotype to presume or expect that girls or women will or should be interested in babies and children. Yet the fact of an apparent present disinterest in and/or dislike of children was cited as a justification for sterilising women with learning difficulties.

(Carson 1989)

The readiness to sterilise mentally handicapped women to protect them from an unwanted pregnancy needs to be carefully considered so that it is not just a measure of convenience for others. There are considerable complex issues surrounding the legal rights and status of different people with learning difficulties that are designed to protect them but which can act as a barrier to their choosing to express their sexuality: 'The mentally retarded person has the same basic rights as other citizens of the same country and same age' (UN 1971).

However, institutional segregation, lack of privacy, lack of appropriate models concerning nudity, social conduct, personal hygiene and appearance can all create barriers to learning about sexuality and standards of acceptable sexual behaviour. The move out of institutions and into the community has been accompanied by a growing belief that sexuality and the choice of parenthood should equally be the right of mentally retarded individuals but the reality is still difficult to achieve.

Even where mentally retarded individuals live in small houses in the community with their own bedrooms, services can discourage sexuality directly and indirectly. They rarely have influence, let alone control over who lives in each house and they are often dependent upon staff for transport which can be used to restrict them from developing relationships outside the home.

(Carson 1989)

Those concerned with the 'normalisation' of people with learning difficulties are placed in a quandary, for even if their right to sexual lives is accepted the practicalities are not straightforward. Those who are the responsibility of guardians and institutions have to be protected from potential abuse – which is an onerous responsibility and an understandable disincentive to encouraging sexuality. If a severely mentally retarded woman becomes pregnant she may well not be able to cope with the stress of pregnancy and childbirth, and the cost and availability of resources to enable her to care for the child may determine how those around her view the outcome.

One of the recurring objections is that a mentally handicapped person cannot understand what sex is and therefore all sexual relationships are potentially exploitative. To counter this there is clear variation in how different individuals are aware of their sexuality. It has been pointed out that there is a difference between understanding and behaviour: just as many people drive cars all their lives with little or no understanding of how a car works, so a mentally handicapped person can be taught to behave sexually in an acceptable manner without understanding some of the complexities of sexuality (Craft 1987). This same principle could be applied to giving birth to and rearing children.

Another objection is that the attempts at expression of sexual interest by mentally handicapped people causes embarrassment and hostility because they do not know what is commonly considered inappropriate. Research has shown that the more normal the environment experienced by people the more normal their behaviour (Craft 1987).

> Unless there are opportunities to watch, copy and obtain feedback from people who are adept in the complex nuances of social behaviour it will not be surprising that skills are not learnt. For so long as their dances, holidays and meals etc. are segregated people with learning difficulties not only do not get any additional help that they might need but get less help and will often learn inappropriate behaviour.
>
> (Carson 1989)

A person who has the mental age of a child cannot take care of children

> The common right for all, regardless of mental age, to enjoy the freedom to procreate and 'bring up' their children would seem to be nothing short of a sign post to disaster.
>
> (Mary Thornley, *The Times* 5/8/87)

It is common to point to the mental age of an individual as indicative of their potential as parents, but this is misleading.

> An intelligence test may conclude that a woman has intellectual abilities normally associated with a four- or five-year-old. Courts cannot justifiably conclude, just from that evidence that she would not be able to look after her child. Certainly four-year-olds do not bear, or, hopefully, have charge of babies. But that is not the point. The court would clearly be in error if it concluded from such a test that the woman had the same physical strength, courage, dexterity or experience as a four-year-old. The intelligence test neither measures these attributes or the ability to look after babies. It is quite possible that a person with such limited intellectual abilities would be incapable of looking after a child properly. But that needs to be tested by behavioral means rather than to be an inappropriate inference from a test that measures something else.
>
> (Carson 1989)

Formal assessments of intelligence do not attempt to measure intellectual capacities that are likely to have a direct influence on parenting skills. The essential point is that intelligence tests are not predictors of social functioning.

> A person may receive extensive education and training in the ways of the world and be able to cope adequately with his or her social world whilst having limited intelligence. Equally a person without a learning difficulty may be open to exploitation and have a significant impairment in social functioning arising from the way he or she was brought up.
>
> (Carson 1989)

So what factors do influence a mentally handicapped person's quality of parenting? Not IQ it seems, but rather the capacity to understand and anticipate social events, to assess the consequences of personal actions, and to organise and plan household management and childcare. Other factors which appear to be significant but are poorly studied are:

- Child characteristics (e.g. age, sex, ordinal position, temperament).
- Family size (e.g. parenting three or more is more stressful than one or two).
- Spouse characteristics (e.g. if spouse has mental health difficulties this can influence quality of care provided by the parent with the learning disability).
- Marital relationship (presence of spouse and quality of marital relationship are known to affect parenting).
- Extended family (level of support, criticism from and conflict with other relatives can all affect parental self-esteem and subsequent functioning).

They cannot be as good parents as more intelligent people

There has been little useful research done in this area, despite the widely held prejudice. The concern has some justification given that 'The cognitive limitations and increased emotional vulnerability associated with mental retardation seem to put mentally retarded people at higher risk of disorders of parenting' (Whitman *et al.* 1989).

The issue of whether mentally retarded people can be as good parents as those with a higher IQ has been addressed by a number of approaches:

- Whether they provide inadequate physical care for their children.
- Whether they need state services to help raise their children.
- Whether children displaying difficulties have mentally retarded parents.
- Whether many children taken into care have mentally retarded parents.
- Whether many abused children have mentally retarded parents.

None of these studies have sought out a large number of mentally retarded parents and examined which are doing well or compared them with other parents in similar socioeconomic settings, nor have they looked at the background or type of preparation for parenthood that any of those parents might have had.

> Although we have been attempting to predict adequacy of parenting by parents with mental retardation (i.e. a positive outcome), such adequacy often has been defined peculiarly as inadequacy of parenting (usually seen as abuse and/or neglect which are negative outcomes). This preoccupation with the prediction of 'inadequacy of parenting' rather than 'adequacy of parenting' by persons with mental retardation has led to a prolonged focus upon the description of negative aspects of parenting by persons with mental retardation. Thus descriptive as well as research reports have invariably reported on how poorly people with mental retardation parent while essentially ignoring any evidence to the contrary and may be part of the self fulfilling prophecy.
>
> (Tymchuk 1992)

Many studies in the past have appeared to show that the high incidence of child removal from mentally retarded parents was due in some way to their deficiency as parents. Many of these studies have now been questioned as methodologically flawed and unrepresentative. Parents identified by childcare authorities as mentally retarded or having mentally retarded children may be more likely to be the subject of intervention (Whitman and Accardo 1990) simply on the basis of the labelling.

Such parents may also be discriminated against in court proceedings because of their inability to present themselves and to communicate well:

> Professionals often respond to parents with unrecognised intellectual limitations in the same way that parents respond to intellectually limited children – with frustration and annoyance. In both cases it is assumed that the individual's failure to cooperate results from an unwillingness to meet expectations, when in fact he or she is unable to do so.
>
> (Valentine 1990)

Parents may become reluctant to seek out or cooperate with professionals for fear of being shouted at or confused – which then becomes a handicap in itself. So it is clearly important for professionals to recognise their influence on the quality of parenting and to understand the skills they need to develop in working with such parents.

Most of the direct observational studies have concentrated on how mothers with mental retardation play with babies and found that they are less involved and sensitive in their play behaviour; they tend to be more directive, punishing more and praising less than mothers of middle socioeconomic status. However, this research is based on a very small group of mothers who were observed for only a few minutes at a time. Other studies have indicated that mentally retarded mothers have difficulty in handling difficult behaviour in their children. The suggestion was that they did not know how or when to reinforce good behaviour instead of just punishing for inappropriate behaviour, nor did they ignore a child instead of reprimanding. Again these statements were made by observing very small numbers of mothers for just a short period of time – but it does seem as if the researchers found what they had expected to find.

Current theories of what children need are arguably based on a middle-class view of family life with children receiving a lot of 'quality interaction' of a certain type from their parents, particularly from their mothers. On these terms the mentally retarded mothers appeared to be less competent than middle-class mothers. But had they been compared to mothers from similar socioeconomic backgrounds, the significance of their mental retardation might be clearer (Dowdney and Skuse 1993).

The following is a sobering reminder of the unfairness of labelling the mentally handicapped as unfit to be parents.

> In my 20 years of psychiatric work with thousands of children and their parents, I have seen percentally [sic] at least as many 'intelligent' adults unfit

to rear their offspring as I have seen such 'feebleminded' adults. I have . . . come to the conclusion that to a large extent independent of IQ, fitness for parenthood is determined by emotional involvements.

(Kanner 1949 quoted in Whitman *et al.* 1989)

The children are at risk of neglect and poor levels of care

Child neglect is commonly associated with mentally retarded parents but the reasons for it are not necessarily simply to do with IQ levels. For example, it is unclear whether the frequency of neglect is any greater than that seen among other poor people.

Many parents with learning difficulties do manage to provide adequate care. This has been discovered almost accidentally by researchers who had set out to discover the degree of inadequacy of mentally retarded parents, but

the emphasis has continued to be upon those families and children who do poorly. Of equal or even greater importance, however, given the inadequate response by society to remedying reasons for such perceived parenting deficiencies, is the identification and reinforcement of reasons why a substantial proportion of the homes are seen as adequate and why a substantial proportion of the children have IQs at least in the normal range. This information is indicative of a substantial proportion of poor people with low IQs assuming individual responsibility, doing reasonably well and whose children also may do well.

(N. Garmezy and M. Rutter quoted in Tymchuk 1992)

Mentally retarded parents have often been found to be lacking in knowledge and skill about health and safety – especially about how to deal with illnesses and emergencies, but these limitations may not be a result of mental retardation:

Such limited knowledge and skill in child healthcare and safety in parents with mental retardation, which are normatively seen as components of adequate parenting within Western society, however appear to be very similar to the levels of knowledge and skill of other poor parents who are not mentally retarded.

(Tymchuk 1992)

Concerns also exist about the ability of parents to be able to take responsible decisions regarding their children's welfare. This has not been widely studied, but the few attempts to do so suggest that while their decision making was less thoughtful and deliberate than those of mothers with higher IQs, they were remarkably similar to those of other poor parents.

Many studies suggest that anyone with an IQ of under 60 is unlikely to be able to take responsibility for children and so the children will be neglected. But recent observers have suggested that the best predictor of neglect is not IQ but the absence of suitable societal or familiar supports which can help prevent neglectful conditions (Tymchuk 1992). They suggest that those who are least likely to be reported for neglect are those with support closely matched to their precise needs including learning style and capacity.

For professionals it is thus particularly important to be aware of the need to assess the availability of social support and environmental stresses.

Critical characteristics of societal supports include their:

- availability (i.e. proximity, transportation provided);
- comprehensiveness;
- frequency and duration;
- longevity;
- place;
- provision by staff with training specifically to work with parents with mental retardation.

(Tymchuk 1992)

The strategy of reducing stress and bolstering social supports can further increase the likelihood that children and families receive the assistance they need to prevent removal of the children, ensure that the individual family members' needs are being met, and accomplish the goals of community participation and least restrictive environment (Valentine 1990). The issue of community participation is an interesting one which I have seen little mention of in the academic literature, but through my own experience of meeting parents with learning difficulties it does seem to be a significant factor in parental self-esteem and fostering a pride and respect amongst their children. The need for continuity and familiarity in the social and physical environment may be particularly important to parents with learning difficulties but they are desirable for all families, particularly those with very young or very elderly members.

Finally, although academics and professionals are not falling over backwards in the rush to say how well some parents do actually manage, a few have at least begun to acknowledge that 'Mentally retarded parents do not constitute a homogeneous class of equally incompetent individuals (Budd and Greenspan 1981).

They will abuse their children

Early studies of children of mentally retarded parents seemed to suggest a high incidence of abuse but these studies are now being questioned for their small size and biased samples.

Abuse is far less common among mentally retarded parents than neglect. IQ by itself is not a predictor either of the occurrence or non-occurrence of purposeful child abuse in parents with mental retardation (Tymchuk 1992). When abuse does occur it is often the result of another person associated with the mother such as her partner or a relative, rather than the mother herself.

Tymchuk points out the lack of studies of mentally retarded parents with regard to the predictors of purposeful abuse in other populations such as being abused as a child, the frequency of stressful events or of a general ability to cope, or such child-related characteristics as temperament, health impairment or disability. Yet all these may have a particular significance in the lives of mentally handicapped people who appear to be at greater risk as children of being abused themselves (Valentine 1990), as well as perhaps being more vulnerable to not being able to cope with stressful events or health impairment in their children.

The connection between intellectual impairment and child abuse is an interesting one as it highlights the essentially two-way nature of parenting: the quality of parenting is in some part related to the nature of the individual child. With reference to mentally handicapped children, it has been suggested that they may be more difficult to look after because the child's responses may not be what the parent expects, the child may require more time and energy and financial commitment, and his special needs may lead to the social isolation of the family as a unit – all these factors heighten the risk of abuse. Parents who might have succeeded in caring for a non-impaired child may not be able to cope with a child with special needs (Valentine 1990). For those who are institutionalised, there is also a high risk of abuse, corporal punishment, misuse of psychotropic drugs, isolation exceeding two hours, restraint by mechanical devices, and lack of attention to the rights and specific needs of individual children. Such children have problems getting protection and help because they may have difficulties in communicating and being taken seriously (Valentine 1990).

As adults, those with a mental handicap are less likely to have high self-esteem, a good network of social supports, to find steady employment or to make stable relationships. These are also common factors amongst abusing parents. All these indicate that a mentally retarded parent may have many risk factors in common with parents who abuse their children but which are socially engendered – not an inevitable consequence of their learning difficulties.

Their children will be retarded

The philosopher John Stuart Mill believed that to bring a child into existence without a fair prospect of being able, not only to provide food for its body but instruction for its mind was a moral crime, 'against the unfortunate offspring and against society'.

(Carey 1991)

This has been a major concern for decades for those who fear the prospect of the feeble-minded spawning more feeble-minded people who will become dependent on the state and dilute the intelligence of the nation. In more recent years the concern has focused on the need to identify children who may be disadvantaged and in need of special attention and services.

There is a common expectation that children of mentally retarded parents will themselves be mentally retarded. Some studies do appear to have shown a higher incidence in children of mental retardation but it is unclear to what extent this is due to hereditary factors, to lack of adequate care by the parents, to inaccurate labelling of the children or to the poor environment available to such families.

Surprisingly there has been little useful research into the outcome of the children of mentally retarded parents. When groups have been identified as having a higher incidence of children with mental retardation there has been little attempt to discern genetic or psychosocial explanations. Nor have I been able to find any detailed studies of children removed from parents with learning disabilities to see how they have fared with their adoptive families.

A British epidemiological study from 1965 suggested that the proportion of mentally retarded children born to parents of whom one was mentally retarded was 15 per cent compared to 1 per cent amongst parents of normal intelligence. If both parents were retarded the figure rose to 40 per cent:

> The current consensus amongst researchers is that while rates of retardation will overall be higher amongst subjects' children, their average IQ will show a regression to the mean. The risk will be markedly higher if both parents are affected. Sometimes this will be due to the transmission of specific inheritable medical conditions; in other cases non-specific genetic factors may be important. The role of psychosocial disadvantage in general, and the effects of a more restrictive and insensitive parenting style in particular, either as independent causal factors or in interaction with the above factors has yet to be elucidated.
>
> (Dowdney and Skuse 1993)

In the absence of more useful research, there is a tendency to assume that the parents' learning disability *per se* will inevitably mean developmental delays in the children. Such assumptions may actually cause the children to be disadvantaged. Many parents with learning difficulties describe their worries about school and many are concerned about being unable to help with their children's reading or understanding the school homework and about not being helped or treated seriously by teachers.

It is interesting to note that many of the education problems that face mentally handicapped parents also apply to other groups of 'normal' intelligence parents, e.g. those from immigrant communities or working parents with limited time. It does call into question the expectations society has of parents as educators of children. Most parents assume responsibility for teaching children practical self-care and health and safety but rely on schools to provide formal education. Other sources of education such as television programmes (*Sesame Street* has been quoted by many parents from different groups) may be as significant to individual children as reading from books.

Their children will be stigmatised

Parents with learning disabilities do not like to identify themselves as such. In societies where intelligence is rated so highly this is hardly surprising. A recent poster campaign for BBC Radio 4, arguably the most influential radio channel in Britain, caused controversy by seemingly bragging that only people with a high IQ could appreciate its output. It was a momentary lapse in the facade that suggests public service broadcasting is intended for all the public, not just the educated middle classes. The campaign was probably a thoughtless rather than deliberate attack on people with low IQs but none the less it adds to marginalisation of people with learning difficulties.

The day-to-day stigmatisation of parents with learning disabilities depends on their communities; the community determines whether the families will be more different or more similar to those around them. There is the risk of stigmatisation but, as with other socially deviant groups, the stigmatisation may in itself not be damaging as much as how it is handled. It is certainly not the fault of the parents if society is so ill-equipped to handle difference but it can none the less cause problems for both the parents and the children. Many parents I have spoken to described their fear of going to any school activity in case they are asked to fill out a form or get involved in a debate where their learning difficulty would be exposed, the constant feeling being that 'everyone else understands what's going on except me'. The fear of stigmatisation can result in not asking for help when their children do need it and may underlie many of their own children's learning difficulties.

Parents with learning difficulties cannot learn to be good parents

The traditional professional response to mentally handicapped parents has been to remove the children at birth or to wait for them to fail and then remove the children. Either way there has been a reluctance to fully address ways in which to equip parents to succeed. Mentally handicapped parents are usually assessed on their current knowledge and skills in parenting rather than their capacity to learn.

This does call into question the 'normal' way in which new parents are supposed to learn: through family experience, through antenatal classes, increasingly through books and peer support – all of which may be inaccessible to people with learning difficulties. Many have not had much opportunity to learn in the context of actual family life, i.e. by watching and participating. Many have problems with traditional sources which depend heavily on the written word or (like television, antenatal teaching or talking with experts such as obstetricians) which require instant assimilation of complex ideas. 'Thus, the most vulnerable prospective parent has the least access to information' (Valentine 1990).

Appropriate and skilled training has yet to be fully recogised as more humane, more effective and cheaper than taking children into care. To compensate for the inaccessibility of the conventional sources, many prospective parents may need to be taught by methods which reproduce the experience that might be gained had they participated in family life first-hand, i.e. with repetition of daily tasks, presence of supportive others, a home environment with continuity of teaching personnel and location and so on.

Because people with learning difficulties are seen to face such a wide range of possible deficits in their parenting skills, what is required to minimise these deficits reveals a lot about what is expected of all parents.

A number of projects to improve the parenting abilities of otherwise high-risk adults are under way in North America and the UK and these are beginning to provide more useful information about what sort of training is needed by parents with learning disabilities.

Among the specific problems encountered were the following: language problems, problems with organising and sequencing, problems of over-generalisation or undergeneralisation, low self-esteem, an inordinate desire to please, inability to read social cues, inability to use nonverbal cues appropriately, untreated medical and social problems, learning-disability problems that further limited skill usage, and a tendency to overtax and ultimately burn out their social support system.

(Whitman *et al.* 1989)

It is clear that to have any effect, parent training of people with learning disabilities needs to simultaneously and intensively address the multiple needs they may have – by means appropriate to their learning abilities, through clearly expressed goals and by supportive trained staff working in a coordinated fashion to boost parental confidence and skills.

Teaching methods found to be successful include professionals modelling good parenting behaviour for the students, role-playing by parents, observing, practising – and, most important, repetition. Parents benefit from plenty of one-to-one attention at home. Group work is valuable in that it can promote socialisation and peer support as well as parent training. Teaching covers areas such as child development and childcare, personal and child hygiene, medical care, nutrition, children's basic needs, parent–child interaction, children's safety, planning of a daily routine and time concepts. The assumption, presumably, is that there exists a cultural consensus about what is desirable in all these areas and that is what is being transmitted.

Many required help with developing pictorial organizational aids centered around their most watched television shows, their favorite radio shows, or some similar theme. For instance one mother knew that the end of *Bewitched* meant it was time for her and her child to meet the transportation van. Another mother was able to match the position of the hands of her electric clock to pictures to know when to give her child medication.

(Whitman *et al.* 1989)

The emphasis is on defining concrete objectives together with the parents and establishing performance indicators to monitor progress. The use of direct instruction, characterised by active practice of each small task and immediate feedback and correction, has been found to be critical to success.

The attitudes of the staff are also critical to the motivation of the parents:

A worker who is responsible to teach and support a family must win the family's trust. The teaching/helping role is completely incompatible with the policing/protecting responsibilities necessary in the child welfare system. We cannot expect parents with disabilities, or any other persons, to enter a trusting relationship if their helper does not fully believe in their ability to succeed as individuals and family units. It is therefore essential to separate all protection responsibilities from the intervention process, and to advocate for the families in their involvement with the child welfare system.

(Pomerantz *et al.* 1990)

Finally, it is important not to expect a once and for all solution to parent training of people with learning difficulties. Children change as they grow, adult circumstances change. For an adult with a learning difficulty many additional resources and appropriate education may be necessary on a long-term basis. What this demonstrates is that parenting is a dynamic rather than a static process of continual development – we all have to be receptive to new information and ongoing challenges as our children and our own circumstances change. How receptive we are to learning depends on the role models we have had, how and where we are taught, by whom and what our motivations are.

To function as completely independent units may not be an option for many families but if the support systems can be maintained there is every possibility that most parents with learning difficulties will bring up their children as well as many other parents. And what of those who cannot?

> There may be a point at which the degree of retardation requires such a high level of support that the practicality (in a given case, and not on the basis of IQ) of parenting by adults with mental retardation is questionable. But the existence and location of cutoff point needs to be proven on a case-by-case basis, and not presumed. A doctrine of fairness does not allow such parents to be treated differently from other parents who neglect, abuse or otherwise mistreat their children.
>
> (Whitman *et al.* 1989)

This is the only feasible response by a civilised society that has rejected the apparently tidy but abhorrent solutions of eugenics.

Having learning difficulties is what makes these parents different from normal parents

As more and more people with learning difficulties become parents their individual strengths (e.g. as substitute parents for certain sorts of children, as has already been noted in Chapter 2) and weaknesses will become clearer – but again we need to be prepared to see the whole picture. In a project funded by the Nuffield Foundation, Wendy and Tim Booth collected the stories of a number of parents with learning difficulties and they sum up their findings to date as follows:

> Parents with learning difficulties do not form a pathological group. Their experiences of childrearing and parenthood show more similarities than differences with ordinary families.
>
> Second, having learning difficulties is not a disqualification from enjoying lasting marriage, bringing up children or leading ordinary family lives, any more than not having learning difficulties is a guarantee of success.
>
> Third, many of the problems experienced by parents with learning difficulties derive more from poverty, poor housing, harassment, victimisation and lack of support, than from their own deficiencies in parental competence.

And last, professionals are a major cause of upset and trouble in the lives of people with learning difficulties.

(Booth and Booth 1992)

This final comment could be interpreted as suggesting that professionals should leave parents with learning difficulties alone but this is clearly not an option in a society which sets itself up to guard children against the inadequacy of their parenting. What is needed is appropriate professional intervention which empowers and equips families to stay together.

USEFUL POINTS TO EMERGE FROM THE EXPERIENCES OF MENTALLY HANDICAPPED PARENTS

The most important point to recognise is that the physical and social environment of western society has become increasingly complex and demands a higher level of ability to think in the abstract and to assess information and risks. We can no longer rely on what we observe to determine our judgements; we have to understand a lot more about what lies behind the immediately observable. Parenting in modern urban societies thus requires a high level of social functioning skills. Literacy is important, whether it involves being able to read and interpret information related to child safety, education, or bus timetables. Such societies can be very disabling environments for those with low literacy and low ability to think in the abstract but, if they live in a supportive environment which can accommodate lack of literacy and a slower pace, many parents with learning difficulties are able to function well.

WHAT THE ASSESSMENT OF MENTALLY HANDICAPPED PARENTS TELLS US ABOUT THE EXPECTATIONS OF FIT PARENTS

Ideal

- Parents need to conform to the dominant culture.
- Middle-class parents who can read and have secure jobs and homes are better than lower-class parents.
- Parents need to have acquired the following skills by the time they have children:
  - Provide adequately nutritious foods.
  - Tell the time.
  - Organise daily household routines.
  - Make judgements about safety.
  - Provide reasonable and consistent discipline with minimal use of physical punishment and with praise for child's compliance.
  - Control anxiety and anger in face of difficult or irritating child behaviours.
  - Recognise and respond to dangerous or high-risk situations.

- Play responsively.
- Make frequent positive remarks to child.
- Be motivated to care.
- Be open to learning and developing.
- Apply rules flexibly to meet their children's developmental needs.
- Provide cognitive stimulation.
- Help with formal education of child.
- Supervise homework.
- Participate in school activities.

Actual

- The skills deemed necessary to raise children well depend on the nature and complexity of the environmental and social demands to which both parents and children are exposed.
- Parents may require training to acquire some of the above skills so that they can be seen to be good enough parents on the terms of the dominant culture. Clear and achievable objectives are critical.
- Parents and children benefit from continuity of location and familiar people around them.
- Parents and children benefit from the acceptance of those of the dominant culture but it may not be critical to the quality of parenting.
- Some parents need more support from friends, family and statutory services than others in order to provide good enough parenting.
- Parental self-esteem is critical to how well they parent.
- Parents' own personal histories are significant in how well they are able to parent.

8   Drug addicted mothers

ADDICT LOSES TEENAGE CHILD

A girl aged 15 has been taken into care after she told her teachers that her mother was a heroin addict. The Berkshire teenager was taking part in a discussion at school about drugs when she staggered her friends and teachers by declaring that her mother was addicted.

She has now been removed from her home. . . . Her parents have not been allowed to see their daughter since she was removed. The mother's doctor said that the woman is a registered drug addict who has a loving relationship with the girl. . . . During the court hearing the mother was told that her daughter had been taken away on 'moral grounds and for her personal safety'.

(The Times 8/12/86)

This case followed hard on the heels of another addict mother losing her appeal to the Law Lords to have her baby returned. The baby had been born suffering from withdrawal symptoms and had been taken into care by the same local authority as the teenage girl reported above. The spokesperson for the Berkshire Social Services division insisted that there was no policy to require social workers to admit a child into care because of a parent's drug taking. The British Association of Social Workers also stated that 'In general we would advocate support through residential and family centres where mother and child could be offered a total care package'.

Many were none the less concerned that such widely publicised removals would reinforce 'the general view that illegal drug users are likely to be out of control of their lives and unfit to be parents'.

The National Local Council Forum on Drug Misuse and the Standing Conference on Drug Abuse issued a report to deal with these concerns, emphasising that drug addiction should never be a reason for legally removing a child from its mother and that parenthood is often an incentive for the drug abuser to reform.

Many people are scathingly dismissive about drug abusing parents' potential for reform. A consultant obstetrician I recently met described the behaviour of addict mothers as irresponsible and reprehensible. It is not difficult to see why, from his perspective. The job of an obstetrician is to help deliver a healthy baby, to save lives of the little ones born premature or ill through no fault of their parents. To see babies born ill through the 'deliberate' actions of their mothers, and to see many of these babies suffer and die is like a kick in the teeth. The fact that these babies often require extra treatment and the use of intensive care units may mean that other babies of 'blameless' parents cannot be treated. The strongest attack was on the fact that these mothers 'don't care'. Their situations are not pleasant to deal with and can make the professional with only a passing, albeit significant, involvement feel angry and helpless.

In spite of attempts to publicise the ill-effects of drug abuse it remains a widespread and ever-growing problem throughout the world, primarily amongst the poor. Surrounding the subject of drug abuse are a whole host of other issues about whether it should be decriminalised, whether drug abusers are simply law-breakers and should be punished or whether they are psychiatrically ill and need medical help.

Men and women who have been abusing drugs do not appear to provide the ideal start in life for their children. Their life-style is perceived as more likely to deviate from the norm of what is acceptable in terms of providing a safe and secure home, in terms of the care they take of themselves and in terms of the family and community support networks they have. In purely medical terms the list of likely problems in both a pregnant mother and her child does not engender optimism for the fitness of the woman as a parent – drug addiction often goes hand-in-hand with poor nutrition and general ill-health, with the danger of HIV and hepatitis all too close and sexually transmitted diseases common. Pregnant women who are drug abusers have a reputation for being unreliable attenders of antenatal appointments, whether because they 'don't care' or because they fear having their babies removed. In Britain at present there is no automatic registration of drug abusers – a doctor is not obliged to notify anyone if he knows a pregnant woman to be a drug addict. The rights of the foetus are not yet considered important enough to compromise the rights of the mother to confidential treatment. Once the baby is born the child has legal rights to protection which may override those rights of his mother to keep him – but by then it may be too late.

The experience of observing a tiny newborn infant suffering the withdrawal symptoms of his mother's drug abuse is a shocking sight. It is as if in the suffering of an innocent and helpless infant, all of society's problems are being reflected back at the observer. It makes us feel sick, and want retribution from the mother. This is an uncomfortable starting point for assessing fitness to parent.

Many professionals argue that addict mothers are too often and for too long given the benefit of the doubt – that the child's future is ransomed in the hope that the mother will shake off her habit and become an acceptable member of the community. They point to the large number of mothers who cannot face up to the void that opens up when they are not on drugs, the mothers who cannot be the good mothers that society wants them to be. No amount of sympathy for their predicament can guarantee a secure future for their children.

These are some of the ethical and emotional eddies that form the backdrop of society's view of drug addicted mothers. Drug addicted parents are deemed unsuitable material for adoption and for assisted reproduction treatment – but few addicts are likely to seek such services. Drug addiction would be a major black mark against anyone fighting for custody of children after the break-up of the parents' relationship. It is certainly a worrying factor in the minds of local authority officials concerned with protecting children. Some social services departments automatically put families known to be drug users on their observation lists. The expectation is that these families are at higher risk of requiring intervention.

As with many marginalised groups there are a number of presumptions that are made about drug abusing parents which need to be examined before any statement can be made to support or refute their fitness to be parents.

They should be punished for both breaking the law and endangering their children's future

In the USA a number of women have been prosecuted for damaging or causing the deaths of their babies through drug abuse during pregnancy. The public cry for blood is strong – a mother's love for her unborn child is seen to be the most sacred bond of all in society; people are horrified when the mother violates this; instead of consuming substances that, through the umbilical cord, are supposed to nurture the growing child, she poisons it instead. Surely, they argue, such women should be locked up and prevented from having the care of any child?

However, despite the fact that using certain drugs is illegal, the realisation was made some time ago that punishing the parents could be counterproductive to protecting their children and much more work has been concerned with understanding the factors that affect parenting ability of drug addicted adults. The American Medical Association recently addressed this issue in a report on legal intervention in pregnancy and identified female substance abusers as having 'high levels of depression, anxiety, sense of powerlessness and low levels of self esteem and self confidence' (Bertin 1993).

Such women do not sit down and think 'shall I protect my foetus or shall I have a good time?' – as is suggested by the moralistic outrage of many observers. Their choices and willpower are limited by their psychological and social needs as well as the physical addiction for the drug. The need for treatment rather than punishment is becoming clear.

This growing number of parents is slowly producing a less judgemental and more supportive approach to treatment and rehabilitation of drug addicts. In the USA and all around the UK, in every major city there exist special medical units to treat drug addicted parents although there are not nearly enough to cope with the demand. Residential units offer places for mothers and their babies together, as it was recognised that the high drop-out rate for mothers alone was because they could not face being cut off from their children. There was also the real risk that going into a residential programme would be seen as evidence that a mother could not take care of her children so they would be removed by the local authority.

Drug abusing parents are all the same

It is increasingly being recognised that the relationship between drug abuse and parenting abilities is complex – drug abuse by parents does not automatically indicate child neglect or abuse. A number of factors are involved and it is only by investigating these that fair assessments can be made. A group of social workers at drug dependency units argue that from their experience

> we consider that some drug misusing parents are good parents in all usual senses. The fact is difficult to accept. The implication of the acknowledgement that drug users can be good parents enables workers to discriminate on the criteria of good enough parenting.
>
> (Dubble *et al.* 1987)

This is an important point: unless society is prepared to acknowledge that drug addiction and good parenting are not mutually exclusive, there cannot be any progress in understanding exactly how to help children and parents. Dubble *et al.* (1987) have identified three patterns of drug abuse, each of which can have specific implications for childcare.

1 Regular and stable – drug use is predictable and sources are regular. (So how do children fit in?)
2 Chaotic – will take any kind of drug in any amount depending on availability, resulting in very erratic behaviour. (What happens to children when parents are on a binge?)
3 Crisis – the person's misuse of drugs is largely precipitated by major life crises. (Often a cry for short-term help.)

They would be better parents if they could give up drugs

It is often implied or made explicit that an addict's chances of retaining care of her child is dependent on agreeing to complete a supervised detoxification programme. Since drug misuse is seen as 'a symptom of, and a solution to, family processes', weaning women off drugs cannot be expected automatically to turn them into fit parents.

Dubble *et al.* (1987) also point out that the effects of withdrawal can have a severe effect on the capacity of parents to tolerate stress and anxiety: 'Some mothers who use amphetamines have told us that they feel livelier and therefore more playful and in tune with their children when using'. These perceptions may well be considered distorted but they clearly do affect attitudes to drug taking and to stopping. So there needs to be an assessment of whether the levels of care are different from when the parent is a non-user.

The addict parent cannot provide a secure home and the child is at risk of neglect

The pattern of drug use may affect the extent to which day-to-day household management is satisfactorily carried out. Activities associated with drug abuse such as prostitution may pose more of a danger to the child's security than the drug itself. To make a useful assessment it is important to separate out the home management from the drug use. Key questions that need to be addressed are, does the child's daily life revolve around the parents' drug use or are the parents ensuring the child's needs come first? Who else is involved in the household and childcare? Is there a drug-free partner or relative?

The addict parent's drug habit is posing a health risk to the child

The dangers during pregnancy of drugs such as heroin, cocaine and marijuana to the foetus have been well documented (e.g. impaired growth, increased risk of respiratory disorders, epilepsy). But all babies do not suffer the negative outcomes that the majority of published research suggests. Here again we need to question the nature of the research and researchers and the bias of those who publish research findings. Research which does not highlight adverse effects of drug use may be less likely to get an airing:

> Of 9 negative abstracts showing no adverse effect only 1 (11 per cent) was accepted, whereas 28 of the 49 positive abstracts were accepted (57 per cent). This difference is significant. Negative studies tended to verify cocaine use more often and to have more cocaine and control cases. This bias against the null hypothesis may lead to a distorted estimation of the teratogenic risk of cocaine.
>
> (Koren *et al.* 1989)

The authors of this study on the reproductive hazards of cocaine conclude that most 'negative studies were not rejected because of scientific flaws, but rather because of bias against their non-adverse message' (Bertin 1993).

Bertin also quotes research (Bingol *et al.* 1987) indicating that babies of middle-class alcoholic women do not display such negative outcomes as those of lower-class alcoholic women. This is revealing, in that it points to the inherent bias of most research into maternal substance abuse which starts with the belief that the substance abuse is the major problem.

> The impulse to control women's conduct to promote fetal and childhood health obscures critically important messages including the significance of socioeconomic factors such as parental education and the overriding importance of postnatal influences. Greater attention to such factors might fuel efforts to improve nutrition, education and economic conditions for infants and parents and would be a more effective way to promote fetal health and early childhood development.
>
> (Bertin 1993)

The health risks in childcare have been more anecdotal. Dubble *et al.* (1987) argue that 'It is important to get away from the narrow "if they leave their drugs around the child may use them" approach'.

The potential health risks may be a direct result of drug abuse, e.g. from used syringes, or indirect, e.g. through neglect of the child. Again it is only by studying the individual family that the real risks can be separated out from the imagined. It often becomes evident that socioeconomic factors are more significant than the drug abuse.

In this section it is worth noting that almost all the criticisms regarding drug addicted parents' health risk to their children is focused on women. Completely absent from the debate is any recognition of the possible effects of drug abuse on the quality of men's sperm, or on the quality of their parenting. Little research attention has focused on the role of men's behaviour in either neonatal outcome or parenting. Tantalising glimpses occasionally emerge – recent studies of children of men working at a nuclear reprocessing plant suggest that male genetic material may be altered by exposure to outside agents. A few other studies have noted the effects of alcohol in male reproduction but this has not received much attention.

> The selective concern about women's conduct is apparent in a [major US DHSS dietary guidelines] report's reference to a study on the effects of alcohol on lactation while omitting mention of a study by the same author reporting an association between fathers' preconception drinking and reduced birth weight.
>
> (Bertin 1993)

There is every reason to believe that, if it is the health of the foetus that society is concerned about, then the father's preconception behaviour may be as significant as that of the mother and worthy of more detailed research. Post-conception, the role of the father and/or other male members of the household are obviously also significant to the health of any babies and children living there. Does substance abuse affect their physical conduct towards the female members of the household and children? Their ability to give financial support and provide security? To provide guidance and good role models? Where is the professional evaluation of drug addicted fathers in their fitness as parents?

The company that a drug addicted mother keeps is unsuitable for a child and may endanger his safety

Again generalisations are unhelpful:

> We know of drug using communities where due to drug dealing, violence, criminality and the consequent acceptance of strangers, children were placed at unacceptable levels of risk, including sexual abuse.

> However health visitors have reported communities where drug taking was an acceptable fact of life. There were fundamental differences to the extent that mothers organised safe childcare arrangements among themselves and that drugdealing criminality and other possible drug related activities did not occur in the community and the presence of strangers was not encouraged.
>
> (Dubble *et al.* 1987)

There is no denying that using an illegal substance predisposes a mother to mixing with what is seen as the darker margins of acceptable society, but this does not necessarily mean that the child will too. Often it is the procurement of the drug that leads to prostitution and violence so, for example, the use of prescription methadone (a heroin substitute) may reduce many of the associated social dangers of drug abuse.

The parent, by participating in an illegal and antisocial activity, is setting a bad example to the child

This is difficult to refute – there is much evidence suggesting that addiction often goes on through generations. Common sense tells us that a child brought up in an environment where drugs are regularly used is more likely to try them himself. What this does not explain is why the need to self-abuse arose in the first place and what factors prevent some children in a family going on to become addicts themselves while others from the same family can remain free.

We also have to ask ourselves to what extent a moralistic approach helps solve the particular situation. Does it imply that all children of parents engaging in illegal/antisocial activities be removed? Clearly the state does not have the resources to do this and nor does it have the evidence that would justify such extreme measures.

The addict parent is incapable of putting her children's needs first

It may seem self-evident that a mother who is abusing drugs is putting her own needs before those of her child, but that does not mean she is incapable of doing so. According to a psychiatrist at the West Midlands Regional Addiction Unit (which offers drug dependents practical support throughout pregnancy, labour and afterwards),

> Drug abuse does not necessarily mean child abuse. We are interested in the mother's rights and to help her be with her child. Generally the drug dependent mother feels a great responsibility towards the child. It is not our intention to take the babies away: quite the opposite.
>
> (Catherine Steven, *Sunday Times* 15/3/87)

To help mothers take responsibility for their children's lives, he suggests they need to be helped to take responsibility for their own first, and this means building a trusting relationship with the mothers, finding out the cause of their drug abuse and tackling that problem. This can take months and sometimes years.

USEFUL POINTS TO EMERGE FROM THE EXPERIENCE OF DRUG ADDICTED MOTHERS

- The overall implications are that to carry out a fair and helpful assessment of parental fitness, a detailed approach is necessary. Drug abuse *per se* is not a justification for labelling a person as unfit to be a parent. The pattern of use, the perception by the parent of its use in relationship to the care of children are all significant factors in assessing fitness.

- Having children is often a major motivation for personal rehabilitation and society needs to support that wherever possible – for the well-being of the parents as well as of the children.

- It is worth noting that while I have focused on illegal drug use in this chapter, many of the same arguments apply to parents abusing legal substances such as alcohol and tobacco which are less socially disapproved of but may be just as dangerous to the child *in utero* and out. Despite the growing evidence for the adverse effects of smoking in pregnancy and the effects of passive smoking (creating respiratory problems and possibly later cancer), few professionals would seriously intervene to protect children of parents who smoke. Could it be that both smoking and drinking are common amongst the people from the professional classes who determine what is socially acceptable?

    The issue of how women conduct themselves in pregnancy is obviously a wider one – excessive dieting or strenuous exercise (the phenomenon of exercise addiction has been recognised) could be added to the list of activities that fit mothers should not undertake in pregnancy. But no one would think to legislate against those.

    It is clear that there are some behaviours which are more acceptable to those who determine social disapproval of parents than others. The sheer numbers of babies born to drug addicted mothers who will need expensive, long-term care points to the real concerns fuelling the bias against their mothers: the expense to the state and the perceived damage to society.

- It will also be noted from this chapter that addicted mothers are deemed more of a concern than fathers – the effects of substance abuse in pregnancy are partly responsible for this but it is also a reinforcement of the expectation that a mother's duty to care is more vital than that of a father. It is expected that the mother will be responsible for a child's health *in utero* and out, so if she is unfit to do this the child is at risk. As Bertin concludes,

    Social tolerance for the choices that men routinely make, even when they advance their own interests at the expense of their children or partners, reveals respect for male decision making and autonomy, even the right to make mistakes. Fathers can be human; mothers must be perfect.

    (Bertin 1993)

- Finally, this chapter shows how focusing attention on the victim of societal processes diverts attention from addressing those problems. Why people become addicted and unable to control their lives is the combination of personal and environmental factors which have disabled them. As the social and environmental demands of modern societies escalate, there will be an increasing number of people who cannot cope. Rather than penalising individuals, perhaps society needs to address the skills and resources that would enable people to feel a sense of control.

WHAT DOES THE ASSESSMENT OF ADDICT PARENTS TELLS US ABOUT FIT PARENTS?

Ideal

- A fit mother nurtures her baby in pregnancy by not engaging in any harmful activity and consuming only substances that will promote the baby's well-being.
- Fit parents have control over their behaviour.
- Fit parents lead morally virtuous lives.
- Fit parents do not expose their children to criminals and strangers.
- Fit parents are capable of putting their children's needs before their own.

Actual

- Addictive behaviour poses a threat to family life but does not rule out good enough parenting.
- People need more education about the effects of an unhealthy life-style on their children before they become parents.
- Parents may need expert treatment and support to enable them to become fit parents.
- Censure of unfit parents does not improve their chances of becoming fit parents.

9   Gay parents

While theorists debate the merits of marriage between gays, many are already living the settled-down life of their 'breeder' peers. That includes children – either through adoption, artificial insemination or arrangements between lesbians and gay 'uncles'. There are an estimated 3 million to 5 million lesbian and gay parents who have had children in the context of a heterosexual relationship. But in the San Francisco area alone, at least 1,000 children have been born to gay or lesbian couples in the last five years. A number of organisations have sprung up to meet their social needs. San Francisco boasts the Lesbian and Gay Parenting Group, storytelling hours for tots at gay bookstores and congregation Sha'ar Zahav, a largely gay synagogue with a Hebrew School for members' children.

(Salholz 1990)

We are a group of women who have chosen to live independently of men and who want to have children. We are going to do this by self-insemination to ensure that we have complete responsibility and control over our fertility. If you agree to be a donor, this would involve going to a pre-arranged venue at short notice. You would then be asked to ejaculate into a clean receptacle. That is all that would be required of you.

(Advertisement placed in *City Limits* London magazine)

In most western countries, the last three decades has seen a gradual emergence into public life of those who are gay or lesbian. There has been increasing tolerance of people who openly wear the badge of homosexuality, to the extent that most heterosexual people do not attempt to interfere as long as it does not encroach on their own lives – that is to say, as long as gay people are discreet and keep their sexuality a private matter. However, any suggestion of openly gay or lesbian adults as parents seems to produce a huge outcry – somehow, having children brings parents into a public arena where their personal lives can be justifiably criticised. All the age-old arguments come flying forth: homosexuality is sinful, perverted, unnatural.

In Britain, the conflicting attitudes of policy makers to homosexuality are reflected on the one hand in many local authority level initiatives to promote tolerance of homosexuality and, on the other, new central government legislation such as Section 28 of the 1988 Local Government Act which reinforced the message of the 1986 Education Act, making it illegal for local authorities to 'promote the teaching in any maintained school of the acceptability of homosexuality as a pretended family relationship'.

Serious problems face the thousands of gay teenagers in schools: 'frequently isolated, sometimes very confused, and . . . often subjected to appalling victimisation. Many young people have even attempted suicide' (report published by NUT, July 1991, quoted by Neil McKenna in the *Independent* 25/11/91).

That homophobic attitudes are allowed to go unchallenged at schools does not bode well for tolerant attitudes to emerge later in life. As Part I has shown, there is still a considerable amount of negative feeling towards gay people when it comes to assessing them as fit to be parents. During the 1980s a number of research projects published findings on lesbian women as mothers, but few people have addressed homosexual fathers as a group worthy of interest. Yet it is clear that men who are known to be gay are unlikely to get custody of their children after a divorce and are also likely to be regarded with grave suspicion if they seek to adopt or foster.

So let us look at what underlies the ambivalence that society feels towards gay parents and look at the extent to which it is justified.

Homosexuality is a psychiatric disorder and so the children will be at risk

A 1992 report from the Vatican stated that it was just to discriminate against homosexuals in the placement of children for adoption as 'homosexual orientation is an objective disorder'. Psychoanalytical theories of how sexuality is acquired long ago labelled homosexuality as a deviant psychiatric trait and, though this has since been discounted, the link has been maintained in the minds of many.

> The last time we tried [to adopt] we were interviewed by a psychiatrist, which at first we did not mind. I later found out that hetero-couples would not have had to undergo this interview. I was very angry.
>
> (Smart 1991)

Recent researchers have suggested that there may be a biological component to determining sexual orientation. There is no clear way of proving the psychoanalytical theories of how homosexuality is caused (e.g. failure to resolve the oedipal phase and thus over-identifying with the mother). Certainly the acquisition of sexual orientation is not clear-cut and until it is understood there is no basis on which to ascribe pathology.

We have to be aware that much of what we label psychiatrically deviant is culturally determined and that as soon as we attach the label 'psychiatric' we engender fear and hostility from those around the labelled person. The label in itself does not help us to understand homosexuality any more, nor does it have any therapeutic value – for example, it does not help 'cure' it. As recently as the 1950s, many homosexuals were subjected to psychiatric treatment to try and make them heterosexual, and many were forced into unhappy marriages so that they could appear 'normal' to society.

It's not what nature intended

Begetting children is at the centre of the family, since family life cannot continue without the begetting of children: and the child is, ipso facto, the harvest of the heterosexual union. That is the way the traditional moral philosophers of the Judeo-Christian ethic phrase it, and that is precisely how the general public wants to keep it; and why 'marriage', children and family will never be accorded to gays in a heterosexual society.

(Kenny 1990)

It has hitherto been impossible for a homosexual or lesbian couple to biologically produce a child themselves – without the intervention or assistance of another person. The sexual organs of a man are clearly designed to fulfil the biological function of reproduction through intercourse with a woman and vice versa. That is biology in purely evolutionary terms. It takes no account of human need for affection and self-fulfilment through relationships of types other than those designed for reproduction. Most heterosexuals do not have sex only to produce children and in western countries most adults do go to great lengths to prevent sex resulting in babies, so tampering with 'what nature intended'.

Furthermore, since nature cannot enable procreation within homosexual relationships the extrapolation is made that it is also unnatural to nurture, i.e. care for, children if you are gay. This argument is reinforced by pointing to the fact that the vast majority of the world's human population engages in heterosexual relations and, where parents live together, it is almost universally the mother and father. It is therefore inferred that this is the natural way of things: the majority do it, so it must be what children need.

A British emeritus professor of education recently argued for discrimination against gay and lesbian applicants for adoption and fostering on the basis that there exist enough 'appropriate' applicants amongst married couples and that when public decisions have to be made about finding substitute parents 'every effort needs to be made to go with the grain of nature' (Whitfield 1991).

However, on the basis that it goes against the grain of nature, people should not fly in aeroplanes, bottlefeed babies, or undertake a whole host of other activities. One of the reasons we indulge in so many unnatural activities in modern society is that we weigh up the pros and cons and decide on the merits of each. We do not watch a baby die of pneumonia because it would be unnatural to give her antibiotics. So invoking nature is an insufficient argument against gays and lesbians as parents. It is also difficult to justify on the grounds that only heterosexual relationships are normal:

Three royal marriages broken, possibly a fourth in trouble; one in three marriages ending in divorce, abortions, unwanted teenage pregnancies, wife bashing, baby bashing, sexual abuse of children by parents, the Director of Public Prosecutions found kerb crawling; prostitution and adultery.

This is the picture which constitutes heterosexuality, held up by churchmen and public moralists as 'normal', in contrast to homosexual love which is 'disordered', 'abnormal', 'immoral' and so on.

As a gay man who has lived for many years in a rich and fruitful loving relationship with a friend, with nothing to hold us together except a bond of love, I cannot help but look on at the 'normal' world with a certain wry amusement.

(Letter from R. Payne, *London Evening Standard* 23/3/91)

Children need a father and a mother as correct gender role models

For children to stand the best chance of thriving in our culture they need, ideally, to experience the unconditional love of a mother and father figure who are committed both to the child and to each other. In this way the youngster daily experiences role models from each gender, helping over a long period, often at the margins of awareness, to promote the emergence of a secure sexual identity.

(Whitfield 1991)

This summarises the commonly held view of how children develop their gender identity – ascribing it solely to the direct and ongoing influence of two opposite-sex parents.

This view leads to a number of fears about the influence of gay parents on children, in particular that the lack of an opposite-sex parent will result in effeminate boys and 'butch' girls.

Gender identity is the child's concept of himself or herself as male or female and tends to define the growing child's sex role behaviour which is what each society designates as appropriate for males and females in a particular culture. Some children consistently report that they would prefer to be a member of the opposite sex and show an overall pattern of opposite-sex behaviour (Golombok *et al.* 1983). Some later undergo sex change operations, many continue to hide their feelings, fearful of ridicule and recrimination. The societal taboos about observing the norms of sex role behaviour are still strong and so there is a fear of producing children with a gender identity that is different from their physical sex. Since the biological components of gender identity are still only poorly under-stood, the finger of blame is pointed at whoever has played the parental role.

A bi-gender model of family life has dominated our cultural expectations for several centuries, if not millennia. The norm that is upheld is the hunter-provider father and the child-nurturing mother. Despite the impact of feminist thought, the vast majority of people still accept this division of sex roles as natural, at least to some extent. It is argued, particularly by religious and political leaders, that for society to be stable and for children to grow up to fulfil society's expectations, they need to be imbued with socially correct gender behaviour from their upbringing. It is inferred from this that the gender role models have to come from a mother and father (no other close adults will do) living together, and, moreover, sharing a sexual relationship with each other.

The gay views on this are, first, who says the traditional gender division is so great that it has to be perpetuated – they put forward the argument that it can prevent men and women from being fully themselves – and second, even if we do accept the differences between genders for growing children, why do they have to come from a heterosexual mother and father living together and sharing the same bed? There is no reason why it may not come from close opposite-sex adult friends, for example. (It is commonly believed that homosexuals must hate members of the opposite sex but homosexuality is only evidence that they love members of their own sex, not that they hate the opposite sex.)

So what is the evidence to support or refute the parental influence on gender acquisition? In the early 1980s a number of studies in the USA and Britain attempted to compare and examine the sex role behaviour of children of lesbian mothers (Golombok *et al.* 1983; Hoeffer 1981) and found no particular differences or preponderance of children with confused gender identities. An examination of preferred toys, games, activities and friendships amongst children in lesbian households and single-parent households found no major differences in sex role behaviour for either boys or girls. In fact the researchers comment that such children are rather traditional in their preferences.

The research to date has its limitations in that it has not compared children born and brought up within gay households with those born and bred by heterosexual couples. The studies have looked only at children of lesbian women who were born to (and spent some of their childhood within) a heterosexual partnership and then suffered the break-up of that relationship and possible repartnering (Tasker and Golombok 1991). They therefore address the issue of whether the absence of a father figure has been significant to the behaviour of the children of lesbian mothers.

The lack of longitudinal research published on the long-term outcomes of children of gay parents is significant but all the short-term studies seem to show no signs for concern over confusion of gender identity and sex role behaviour. Parents do not appear to play as significant a role as is commonly held. Instead they suggest that gender identity has other more important influences: perhaps these are biological in origin or come from the wider society. (It is worth noting that many heterosexual parents who have had several same-sex siblings describe the huge variation of sex role behaviours – clearly the parental influence is not all-powerful.) As the children of the first openly gay generation of parents enter adulthood, more and more useful knowledge should emerge.

Children brought up in gay households will become confused about their own sexuality

There is a widespread fear of 'contamination' of children by gay adults. A prominent tabloid newspaper columnist recently said on television that he was disgusted by the fact that Judy Nelson (tennis star Martina Navratilova's ex-lover) allowed herself to be photographed with her two sons after a court case in which she successfully sued Ms Navratilova for alimony. He opined that she had no right to include her children in a lesbian domestic life and that they should remain with the father, her former husband.

No study has shown any connection between the sexual orientation of the parents and that of the children. The fear that homosexual parents will lead to homosexual children is clearly without much foundation: most homosexuals have heterosexual parents. Studies suggest that sexual orientation occurs at a very early age, so parents' homosexuality can be ruled out as an issue.

The impact of parents' sexuality is not clear. Studies have not examined the children born by AID or the variety of experiences of gay parent families – in particular, how the child finds out about his parent's sexual identity and his own origins. There is some suggestion that

> the mother's openness with her child and the extent to which she understands any difficulties which the child may have with her sexuality, for example, in presenting it to friends at school, are associated with a good parent–child relationship which provides a solid base for the child.
>
> (Pennington quoted in Tasker and Golombok 1991)

(This echoes the experience of children of parents from other socially 'deviant' groups – the quality of a relationship determines whether or not the 'deviancy' is a problem for the child.) What may be more significant to the child's welfare is that the parents are happy and have a close, satisfying relationship in their lives.

> I take the view that there are three main situations everyone must solve in life: the means of financial support; intimacy or sexual relationships; a social network and friends. If these are more or less solved it is possible to enjoy a normal existence. How we find solutions is up to us and in no way do the solutions bear on parenting skills. Our own experience proves that this is so.
>
> (Smart 1991)

Furthermore, as far as providing a good role model for sexuality, the quality of the sexual relationship between a child's parents may be more important than whether it is a homosexual or heterosexual one: 'A child might also learn a lot from lesbian parents. If their relationship demonstrates sensuality and loving exchange then the child will be picking up extremely important values' (Paul van Heewyck quoted by Liz Hunt and Jack O'Sullivan, *Independent* 13/3/91).

Children of gay parents will suffer from the stigma of having parents who are different

LESBIAN CASE BOY'S FUTURE SET FOR REVIEW

> The future of a 10 year old boy placed by a local authority in the care of his jailed mother's lesbian lover will be decided by a High Court judge. . . .

'The newspapers and the public were concerned about the principles on which the local authority had placed the boy with this woman' the judge said.

Although the local authority considered his future secure, stable and satisfactory 'there would now be a review'. The judge said that as a result of the press reports, the woman and the boy had been pestered by reporters.

(Independent 16/4/92)

This is a transparent example of stigmatisation changing the outcome of a gay parent–child relationship. Homosexual people like those with a disability are still seen as a pathological group who are shunned by society and thus many are forced to hide behind the cloak of secrecy. But having children does force parents into contact with many more people and so the impact of stigmatisation is potentially very significant.

In a recent custody case in which custody of a young girl was awarded to her mother, a rehearing was ordered to address specifically the relevance of the mother's lesbian relationship. The Official Solicitor sought advice from a psychiatrist who was asked to address, amongst others, the question of whether the child in a homosexual home would be likely to suffer taunting from his or her peers.

That was a possibility, but children can be discriminated against for all sorts of reasons, and it was a matter of how best to manage that. The mother (who together with the other adults involved had agreed to accept expert help in ways of explaining the situation to the child) would be the person best able to explain the situation, and other people's attitudes, and she would most easily be able to do this if she were caring for the child.

(C v. C (no. 2) Adoption & Fostering 1992 vol. 16, no. 2)

The longer that society treats homosexuality as abnormal and forces those who are gay and lesbian to hide their sexuality, the more ammunition this gives to those who wish to ostracise them, but it also may actively prevent good parenting.

- Enforced secrecy may mean that one partner's true role is disregarded by outsiders:

  Katyie and Barbara's main problems so far have revolved round the authorities' difficulties in recognising both women as Isaac's parents. 'When Isaac had to go to hospital, Barbara had to go home and I just stayed there. That was horrible because I couldn't get any support from Barbara'. Barbara was regarded as 'just a friend'.

  (Egerton 1990)

- Stigmatisation may hamper a gay person's own identity as a parent:

  Homosexual males who are fathers face a special set of problems in the area of self and social acceptance that is considerably more complex than that confronted by most homosexual males or by most fathers. The acquiring of both identity as a gay and an identity as a father involves an active process requiring conscious effort. Identity development occurs within a cultural and social milieu that, for most individuals, facilitates the process. This is not the case, however, for homosexual men, who are reared in a heterosexual social context that is laden with antihomosexuality. Homosexuals must rid themselves of society's heterosexual expectations, they must also overturn their own introjected negative stereotype of homosexuality.

(Bozett 1981)

Gay fathers have problems being accepted not only by the heterosexual world as parents, but also by the gay community for not being unattached and free of what are seen as heterosexual commitments: 'Many gay men are intolerant of children: having children is a status passage in the heterosexual world. In the homosexual world it is often a stigma' (Bozett 1981).

Bozett noted that gay fathers who were homosexually active before marriage reconciled their gay and father identities more readily than those who were not:

Gay fathers who first began to act on their homosexual desires after marriage had considerable difficulty resolving what initially appeared to them to be an irresolvable identity conflict. They perceived their gay identity as hopelessly incompatible with their fathering role. The result was serious role conflict and inner turmoil.

Resolution to this conflict involves 'coming out' and being accepted by intimates: 'Self acceptance as gay almost demands disclosure of the homosexual identity. Disclosure defines the self to others. It also helps to confirm one's identity to oneself.'

These observations of gay men as fathers have significant resonances with those of other stigmatised groups – in particular disabled parents. Being gay and a father, being disabled and a parent: both can seem like a contradiction in terms not just to outsiders but to many gay or disabled people – such is the extent that they have internalised society's negative social expectations of them. The problem of resolving this identity conflict is largely left to the individual but it may well be significant in affecting parenting capacity.

It has been suggested (Cosis Brown 1991) that potential homosexual adopters and foster carers should be assessed like all other applicants; additionally, however, assessors should explore how comfortable these adopters and carers are with their sexual orientation, what support or opposition there is from their own families, how they deal with homophobia and how they would deal with the possible stigmatisation of the children. Those who have resolved their identities and coped with the stigmatisation may be a particularly valuable resource:

Coping with stigma is often a strengthening, enriching process, as well as a harrowing one. We need to be recruiting people who have developed through their experiences, and not those who have been crushed by them.

(Cosis Brown 1991)

The notion that there may be a positive side to the stigmatisation coin is a promising one – a few other glimpses of this occasionally emerge:

A great deal of research into children of lesbian parents has focused on their similarity with other children in terms of gender role development, peer group popularity and social adjustment. While this research has been invaluable in the context of courtroom strategies in custody cases, its tendency to minimise the meaning of difference poorly equips children either to deal with oppression or to develop any pride in the specialness of their origins.

As Laura says, 'I've never felt the same as kids from traditional families. Ultimately, I think I have got an enormous strength out of being different. Discrimination teaches you some precious lessons. There are no perfect families of whatever composition. Lesbian mothers should not have to prove themselves to be better than any one else.'

(Egerton 1990)

Finally, as with disabled people, there is also a sense that having children is seen as a 'normalising' process which reassures others and can be a road out of isolation and in itself a step towards being integrated into a community:

One unexpected positive result of motherhood, with all its contradictions, is that I do feel generally more rooted in that I can now relate to a larger number of women and men who also carry the burden of child-rearing responsibilities. From those early days when I was feted with gifts and congratulations in the maternity ward, I realised that I was entering into a new relationship with the community. As I was waved down the hospital steps surrounded by friends and whisked away in a high status car to a champagne homecoming, I remember thinking that this is what it must be like to get married.

From being a single, childless lesbian in a position systematically marginalised by society, it seemed that I was suddenly being received everywhere by warm smiling faces.

(Walker 1992)

Children in gay households may be abused by their parents or parents' gay friends

Homosexuality is frequently linked in the public mind with promiscuity, rootlessness, selfishness and a whole host of other negative characteristics. The fear of sexual abuse is just an extension of this. This is a fear fuelled by ignorance and a general increased awareness of the extent of childhood abuse. In a review of the research to date on homosexual parents King and Pattison (1991) conclude:

Despite popular confusion between (particularly male) homosexuality and paedophilia there is no evidence for any connection between the two. Children are at just as much risk of sexual assault by a heterosexual parent or step parent as by a homosexual counterpart.

The fear of the sexuality of gay people is significant. It raises an interesting and more important issue of the extent to which sexual activity is seen to dominate a gay person's life above all other aspects of daily life. A solicitor who specialises in lesbian custody cases noted the prurient obsession in the courts with sex:

> I've never yet had a case where a lesbian mother hasn't been asked in detail about her sex life. She recalls questions like: 'Will you have sex in front of the children?' 'Do you make a noise when you have sex? Do you use appliances?' (The witness reportedly replied: 'We've got a Hoover.')
>
> (Reported by Helen Garlick, *Guardian* 5/12/90)

It is at least partly a problem of labelling someone on the basis of their sexuality – that label then comes to replace every other personality trait in the eyes of others. There probably are homosexuals (just as there are heterosexuals) for whom sexual activity is the most overwhelmingly important feature of their lives, but there is no reason to suppose that this is the case for all gay people.

> Another social worker, Jean, adds that once a couple admit they are gay or lesbian, questions of their lifestyle start to enter into the debate. 'We don't have that argument if we are talking about straight couples. We talk about whether they have good parenting skills.'
>
> (*Social Work Today* 18/8/86)

All gays and lesbians are the same

> Heterosexuals seem to hate, fear and be fascinated by homosexuality. Those feelings often lead to stereotypes and the inability to see the individual rather than the label.
>
> (Cosis Brown 1991)

It can be seen from this chapter that there is a tendency to treat all gay people as the same, irrespective of other aspects of their individual lives. This can obscure understanding of other issues in the lives of the families concerned.

> We should cease regarding lesbian households as all the same. Like heterosexual households they differ greatly. Perhaps it is the quality of the family relationships and the pattern of upbringing that matters for psychosexual development and not the sexual orientation of the mother.
>
> (Susan Golombok quoted by Adam Sage, *Independent on Sunday* 10/3/91)

Interesting work is gradually emerging as the first generation of children born to openly gay parents come into adulthood and can be asked to reflect on their childhood. What they highlight is the variety of experience.

USEFUL POINTS TO NOTE FROM THE EXPERIENCES OF GAY PARENTS

- Many similarities with other stigmatised groups.
- Stigmatisation may undermine parenting abilities.
- Dealing with stigmatisation can be a source of strength.

- Gender role expectations are powerful cultural controls on how we raise our children – gender identity is not solely the parents' influence.
- A close relationship with another adult, aside from the child's prime care-giver, may be what is important, rather than the sex of the second caretaker.
- The importance of the role of sexuality in parenting – both as it is perceived by society and in its effect on development of a sense of self. How we feel about ourselves physically and sexually is likely to have profound impli-cations for the development of children in our care. How children feel about themselves physically and sexually will also have implications for how they relate to others and society. This is all part of developing a good enough sense of self and helping this development is one of the major tasks for prospective carers (Cosis Brown 1992). For children who have been sexually abused, the quality of understanding, or for those who as adolescents are grappling with their sexual identities, the role of the carer's sexuality, may be particularly significant. Some gay parents may have particular advantages over hetero-sexual parents for individual children in these situations. Being treated as different means that many gay people have spent a lot more time than most thinking about the issues of sexuality in our society.

WHAT THE ASSESSMENT OF GAY PARENTS TELLS US ABOUT THE EXPECTATIONS OF FIT PARENTING

Ideal

- Parenthood is not a private activity but one which brings adults into the realm of society's arena.
- Should conform to the majority norm.
- Should be two parents of the opposite sex, providing clear gender role models and sharing the same bed.
- Should not draw undue attention to their sexuality but should behave in such a way as to ensure their children grow up heterosexual.
- Their pursuit of personal happiness should not be at the risk of endangering their children's need for parents who conform.

Actual

- The sexuality of the parents is not in itself relevant to whether children have a physically and emotionally healthy upbringing.
- The existence and nature of a sexual relationship between parents is not necessarily significant to the child–parent relationship.
- The quality of the parents' affective relationships are more important than the form of those relationships.
- While it is preferable that parents place a high priority on their children's needs these are not exclusive to considering their own needs for personal fulfilment in whatever sort of adult relationships they desire. Common sense

suggests that people who are contented in themselves are more likely to be able to be generous and supportive to others, particularly children.

- The social stigma attached to parents who are different from society's perceived norms is slowly waning as more and more different groups openly display their parenting styles.
- Parents need to be able to facilitate the development of a secure sexuality in their children whether they develop into hetero-, bi- or homosexual adults.

10 Teenage mothers

Teenage girls are more likely to become mothers than ever before, with one in 20 in some of Britain's towns and cities becoming pregnant this year. Conception rates among 14 year olds have risen nearly 50 per cent in a decade.

. . . Leading campaigners are to call for an inquiry. 'We are extremely concerned,' said Doreen Massey, director of the Family Planning Association. 'We would like an investigation, which we hope would lead to greater provision of sex education in schools and family planning services for young people'.

Typical of the teenage mothers is Daniella who was 14 when her first sexual relationship led to pregnancy. She had Chloe when she was 15. After the birth she suffered a year of depression, partly because the father had gone off with another girl, making her pregnant too.

Now 16 she lives with her baby in a home for young mothers. She loves Chloe, a blonde toddler with an appetite for dancing to acid house music. But if she had her time again she would not have a child so young: 'You've got the rest of your life to get pregnant'.

(Tim Rayment and Grace Bradberry, *Sunday Times* 5/1/92)

The age at which people should become first-time parents has traditionally been deemed by society to fall between 21 and around 35. Even today baby adoptions outside these ages are virtually impossible and the option of fertility treatment on the NHS remote. But things are changing: more and more people are becoming parents outside these margins and are forcing society to re-examine the arguments that had previously been used against them. Below the lower age margin teenage conception rates are on a steeply upward curve. In early 1992, the papers carried reports of the youngest known father in Britain – a thirteen year old who had impregnated a girl not much older than himself. Only a few weeks earlier the papers reported the case of a 50 year old woman who had just given birth to her first child as a result of private fertility treatment. These may be extremes but there is no doubt that more and more teenagers and more and more women over 36 are becoming first-time mothers. The two groups have been stigmatised for different reasons but both give interesting insights into why age has been seen to be significant in who is fit to be a parent.

Teenage mothers have been the subject of a considerable volume of research and attention. As soon as the rate of teenage pregnancy began to rise at the end of the 1960s, alarm bells started to ring for those concerned with the cost to the state of a growing body of expensive consumers of state resources. A veritable explosion of research into teenage pregnancy and motherhood was launched, apparently to try and understand better the problems such mothers and their children face but implicitly attempting to find ways in which to stop it – or at least prevent it from incurring cost to the state.

Unlike older mothers, teenage mothers are more likely to be from poorer backgrounds and to have lower educational attainment. This contrast is significant for a number of reasons and underlines the fact that those parents who are poorer and on state benefits are more subject to investigation than the professional classes.

In this chapter I will look at teenage mothers and the assumptions that underlie society's disapproval of them.

Teenagers should not be having sex

Teenage mothers are explicit evidence of the fact that teenagers do have sex. In Britain, and even more so in the USA, despite the prevalence of sexually explicit media images, there is still a widespread feeling that teenagers are too young to have sex but if they are then they should be discreet about it. This attitude leads to an ambivalence about providing information and ready access to contraception. The argument seems to be that since they should not have sex, they will not need sex education or contraception advice and, if you offer it, it will only encourage them to go off and try it out. Government policies reflect the lobbying of powerful religious groups who oppose sex education in schools. The fact that there is peer pressure to have sex and to emulate the adult behaviour that is so clearly on display all around them means that, in the West, many people's first experience of sex takes place during their teens. Since this is also a time of developing self-identity and emotional vulnerability, sex is often seen as a way of feeling wanted, loved, admired by one's peers (Allen-Meares 1991).

It may also be that the teenager is fully aware of what she feels and is making a responsible decision about her actions. Not all teenage pregnancy is thoughtless or careless. We should also remember that while we rightly identify teenagers as a vulnerable group in need of special care and attention, many adults over the age of 19 having sex are not emotionally mature, married or in good jobs. So the moralistic disapproval of teenage mothers is not a useful one in terms of assessing their fitness to be parents.

Teenagers are only children, so cannot take care of children themselves

Daniella's bedroom is a teenager's, decorated with posters of the supermodels; her routine is a parent's.

'It's made me grow up really quickly,' she said, as Chloe slid off to the kitchen with one foot in a plastic fish tank. 'I feel like I'm an old woman. I feel about 23.'

(Tim Rayment and Grace Bradberry, *Sunday Times* 5/1/92)

The teenage pregnancy rate for under-16s has risen steeply in the past decade. A teenager of 13 becoming pregnant is perhaps more obviously a child than a 17 year old and as such more obviously idealised as an innocent in need of protection – certainly not capable of caring for a child herself. For older teenagers this view is less clear-cut. To some extent there is an imposition of the adult view of children on teenagers – a view that adults can vary to suit themselves. Many people hire teenage babysitters or nannies to look after their children full time, so clearly age alone is not the main factor.

Underlying this objection is the feeling that teenagers should be kept in line by their parents and other adult authority figures, so their 'mistake' is seen as also the failure of those adults around them. This probably explains the fact that so many parents still disown their pregnant teenage daughters.

Once such girls become homeless their age plays a role in how the state responds to them. Over-16 year olds have to be accommodated by the local authority – perhaps in a hostel or bed and breakfast accommodation (which in itself is likely to be a less than ideal setting for fit parenting to develop). If the pregnant teenager is under 16 and homeless she is liable to be taken into care herself. (Under-16s are not entitled to benefit payments either.)

Teenage mothers are often criticised for deliberately becoming pregnant because they think it will be a short-cut to adulthood, to being recognised and respected by other adults and having a child of their own who will love them uncritically and give them a role in life. These childish fantasies of motherhood may seem naive and certainly need tempering with information about the reality of full-time motherhood, but it should be remembered that many adults over 20 harbour similar fantasies. Motherhood is seen in our society as an essential step to becoming a 'normal' adult woman. The social and cultural backdrop to teenagers' views of parenthood are increasingly confused – the prospects of secure employment or marriage are probably more distant for a 13 year old now than in the past with changing expectations of relationships, availability of affordable housing, media images of what life-styles are desirable, to name but a few elements which have undergone significant changes in the past three decades (Gelman 1990).

This raises the issue about what leads to emotional maturity: at what stage does a teenager stop being a child and become capable of taking a responsible decision about becoming a parent? How can society ensure that teenagers leave childhood with a sense of self-worth and understanding of themselves that prepares them to make the best decisions?

Babies should be planned

With the advent of medical forms of contraception and the contemporaneous growth of feminist thinking about women's right to control their childbearing, planned pregnancy has come to be seen as the responsible way to embark on motherhood. The fact that most teenage pregnancies are unplanned thus automatically relegates teenage mothers to a lower status as suitable parenting material (and also explains why older women – who are more likely to have carefully planned the commencement of their childbearing – are more highly regarded).

Teenage mothers are likely to be single, so they are depriving the child of a father

While teenage motherhood has been a common and acceptable feature throughout the centuries and remains so in many other parts of the world, it is the dramatic increase in the rate of single motherhood that has caused political concern in western countries. All the arguments against single parents (see Chapters 12 and 13) are applied to teenage mothers. Often the two terms are treated as synonymous, so it should be pointed out that a significant minority of teenage mothers are married or cohabiting with their partners.

Teenage mothers are unable to be economically self-reliant, so they are inflicting poverty on their children and becoming a burden to the state

That teenage mothers are predominantly dependent on state benefits is certainly the case. Even if the fathers are keen to be supportive they are less likely to be in adequately paid employment at this age. But it is important to look at other factors. For example, pregnancy often precipitates an end to formal education or becomes a barrier to training for employment.

As the stigma falls away there are occasional glimpses of how things might be. A recent newspaper report ('Three A-levels and a baby') featured a school whose headmistress had made a determined effort to support a pregnant teenager in completing her studies. As a result she has been able to plan out her life in terms of how her education and job will combine with bringing up her son.

> I've really got to plan things now, instead of just drifting along. Joshua made the exams much more important. If I'd been doing them just for myself I wouldn't have cared whether I failed, but I was doing them for him.
>
> (Reported by Celia Dodd, *Independent* 21/1/92)

The lack of affordable childcare means that women who become mothers in their teens are less likely to be able to become economically self-reliant. But it is also clear that many of the teenage girls are from a background that suggests they are likely to need state benefits, whether or not they become mothers. It is also important to note that poverty is not confined to teenage mothers: women over 20, whether single or married, often find that becoming mothers without access to jobs and childcare imposes a lower standard of living on them. So the underlying objection is not to teenage mothers *per se* but to the notion that anyone who is not economically independent should have the right to bear children.

Teenage mothers are less competent at parenting than older mothers; if they waited until they were over 19 they would make better mothers

At a recent London conference organised by the Trust for the Study of Adolescence, results of two separate long-term studies of teenage mothers were presented. Although they both found that poverty and housing were major concerns for the mothers, they also found that the majority were happy with their role as mothers and their children showed no differences in development to those of older mothers.

Ann Phoenix, a researcher at the Thomas Coram Research Unit of the University of London who conducted the survey, 'argues that the portrayal of teenage mothers as a distinct social problem may be due more to "moral panics" in society than to their parenting skills' (quoted by Judy Jones, *Independent* 12/5/92).

Her survey findings and the media reports that ensued are in sharp contrast to the prevailing assumptions about teenage mothers and their children. Over the past twenty years, studies have purported to prove that children of teenage mothers were socially, emotionally and intellectually more disadvantaged than those of older mothers; that teenage mothers were more authoritarian in their child-rearing style, less responsive and communicative, more likely to neglect their children and so on (Culp *et al.* 1991; Furstenberg *et al.* 1987).

Recently some of these research findings have been more closely re-examined and their validity questioned:

Studies which attempt to relate differences between mothers who are under 20 and other groups, whether other teenagers or older mothers, face the problem that maternal age is confounded with other psychological, social and economic factors which are likely to influence the results of any comparison. . . .

For example, from longitudinal study of all children born in a particular week in 1970 in the UK, Butler and colleagues (1981) have produced a report on the characteristics of mothers under 20 and their children. They report that these children are more likely to be of low birthweight, to suffer foetal distress and to be either premature or postmature. In their first 5 years they were about twice as likely to be admitted to hospital for an accident or gastroenteritis than older mothers' children and on verbal and non-verbal ability tests and parental questionnaires of behaviour problems they scored less well. However when account was taken of factors other than age, this picture changed. For example, when parity was taken into account (i.e. first born/second born etc.) there was no more likelihood of children of teenage mothers suffering foetal distress or being of low birthweight than children of older mothers. Where accidents were concerned, Taylor *et al.* (1983) report that the age of the mother was not the most significant factor, the number of children in the household was and several other factors apart from age were also highly correlated with rate of accidents. Wadsworth and colleagues (1984) found that the deficit in non-verbal test performance of children of mothers under 20 disappeared and the differences in verbal test performance and behaviour questionnaire results were reduced if social disadvantage and parity were taken into account. Broman (1981) analysed longitudinal data from the national Collaborative Perinatal Project conducted in the USA. He found that differences in intellectual performance up to 7 years between children of younger and older mothers were largely accounted for by differences in socio-economic status, ethnicity and birth order. Similarly, Belmont *et al.* (1981) using data from several national studies in the USA found that the differences between the children of teenage and older mothers, in intellectual performance over the age range 6 to 17 years were explained more appropriately by factors other than maternal age.

(Melhuish and Phoenix 1988)

I have quoted this at such length because it very precisely illustrates the care that has to be taken in drawing conclusions from research based on subjective premises. The stigmatisation that results from negative findings has a detrimental effect on teenage mothers which adds to other problems that they may have.

It is also being increasingly recognised that simply deferring parenthood until beyond the age of 19 would not necessarily improve many women's socio-economic circumstances or mothering abilities. Pre-existing differences in women's backgrounds may play a more significant role in their mothering at whatever age it takes place. Certainly the evidence for poor mothering is not conclusively linked to young age.

Having a baby while in your teens spells long-term disaster for the child and for the mother

Teenage mothers have been regularly blamed for producing delinquents and social misfits and daughters who will themselves become young mothers and perpetuate the cycle of disadvantage. Most of the research purporting to prove this focused on the mother and child in the child's first years and noted that there were often problems for adolescent mothers in adjusting to parenthood and inferred negative long-term outcomes. However, as Furstenburg states,

A full and fair assessment requires a further examination of adolescent mothers in later life. Unfortunately very few studies have followed up teenage mothers long enough to observe changes in the adaptation to early child-bearing over the life course.

(Furstenberg *et al.* 1987)

This plea for longitudinal research which embraces the diversity of outcomes is one which we will see recurring in other chapters.

More recently, a number of workers have started to question the notion of teenage mothers as a social problem, pointing to the large numbers who do manage well. Increasingly, there are reports which highlight the fact that the majority of teenage mothers and their children do not show the disastrous negative outcomes that have been so widely publicised.

Teenage mothers are all the same

Treating mothers under 20 as a single group in research studies implies a degree of homogeneity which is not appropriate, and in fact hides an enormous degree of variability. Women included in such a category differ in colour, ethnicity, household composition, employment and educational histories as well as marital status. In addition, the age range covered by the term teenage mother (13 to 19) is a period of life when there is tremendous change taking place at a psychological and social level.

. . . . It would be more productive to use the variability within the group of mothers under 20 to gain a better understanding of the range and operation of potent factors in their lives.

(Melhuish and Phoenix 1988)

This then is the crux of the matter. It is not the age of the individual but the many aspects of her background and the environment in which a woman becomes a mother that are critical to the outcome for herself and her children and which need further study.

WHAT ASSESSMENT OF TEENAGE MOTHERS TELLS US ABOUT FIT PARENTS

Ideal

- Twenty years old is the minimum age for becoming a mother.
- People need to be emotionally mature before becoming parents.
- People need to be financially secure before becoming parents.
- Conception of children should follow marriage and a period of setting up home.
- People need to be in a secure long-term relationship before becoming parents.
- People need to have established a home before they become pregnant.
- Parenthood should be a carefully exercised choice, not an accident.

Actual

- Age itself does not determine the success of the parenting.
- Parents' emotional maturity and financial security are desirable but cannot be guaranteed at any age.

- There is a need to temper the myths of romance and parenthood with information about the reality of adult relationships and parenthood.
- Support networks can make a big difference to the success of a parent, whatever the age.
- The complexity of the physical and social environment demands the acquisition of certain skills before parenting can be good enough.

11 Older mothers

TEST TUBE ROW AS MOTHER, 50, HAS BABY BOY

The controversy within the medical profession over infertility treatment for older women deepened today after it was revealed that a patient of 50 gave birth to a boy last year and another is expecting her first baby in June.

. . . Dr Abdalla refused to give any information about the women, except that both are 'English and middle-class' and were 49 when they became pregnant.

. . . 'You have to consider each case on its merits. It's not only a medical question but a moral and social problem.'

But some doctors are worried that ethical considerations are being neglected. Dr Gerald Swyer, a pioneer of IVF treatment, said 'It's very worrying. The obvious problem is that of very aged parents – when the child is 10 they will be 60.'

(Martin Delgado, *London Evening Standard* 9/3/92)

Having children in later life is regarded as inappropriate and often provokes hostility – if you are a woman. More and more women are putting off childbearing until their thirties – and then sometimes discovering that it takes longer to become pregnant. Men and women are also likely to have children later as a result of changing relationships: the breakdown of one followed perhaps by a gap before another stable relationship is formed can add several years to the time a person first becomes a parent. Once they become pregnant, older women and their babies are labelled as a high risk and subject to more medical intervention and supervision than younger mothers, with more likelihood of being offered abortions.

Prior to the 1920s there was little stigma attached to having children later in adult life – there were probably many 50 year olds caring for young offspring. Most women continued their childbearing for as long as they were fertile because lack of effective contraception gave married women little alternative. The development and social acceptance of modern contraceptive methods and the increase in medical involvement in obstetric care has shifted attitudes towards older mothers. Doctors started recording the ill health and complications they observed in older mothers and their newborn babies and advised smaller, planned families. The motivation was to relieve older women of the burden of continued childbearing and the poverty of large families.

Other events played a part – two world wars encouraged women to enter the workforce and enforced delayed childbearing on the many women whose husbands did return. The phenomenon of older women having their first babies in their thirties and forties took place under the supervision of the newly vigilant medical profession of post-war Britain. The term 'elderly primigravidae' was coined by two American obstetricians (Waters and Wager 1950) to describe women over the age of 35 in their first pregnancies who they found to have more complicated pregnancies and more problems with their newborn. The elderly primigravida went down in the medical textbooks as in need of extra supervision. The 1950s saw a setback for the emancipation of women – they were encouraged to return to domestic lives and to leave the jobs for the men who had returned from the war. The proper way then for women to do things was to marry and have children young and to devote their whole life to home and family. Thus the medical and social changes conspired to stigmatise older mothers.

However, in most parts of the western world, the birth rate for women over 35 has been steadily increasing in the last two decades and breaking down some of the barriers of prejudice. The age which is regarded as old is steadily being pushed upward. The well-publicised reports of a few technology-assisted, post-menopausal women giving birth (currently the oldest reported is a 62 year old Italian woman) have provided us with a real opportunity to think hard about what the rights and wrongs might be for older women as mothers.

As more and more women do have babies later in life and as the need for substitute parents for the growing number of older children also means that more older parents are becoming valued, a body of research questioning the risks and objections has slowly started to emerge, mostly from North America where the trend was noticed earlier than in the UK. It is still a tiny amount compared with teenage mothers but significant none the less.

Menopausal women should not be having sex

A number of women felt that their teenage children would feel embarrassed by an obvious sign of their parents' sexual activity.

(Berryman and Windridge 1991)

Since many children are brought up by their grandmothers and many foster mothers are older women, age alone is clearly not the only objectionable factor to older women caring for children. Sexuality and fertility are closely entwined in the minds of most and the stories of women over 40 having babies has brought out into the open the sexuality of older women. There has never been any serious objection to older fathers – siring children into their seventies, men receive nothing but admiring compliments for having maintained their virility – but there is often an underlying disapproval of the sexuality of older women. Older women are supposed to take on the role of benign grandmother figures who knit socks and organise church fetes. In fact some (male) pioneers of treatments designed to reverse the menopause argue that all they are doing is redressing the inherently sexist inequality of natural design.

Older women have more medical complications in pregnancy and labour

This has been the underlying objection to older women as mothers since the 1950s. The list of complications varies according to different sources – hypertension in pregnancy (toxaemia), placental complications, premature labour, prolonged labour, delivery by Caesarean section, perinatal mortality, maternal mortality, neonatal mortality, low Apgar scores, low birthweight and so on. With a list this long it is no wonder that most doctors regard any pregnant woman over 40 as a walking obstetric hazard!

But how valid are these concerns about older mothers? Mansfield (1988) reviewed 104 studies which purported to show the medical risks facing older women and their babies and concluded that most of the studies were methodologically flawed and therefore their findings were of questionable value. Others have suggested that, because of better diet and general health, the findings of studies in the past cannot be applied to women today.

Berkowitz *et al.*, in a study of urban middle-class college-educated women, compared older first-time pregnant women with younger first-time pregnant women and found that some increase in complications during pregnancy was apparent but most could be managed well by current medical practice. Their study failed to confirm any increased risk to the neonatal outcome. As for Caesarean section rates, while they confirmed that this was higher among older women there did not seem to be any single medical explanation, and they wondered whether it might be a case of over-cautious obstetric care, or as Berryman quotes obstetrician Wendy Savage, 'if you're surrounded by people who don't expect your body to work, it won't!'.

Certainly it seems that as older motherhood becomes more socially acceptable, the medical community is changing its message to approving older motherhood – but only under strict medical supervision.

They will be guilty of producing deformed babies

The evidence which suggests that the risk of genetic abnormalities and neonatal complications increases with maternal age places a great burden of responsibility on the mother. As women are held more and more responsible for planning their fertility it follows that women over 35 choosing to become pregnant or to continue with an unplanned pregnancy must be taking an irresponsible risk with the well-being of their unborn babies. The growing availability of a whole host of medical screen- ing procedures and abortions doubles the pressure on women to produce perfect babies or not at all.

There are two counter arguments:

1 The medical argument, which is now refuting the over-alarmist predictions about risks of deformity and also offering reassurance in the form of medical expertise in 'dealing with deformity'. The probabilities for genetic abnormality are thought not to be so weighted against older mothers as was previously believed. Greater medical supervision and intervention both inside and outside the womb is also thought to be able to minimise the risks of handicap to the child and increasingly women are taking up the option to abort foetuses identified as deformed.

> Teratologist Robert L. Brent has written that: 'Nature does eliminate most abnormal embryos spontaneously and it is very likely that by the year 2000, biomedical science will have available electronic, biochemical, and genetic techniques to evaluate the status of every embryo at very early stages of gestation.' In other words, Solomon might have had it much easier with his moral decision making. What wisdom will help us evaluate who is to be born and who aborted?
>
> (Carey 1991)

2 The humanitarian argument, which says having babies who are born with a deformity should not be seen as such a failure. Unfortunately the stigma attached to physical difference combined with the pressure on women to produce perfect babies creates unrealistic and hostile perspectives of normality. There is also sometimes the sense that if nature were allowed to take its course, some babies with very severe problems would die *in utero* or soon after birth. But the availability of medical techniques means that doctors may fight for the life of a baby but once that life has been saved, the parents are left with little support to handle the ensuing problems that may accompany looking after a child with a deformity or disability – for both are isolating and problematic in our society.

Many parents do develop rewarding relationships with their children and are able to say honestly, 'we are glad that our child is as he is – we would not want him to be any different'. Their commonest regret is not for their children's difference so much as for the lack of appropriate facilities and understanding which would permit those children to fulfil their potential and participate on equal terms with the rest of society.

Older mothers cannot cope with the physical demands of child-rearing

There is a commonly held feeling that older people do not have the stamina to cope with caring for children. Tiredness is an omnipresent feature of child-rearing for the majority of western parents young or old, and certainly there does not seem to be any substantial evidence to suggest that mothers over 40 suffer more.

> I have enormous stamina. I have had dozens of tests that show I am perfectly healthy. My mother lived until she was 86 and I expect to live at least until the

child is 20. I have a guardian for the child should I fall ill or die. I passionately want it. This child would be surrounded by love – from me and my friends.

(A 56 year old woman seeking fertility treatment abroad after being turned down by British clinics quoted by Lorraine Fraser, *Mail on Sunday* 5/7/92)

While stamina and fitness may generally decline with advancing age, there is no accounting for individual variation. There is also the trend of people remaining fitter for longer as they have become more conscious about exercise and diet. There are many 40 year olds who are as fit as many 25 year olds, so age in itself is not an indicator of fitness and stamina.

In adoption, where older age is often regarded as significant, it is interesting to note the ambiguities:

One of my colleagues described to me the doubts expressed by one local authority panel about the capability of a 50 year old wife to care for a nine year old boy, although this woman had her own 12 year old, and regularly child-minded pre-school children during the assessment period. Although parenting experience is highly valued people are somehow supposed to have gained it without aging too much in the process.

(Caine 1990)

Many people who choose parenting in middle or older age are likely to have spent more time considering their fitness and general health – they may be self-selected in that only those who feel they are fit actually go ahead. Many have already had children and have learnt how to organise life and pace themselves so as to make better use of their energy resources.

The age gap is unfair to children

Hasn't a baby a right to a mother of a reasonable age?

(Katherine Whitehorn, *Observer* 16/8//92)

Critics often argue that children will suffer the stigma of having a granny-like figure at the school gate – but this is not necessarily a major problem as more and more older women do become mothers. There is of course no law which says children have any right to youthful-looking parents. Others contend that if the generation gap is so much greater it will cause problems of lack of under-standing, but this depends so much on the individuals concerned.

Finally, it is suggested that it is unfair that the parents have less of a lifespan left to devote to children. This may undoubtedly be a concern for parents over 50 but it has to be remembered that no one can guarantee they will live to see their children grow into adults or not become in need of care themselves. Older mothers are less likely to have the support of their own parents to help with the care of the children, and the children may be less likely to know their grandparents.

Older mothers will find it more difficult to adjust to their role

For those who have their first child in later life, some may feel less prepared to allow their lives to revolve around the demands of children. But there are others who feel that they have more patience as well as greater maturity, stability and financial security:

> 'I'd have probably strangled him when I was younger, as I've grown older I've mellowed.'
> 'The child isn't going to come between us and break us up, now.'
> 'You're earning decent money, you're well on the way to paying for the house and therefore you're better off and can give the child more.'
>
> (Caine 1990)

For those parents for whom it is not a first child, they may be better adjusted already to the role, having seen the progress of their other children. There is a small but growing body of research which suggests that older women may in fact be 'better' mothers than younger women because they are likely to have more confidence in themselves and to choose more willingly to have children when circumstances feel right to them; they are more likely to have a partner, more information and experience from having seen contemporaries becoming parents, and more likely to be relaxed about parenthood because they have done other things already. There are some suggestions that children are actually at an advantage with older mothers (e.g. better intellectual development of the children and more responsiveness to their babies' cues). Certainly older parents are more likely to have material, domestic and educational circumstances which enable good enough child-rearing as perceived by the professionals.

They're all selfish professional women who carefully plan babies around career moves

COUPLES DELAY FAMILY LIFE TO BOOST CAREERS
FERTILITY RATE SOARS AMONG WOMEN AGED OVER 30

The change is seen as largely the result of highly educated women, whose husbands or partners are professional men on high salaries, delaying child-bearing.

> (*The Times* Population Trends, 67, 18/3/92)

Underlying the career woman stereotype is the criticism that older mothers are more selfish and have children to suit their own whims. While the career woman stereotype may be more accurate for older mothers in the USA, it seems to paint an incomplete picture of older mothers in the UK. Berryman and Windridge's survey (1991) found that many of the older mothers already had children and found that planned motherhood was a myth for this age group. Women who volunteered to participate in her research were not predominantly professional women whose career was particularly important to them at the time they became mothers and half of the pregnancies were unplanned. This surprising fact may at least partly be explained by the misleading popular belief that fertility declines with age – perhaps not so for women who have already had children.

But certainly the subject is one that is frequently associated with professional women and as such receives a lot of media coverage – they are after all the wealthier consumers that newspapers and commercial television companies want to target. This attention focuses on the first-time mothers having their babies late in their professional lives and on the whole promoting the 'Having it all' philosophy of the successful late-twentieth-century woman: successful job, successful partner, successful pregnancies and successful juggling of the ensuing home and work life. Every other newspaper seems to carry regular profiles of celebrities and journalists describing the joys of late motherhood.

Many older first-time mothers come from affluent sections of the population and many will have careers and professional jobs – this includes many of the professions hitherto involved in assessment. Their age and status mean that they are likely to be better informed about pregnancy and childcare and more assertive in their dealings with professionals. (Many of the improvements in maternity services have been brought about by the campaigning of such mothers.)

Thus their voice is being heard and their experiences of parenthood are being witnessed by all those who have previously sought to criticise older parents. The result appears to be little official cause for concern. The overall picture is that it has become socially acceptable to start having children later in life and, as older parents do not generally become an added cost to the state, there is minimal research or attention devoted to them. If the number of post-menopausal women having babies escalates, I suspect we will see a flurry of research into *their* pregnancy and parenting behaviours and outcomes.

WHAT ASSESSMENT OF OLDER MOTHERS TELLS US ABOUT FIT PARENTS

Ideal

- Mothers should have their children before the age of 36.
- Mothers are responsible for producing healthy babies.
- Parents should be young enough to be able to cope with the physical demands of child-rearing and old enough to understand the responsibility it entails.

Actual

- There is a balance to be struck between the ideal time in terms of physical fitness and the ideal time as far as emotional and economic readiness is concerned.
- There are no guarantees in life; disability and illness may affect children whatever the age of the mother.

- Self-confidence and a sense of control over one's own life are important aspects of good parenting – thus the more experience one has, the more capable one is of making choices about parenthood and to deal with the ups and down of family life.
- There is no right time to have a child but if someone believes they have made the choice at the right time it is more likely to be so.
- Parents have different qualities to offer at different stages of their own lives.

12 Single mothers

SINGLE PARENTS 'CRIPPLE LIVES'.

(© The Telegraph plc, London 2/8/91)

We must face the truth about these tragic children.
One parent families bring misery for parents, young people. . . and society.

(*Daily Mail* 2/8/91)

The above article was accompanied by a photograph *posed by models*, of a well-dressed mother in a booklined room sitting with her daughter, both looking wistfully into the distance. Its message was clear: even well-heeled single mothers are pitiable and undesirable parents. Single parents are selfish, immoral scroungers off the welfare state whose children are deprived and destined to a life of disadvantage. However, what was once viewed as a morally reprehensible aberration of a particular subculture is now increasingly becoming commonplace in western societies throughout all classes.

Since the 1970s the number of single-parent families has more than doubled (Population Trends 67 1992), bringing widespread consternation. The reasons for this rise is the high break-up of relationships combined with the falling social stigma of lone parenting. But the causes behind the high break-up of relationships are in themselves more complex. For example, there are now far greater expectations of relationships to be personally fulfilling, there is more acceptance of sex outside of marriage, the availability of contraception gives perhaps a false sense of control, more social mobility and personal isolation reduce the effects of stigma as a means for social control but also as a source of support for troubled relationships, the influence of religious codes on family life is falling away, and more pressures on individuals as consumers and workers has led to a confusion about the relative importance of marriage and children.

The vast majority (about 90 per cent) of single-parent families are headed by women, so the focus of the criticisms of single parents has been on single mothers. Lone fathers have been less scrutinised but I will consider them separately in Chapter 13.

Single mothers are all the same

The assumption as with the other groups is that all single mothers share the same essential characteristics which are responsible for the problems they cause to society and to their children. But single mothers come in many different forms. Old, young, rich, poor, happy to be single, depressed to be single, in supportive communities or isolated, temporarily single or long-term single. Their children may or may not have some sort of relationship with the man who is their biological father. The only thing they all have in common is an absence of an ongoing partnership with another adult in the household where the children are being raised.

How society regards single parents depends on how much they can be held responsible for having brought about this generally undesirable deviancy from the two-parent norm. A small proportion are single parents because of the death of the spouse. These people seem to be above disapproval because they can in no way be seen as having chosen their single-parenthood status. Their position is regrettable but could not have been avoided, so society tolerates it as long as such parents behave appropriately (e.g. widows should not invite new lovers into the home too soon).

The largest group of single parents are those who care for the children born of an adult relationship that has broken up. Society is ambivalent about this group. There is a considerable lobby that believes such parents have only themselves to blame for either getting pregnant outside a stable relationship or not enduring an unsatisfactory relationship 'for the sake of the children'. Those holding this view disapprove of the burden these parents become for society and generally predict doom and gloom for their children – pointing out the greater number of such children offending and going into care. The opposing lobby counters that freedom of the individual is paramount, particularly for women to escape unhappy relationships. They also argue that all the evidence suggests that an unhappy home resulting from warring partners is more detrimental to a child's well-being than a happy home run by one parent alone. The result of the ambivalence is a general feeling that such single parenthood is a regrettable but unavoidable feature of modern society.

Finally, there is a tiny but increasing group of women who are choosing to become single parents, perhaps through fertility treatment or adoption or through sexual intercourse with men with whom they never intend to have ongoing relationships. These are the women who cause sections of society to throw up their hands in horror mainly because they are seen as deliberately imposing single parenthood on their children. They are entering a situation which is avoidable and therefore, the argument goes, should be avoided. Ironically it is precisely this group that is also pioneering a different way of looking at single parents as better than 'second-best', perhaps even better than the reality of many two-parent families. Some argue that their children have not had to suffer the trauma of divorce or bereavement, that their children were planned and wanted and so are unlikely to be disadvantaged.

Single women should not be having sex

This may seem outdated given the sexual norms of modern western society, but there is still an underlying objection to women having sex outside marriage, and having babies outside marriage is an obvious reminder of the fact that sex has taken place. There is no doubt that the stigma against single mothers is shifting but it does still exist and there is a tendency to label single mothers as, at worst, promiscuous or, at best, careless. It is interesting to note that the moral outrage is directed almost entirely at women, not at the men who impregnated them, or whose adultery led to the break-up of a family.

Women should be having sex to be fit mothers

OUTLAW VIRGIN BIRTHS SAY MPs

Outraged MPs today demanded action to halt virgin births after it was revealed that a woman who has never had sex is undergoing artificial insemination.
(David Shaw and Tim Barlass, *London Evening Standard* 11/3/91)

This example of the spate of headlines over the so-called virgin births is interesting in that it highlights the expectation that parents are supposed to be having an ongoing sexual relationship with each other in order to be fit parents, yet no one asks most couples about the state of their sexual relationship because a pregnancy makes it self-evident that sex has taken place at least once. It raises all sorts of issues about what role the adults' sexual relationship plays in parenting and what form it needs to take in order to fulfil society's expectations.

Various (male) psychoanalysts were asked for their opinions as a result of this publicity and came up with a range of opinions:

A good sex life bonds the parents. They will get a lot of pleasure from it and it makes for a stable home. If they are not enjoying themselves, the sexual energies are still there. They are just not getting discharged to earth. That means the parents are far more likely to get into an overbearing relationship with their children. In extreme cases, that can take the form of overt incest, but in lesser cases, where for example, the mother is sexually dissatisfied with the father, she is likely to have too intense a relationship with a son, clinging to him too tightly.
(Robin Skynner quoted by Liz Hunt and Jack O'Sullivan,
Independent 13/3/91)

Homespun hogwash or clinically proven wisdom? These sorts of assertions are untestable but are given authority by the status of the professionals who utter them. A female research psychotherapist disagreed:

'I heard one psychologist refer to these women as borderline psychotic because of their decision not to have sex with a man. That is outrageous.' She argues that it is a mistake to always associate sexuality with genital sex.

'Human beings express their sexuality in many different ways'. . . she also contends that choosing virginity is often a valid criticism of many heterosexual relationships which end in divorce.

(Quoted by Liz Hunt and Jack O'Sullivan, *Independent* 13/3/91)

It may be that some, perhaps many, women do not attach as much significance to genital sex as do most men so that the decision to have a child by artificial insemination is less shocking to them than to outside observers. Certainly it seems that the official view is becoming less disapproving:

The range of a woman's sexual experience does not affect her ability to be a good parent, according to the British Pregnancy Advisory Service, though whether she is in a relationship naturally affects the baby's upbringing.

(Quoted by Judy Sadgrove, *Guardian* 13/6/91)

Again we note that a man's sexual proclivities are not under scrutiny – he can be as promiscuous or as monastic as he chooses.

Choosing to become a lone parent is selfish

ARCHBISHOP CONDEMNS 'SELFISH' SINGLE MOTHERS

The Archbishop of York launched an attack yesterday on women who choose to be single parents. Dr John Hapgood insisted: 'Every child needs a man about the house.' He said the targets of his criticism ranged 'from naive young girls who think that by becoming pregnant they can gain some significance for themselves and perhaps even get on the housing list, to self sufficient career women who want babies but not men.' They were 'playing truant' from the challenging relationships which give children vital role models.

'A child wanted because the parent wants someone to love, wanted as an act of defiance, wanted in extreme cases as a kind of accessory, has to carry too much of the emotional burden of its parent's needs.'

(Joanna Walters and Jo Haynes, *Daily Mail* 1/12/90)

This type of article regularly features in the Press, the spokespeople for these views usually being politicians or church leaders. What is interesting is that they all treat such parents as errant children themselves and limit their criticisms to a group which is unlikely to be their main constituency – i.e. 'safe' targets. There seems to be no room for promoting tolerance or trying to understand underlying causes that may be the responsibility of the wider community. (For example, it could be argued that better and more widespread sex education for children might engender a more 'responsible' attitude to parenthood, yet both right-wing political parties and the Church have been reluctant to promote these.) As well as the articles criticising 'selfish' single parents there has been a steady stream of articles on the problems of all single-parent families who are seen as a burden on the state and whose children are portrayed as doomed to social and academic failure.

Slowly, the voice of the 'selfish' single parents is being heard. It is only a whisper so far but it is interesting to note the publication of such books as *Alone Together* (Morris 1992) and occasional articles:

IF COUPLES CAN BE SELFISH, WHY CAN'T I

I tried long and hard to analyze why having children alone often led to the accusation of selfishness, while having them as a couple did not. Were there any unselfish reasons for having children? The human race is not in jeopardy, I did not already have a child who would benefit from having a sibling, I could not know I would produce a child who would find the cure for cancer. It seems to me that having children is always selfish.

(C. Abbott in the *Independent* 12/5/92)

A young male psychiatrist once told me that a child needs two parents. He seemed to have an irrationally fixed idea about the quantity rather than the quality of parenting. If I believed that the traditional family of mum, dad and 1.8 children was the only guaranteed recipe for success, then I would have to admit that I had been selfish in deciding to have a child on my own. But this so obviously is not the truth that there is no case to answer. Who are the people who call single women who choose to parent selfish? Certainly none of my friends, colleagues or acquaintances, all of whom say admiringly that they don't think they could take on the hard work involved.

(Walker 1992)

Single parents are treating children as commodities

God instituted the family when he created Adam and Eve and told them to go forth and multiply. The decision to bring children into this world by artificial insemination is a dangerous road to travel – and gives further sanction to the ideal of the 'fatherless' family. Children aren't toys to be bought just because an individual desires them.

(Marcia Dixon in *The Voice* 19/3/91)

The notion that children should be a gift that only the normal married couple deserve to receive is a widespread one. While the fear of children being treated as consumer goods may be a justifiable one, it should be remembered that society does not vet the motives of those couples who want children and who have their own 'production lines'. On the contrary, we encourage all parents to consider parenting as a consumer exercise, e.g. assessing the financial implications of having a child and to some extent its cost-effectiveness as far as giving up one's salary, school fees, etc. This sort of equation determines the size of most people's families in the West. It is therefore not such a surprising extrapolation for some parents to want a child as they would want a pet. Rather than disapprove of single parents for wanting a child, perhaps we should be encouraging all would-be parents to think more carefully about the responsibilities and realities of bringing up children.

Why does anyone want children? The notion of choice needs to be understood in the context of the external factors that are at play. The desire to have children is a complex mixture of internal expectations and external pressures. There is undoubtedly a prevalent and potent family ideal which appears to promise security, status and normality in an increasing unstable and unpredictable world but also a desire to care for and nurture a new human being. While most people seek to emulate the ideal in partnership with another adult, where that is not possible or desired many are prepared to accept the nearest version. The criticism that children are not consumer goods and should not be treated as such by would-be parents is easy to express but difficult to counter in western societies which are increasingly about 'what you own', not 'who you are'.

For single women who become pregnant, the 'choice' they have made may represent their immaturity and selfishness. It may also be a response to deliberately defining a future for themselves when no other seems attractive or possible. In a society that is increasingly fragmented and in which expectations of individual happiness are so high, forging permanent relationships is difficult. The taboos have gone – it no longer carries the social stigma of thirty years ago. If a boy gets a girl pregnant, he is no longer expected to do the 'honourable' thing and marry her – in fact, even if he wants to, she may refuse, preferring to bring up the child without the encumbrance of a relationship she does not want. If there is little prospect of finding a suitable, unattached and willing partner with whom to travel the conventional road to parenthood, it is not surprising that the urge to procreate will sometimes be channelled instead into single parenthood.

Children need fathers to develop normally

A foster placement panel in which I was involved 10 years ago looked at a report on a prospective single carer. This was still uncharted territory. The lines were drawn between those who felt individuals had to be assessed on their own merits and those who felt children should only be placed in normal two parent families. Both sides were searching for theories to back their positions. One participant intervened: 'what about the oedipal complex, how could there possibly be a healthy resolution of the oedipal phase?' The intervention was successful. We didn't know. No-one challenged this intervention as being outside the capabilities and expertise of those present. We were just silent.

(Cosis Brown 1992)

The question is really 'what is it that a man is supposed to be providing and how many are actually doing so in dual-parent families?' Much of late twentieth-century analysis of how children develop has been based on the notion that boys imitate their fathers and so grow up to be normal males and girls imitate their mothers in order to learn to be normal women. Without any formal testing, this assumption was held to be the truth and is still widely regarded as such – perhaps because it seems to fit in with what most people would expect. The presence of a father and mother has thus been considered essential to healthy psychosexual development and the absence of a same-sex role model is seen as risking future deviancy. As we have seen in the research with lesbian mothers, it is only since the prevalence of single-parent households has become more widespread that scientists have actually tried to test this assumption. The research that has subsequently taken place with children in single-parent homes has failed to show any such deviancy or confusion over sex roles (e.g. there is no increased effeminacy in boys raised by single mothers) (Golombok *et al.* 1983; Schaffer 1990), so we need to address what else it is that two parents are supposed to be providing.

The Archbishop of York's assertion that every family needs a man about the house suggests that the man should be doing more than coming home to eat, watch television and read the newspaper before going to bed. The following criteria seem to be the common expectations of the traditional father:

- Provide the family name and status.
- Protect the family unit.
- Provide leadership for the family.
- Provide the income to support the household and keep it from becoming dependent on the state.
- Discipline the children.
- Support the mother in child-rearing activities.
- Support the mother in domestic chores and home maintenance.

When considering the fitness of single mothers it is interesting to consider how many of these roles modern men actually fulfil and how many could be done by people other than the father.

There is no doubt that women are increasingly taking on the roles held by men in the past (e.g. earning income) but there is less evidence that men are taking significantly more interest in child-rearing and household chores (Henwood *et al.* 1987).

That two parents are prerequisites as healthy role models suggests that the relationship between them is also an important one. Indeed, that children should be the fruit of such a lifelong union underlies most religious teaching on who is fit to be a parent. As parents we are expected to provide a desirable model for our children's future relationships: to show affection and support towards each other, and to work together as a team to run the family unit within the wider community.

The argument cannot be refuted: if all that society wants future generations to aim for is dual-parent families, it has to argue that present parents must set the correct example. Scientific evidence cannot be invoked but it is common knowledge that the presence of two parents does not guarantee that they will have a loving or secure relationship worthy of emulation. It should also be remembered that even in two-parent households it is often only one parent who does most of the caring of the children – either because of the father's employment or because of the poor relationship between parents. In particular it is the women who are deliberately becoming single and without the break-up of a prior relationship to deal with are proving that single parenthood does not lead to social or emotional disadvantage any more than do two-parent families.

Defining single mothers in terms of their lack of a male partner obscures the actual number of care-givers with whom the child may or may not have a relationship, e.g. grandmothers, aunts, childminders, etc. Observation of a wide variety of family set-ups demonstrates that what children ideally need are a number of interested and committed adults who provide love, care and support. The success of a single parent is largely affected by the same sorts of factors as other parents, e.g. what other support she has available both in terms of childcare and for herself.

Children of single-parent households are more likely than those of two-parent households to become delinquents, to go into care, to do poorly in academic and professional terms

> Peter Dawson, general secretary of the Professional Association of Teachers, told his annual conference that it was 'a matter of fact' that children from single parents families were more likely to do badly at school . . . more likely to be poorly fed and clothed, ill-treated at home, and to get into trouble with the law.
>
> (Donald MacLeod, *Independent* 12/8/91)

This sort of argument is what philosophers call 'the fallacy of the excluded middle' (e.g. The Dutch have a queen, I have a queen, therefore I am a Dutchman):

> Some children are deprived.
> Some children who are deprived come from single-parent households.
> Therefore all single-parent households result in deprived children.

The mistake is to confuse correlation with cause. These correlations have long been recognised and cited as evidence of the undesirability of single parenthood.

> Boys can generally only be civilised by firm and caring fathers. The banishment of the father means that boys take their values from their aggressive and often brutal peer groups and are prepared for a life of violent crime, of football hooliganism, mugging and inner city revolt.
>
> (R. Boyson quoted by David Hencke, *Guardian* 10/10/86)

The socialisation and disciplining role of fathers appears to underlie most of the concerns about their absence. Yet how many modern fathers fulfil that role – how many of them can fit in much firm and caring modelling after long hours at work away from the home? And even if they are present is it really true that it is fathers rather than mothers who provide the discipline required?

Is it even true that only boys from single-parent homes fail in school, turn to crime or football hooliganism? It is too easy to exploit people's fears and turn a particular group into monsters. Many young men who commit crimes are from single-parent homes but their proportions are often in line with what would be expected, given the demographic make-up of a particular area. But more significant is what has led to their delinquency. Is it the mere absence of the father?

Or is it their socioeconomic status which gives them little sense of self-worth in society? Or is it the effects of the parents' unsatisfactory relationship prior to the father's departure? Or the fact that their fathers have disappeared out of their lives leaving them feeling rejected and confused? Certainly the evidence emerging from longitudinal and comparative studies suggests that these might be the real answers (Berman and Pedersen 1987).

Nearly half of all absent fathers whose children live alone with their mothers have lost contact with the family. Recent moves to force all fathers to pay more towards their children's maintenance will not lead to greater involvement with their children. All the evidence from children of divorced parents suggests that what children want and need is ongoing and stable relationships with adults whom they have known as parents. However, for those who have never had such a relationship with a father, the long-term effects are not self-evident at all.

There has been no research that has proved that single parenthood of itself causes such negative outcomes. There are certain factors more commonly associated with single parenthood than dual parenthood which are the more likely culprits: poverty, poor accommodation, more likelihood of domestic impermanency, poor support networks and so on. But all these factors would not automatically be put right simply by having a second parent living with the family unit. The welfare of the child is more at risk in a single-parent household: if the parent dies or becomes incapacitated the child is at greater risk of losing his security than if he had two parents but this again points to the fragility of family units with little external support.

If a single parent is materially self-sufficient, well supported and committed to the welfare of the child, is there any reason to believe that the child will be disadvantaged? Will the new breed of 'selfish' career women who chose to become single parents and raise the child with the assistance of a nanny or relative, show up the real differences? Increasing numbers of children of single parents are speaking up for themselves and refuting the assumption of disadvantage. More detailed studies of their experiences are also emerging.

A number of longitudinal studies of very large numbers of children have found that when socioeconomic status is taken into account there is no indication of lower IQ in father-absent children (Berman and Pedersen 1987). By focusing on father absence as the cause of delinquency and poor school achievement we obscure some real and important concerns about what parents and children actually need and the role that society at large plays in ensuring that these needs are met. We perpetuate the unfounded belief that fathers alone are responsible for socialising their children and ignore the role that children's inherent temperament plays in eliciting certain responses from those around them and also the significance of the role that other societal influences play, such as school, television and peers. And as far as research into fathers is concerned it has until quite recently been focused purely in terms of what men do not do by being absent rather than what they do when they are present and how. Fathers have thus remained as rather two-dimensional cutouts, invisible as long as they provide financial support and keep their children in check.

Single-parent families cannot be financially self-sufficient

There exist many single mothers who are not dependent on the state for their income, many of whom are determined and able to combine work with bringing up their children.

However, for a large majority of single-parent families, most of whom are headed by lone mothers, poverty is a very major factor in their lives. Some have chosen to fund their child-rearing through state benefits as a political statement against male domination and unequal distribution of opportunities and wealth but most have found themselves forced into dependency on the state. The absence of affordable childcare and availability of flexible and well-paid employment relegates many single mothers to a lifetime of poverty with all its repercussions on self-esteem and material deprivation and low social status. But they are not alone in these needs – mothers of every type share them, so it is wrong to single out lone mothers as somehow guilty of self-inflicted poverty. Again the presence of a father would not necessarily solve their economic problems.

The child will face social stigma

Me
Statistically, how unusual is it for a single person to apply to become a foster parent?

Social worker
Do you feel unusual?

Appreciation of irony was not his strong point either. I gave him a photograph of myself sunbathing in a bikini and looking extremely youthful to show to the foster child.

Me
And here's a picture of foster mother on her holiday.

Social worker
Oh, so you see yourself as a mother, do you?

. . . After we had discussed my personal relationships in some depth, he felt able to cope with my 'unconventional' lifestyle and we considered whether this might be a 'problem' for a foster child.

(Blunden 1988)

That single mothers are stigmatised is a common reason for withholding treatment for childlessness or acceptance of adoption applications, but few attempts seem to be made to evaluate how much of a stigma it actually is for the individual concerned. The stigma varies so much, depending on the circles one moves in, that it cannot be held as an absolute. With divorce rates being as high as they are and increasing, the numbers of children living in single-parent households for at least some of their childhood are about the same as those who will live in two-parent homes all their lives. The stigma is therefore not based on rarity or belonging to a minority. As with other groups the stigmatisation can itself be a source of anxiety: 'I felt under pressure to be an exemplary mother (a pressure I had not experienced within the respectability of a destructive marriage) and I knew our survival depended on it' (Morris 1992).

Another mother discovered the powerlessness that being scrutinised brought, whereas before her daughter had been born she

> would never have been scared of health and social services professionals, reacted with fear, when her health visitor accused her of ignoring her daughter's immunisation appointment. 'Instead of responding with all the middleclass outrage I could muster . . . I shuffled my feet and promised to go next week. I went . . . because I was scared they might take Ella away from me. The state terrified me and I wasn't used to feeling that scared . . . social workers, health workers were dangerous for the first time.
>
> (Eileen Phillips quoted in Morris 1992)

To counter the stigma, we need to know what it is about two-parent homes that enables some children to do well in life – is it really just having two parents and being in a family that is regarded as normal? Or, as is increasingly being suggested, is it to do with feeling secure, having good self-esteem, having stable emotional relationships and a stable home life with adequate material comforts? All of these things may be possible in a single-parent household.

USEFUL POINTS TO EMERGE FROM EXPERIENCES OF SINGLE MOTHERS

I have been interested to find that, as with other marginalised groups, as single mothers become more common and their own voices are heard, statutory bodies are beginning to accept their existence and there are even inklings of a recognition of the possible particular strengths that may make them superior to standard couples:

> Many of the older children to be placed had explicitly requested a single foster parent, to act as an adult 'friend', with no competition for attention from a spouse or partner. Increasingly, social workers are pleased to welcome the single applicant for another reason: there is likely to be no conflict between the foster parent's commitment to fostering and his or her other domestic responsibilities. The question of one person being asked to acquiesce in another person's decision cannot arise and the childless, single applicant is especially desired since the placement cannot break down because of difficulties between the natural and fostered child.
>
> (Blunden 1988)

One of the recurring problems that has been identified in this book has been the need for good support structures. It may be that single parents are actually pioneering a new approach to parenting which creates a more open family:

I know for Lucy and me, being a single parent family works well. My unusual circumstances have opened the door for many people to become closely involved, and I often think we are like a nineteen parent family. Everyone concerned feels they have been enriched by the experience, and we have never lost sight of the fact that the main thing about becoming a parent, under any circumstances, is that you get to give life to a new, unique and priceless human being. In a society which really valued young people, parents would not be relegated to the same status as pet owners, as we currently are, but would be given every assistance necessary to do a good job despite any unfavourable circumstances. Single parents would not be seen as deviants, failures or social problems, but as people to be cherished and supported as life givers, not resource takers.

(Mason 1992)

As with many of the previous groups, this is a reminder that the pioneers of new ways of living have much that is of value to offer the rest of society.

WHAT ASSESSMENT OF SINGLE PARENTS TELLS US ABOUT FIT PARENTS

Ideal

- Only two-parent families are normal.
- A child needs two parents living in the same house for correct role models.
- Parents should not treat children as consumer goods.
- Parents should put the security and future needs of their children before their own personal happiness.
- Children need two parents with clearly defined and complementary roles working in partnership. A father's role is to be the provider and protector to his children. A mother's role is to nurture and care for them. A father's arena is the outside world of work and politics, the mother's is the home and the daily activities of her children.

Actual

- It is not the quantity but the quality of parenting that is important to a child.
- Parents in difficult circumstances need support, not hostility to do their important job well.
- Parenting success depends on support networks and financial security.
- A parent's emotional well-being affects the child's emotional well-being – their needs are thus linked, not separate.
- Socioeconomic class affects the extent of stigmatisation of deviant parents by professionals.
- Single parents may be particularly suitable for certain children who need more undivided attention.

13 Lone fathers

HAVING A BABY WITHOUT A WOMAN

In Sweden of today where marriage is a fast disappearing institution and where women are shunning emotional commitment, there are a growing number of men like Jonas. Unable to find a woman to share their lives, they are experiencing a yearning that has traditionally been felt by single childless women: they ache for a baby. Jonas has found a solution. 'I have a friend who will bear my child for me'. The pair like and admire one another but they are absolutely not in love. They will not live together after the birth. . . .

Jonas easily imagines taking care of the baby on his own and he fantasises openly about being a father.'There is nothing better than holding a baby in your arms. That feeling beats everything. I have a dream that if I can have a little girl I would teach her swimming and then in the wintertime I'd teach her to ski. It would only be the two of us and I know already how happy I would be. I think it is OK to produce a baby this way.'

(Jessica Davies and Maria Scherer, *Daily Mail* 9/5/91)

In Sweden, men have been sharing the parenting role for long enough for society to find it acceptable that they should also wish to be fathers alone. But in Britain as in most countries, despite some shifts in attitudes to male/female roles, lone men are still at the margins of what is considered appropriate material for fit parenting and this has a direct effect on those lone fathers who do exist as well as on those lone men who want to become fathers.

The lone man is seen at best as incompetent in the home, at worst a sexual threat to his children. Physical care of a child, as opposed to just providing sperm, has never been seen as the *sine qua non* of fatherhood. Their biological role has been to inseminate as widely as possible and therefore the common perception is that they are only held in tow by the combined efforts of the mother of their children and societal pressure but, if they could follow their natural urge, they would pursue an unfettered and promiscuous wanderlust. Thus, unlike mothers, the biological and social roles have never automatically gone hand in hand. Few men have lone fatherhood thrust upon them (i.e. through being widowed or deserted by the mother) and traditionally, few have demanded more than nominal access. So when lone men ask to adopt or want to get custody of children they have sired, society regards them with a certain suspicion.

As with single women, lone men comprise a spectrum from those who actively seek lone parenthood to those who have lone parenthood thrust upon them unwillingly. The situation of each is a complex mixture of circumstances and expectations and cannot easily be generalised. Men tend to become lone parents only when there is no other choice available to the children, i.e. their mother dies, leaves home or becomes severely incapacitated through illness or disability. In the case of single men seeking to adopt, their chances are fairly minimal. Most agencies are conscious of the furore such placements attract and while they may use single men as a fostering resource for older boys for whom they have no alternatives, they are likely to avoid long-term placements. The main reasons are seen as prejudice against single men, problems of balancing work and childcare, and their sexuality (Caine 1990).

But the number of lone fathers raising their own children is increasing in many western countries. In the UK it is estimated that the numbers of lone father-headed households are in the order of 100,000 and in the USA nearly 1.5 million. Most of these become lone fathers after a divorce. In the USA, as increasingly in Britain, there has been a trend towards less gender-based court decisions and women are no longer as stigmatised if they do not remain their children's prime carer. More men have been getting involved in sharing childcare with their partners and so it does not seem as major a switch to become the main carer as it would have done thirty years ago. As their numbers increase, academics are turning the spotlight on to this new group of deviant parents to see how they are faring. Unlike most of the other groups so far considered, lone fathers tend not to become dependent on state welfare benefits so they are not subject to the same sort of scrutiny as lone mothers. The objections tend to focus more on the incongruity of 'men as mothers'.

It is not natural – men should be out in the world of work, creating the correct role model for their children of what it is to be male

The words of Sir George Baker, president of the Family Division of the High Court, were probably as close to the real state of the nation's thinking, when he said: 'There is I think in the minds of most people, something not very satisfactory in the idea of a young man giving up all to look after a baby.'

(Charles Langley, *Independent* 21/11/88)

The implication is that they are deviants from the accepted norm of maleness – and therefore unable to provide the 'right' role model to their children. It is a threatening thought to many that the hunter-gatherer is turning soft – who will be providing the macho men to populate the armies of the future if men start abandoning their aggressive, competitive roles honed in each other's company and turn instead to nappy changing, cooking and wiping fevered brows? There is no doubt that such a prospect shakes the foundations of so many deeply rooted attitudes – to male–female relationships, to work, to politics – that it is difficult to see the matter being resolved conclusively. In Sweden, the breakdown of traditional roles has brought confusion and disillusionment:

> We have forgotten how to be real men and real women. Of course it is good that women should have equal rights at work and that men are more involved with their children – but you have to know how to play the old fashioned male/female roles as well. Men here have become very soft, very feminine . . . they lack the sense of responsibility that a woman wants in a man.
>
> (Jessica Davis and Maria Scherer, *Daily Mail* 9/5/91)

Society needs to face up to whether its expectations of masculinity and femininity are outmoded and ask what sort of society it really needs in the future. Many suggest that the prospect of a world populated by caring, sharing men is a lot brighter than what we have at present.

> In the past, men who were sensitive and caring were seen as wet and wimpish, but as Jeffrey Richards, Professor of Cultural History at Lancaster University says: 'In the long run, if civilisation is to survive and violence is to be contained, it is the wimps and the wets who must inherit the earth.'
>
> (A. Katz in the *Independent* 29/4/92)

A father's role is to earn the family's upkeep

FATHER WINS FIGHT FOR MAINTENANCE

A father has won a six year battle to make his former common-law wife pay him maintenance for bringing up their son. Magistrates at Blackburn, Lancashire made legal history by ordering the mother of the ten year old boy to pay the father £15 a week. [The mother] a health visitor who now lives with another man on £907 a month take home pay with a low start mortgage in a detached house told the court she was old fashioned. 'I really don't feel a woman is in a position to pay. The man is the bread winner.' [The father] described the amount of the maintenance awarded as disgusting.

(*Guardian* 16/11/89)

As we have seen, men's role in western society is to earn money and their role as fathers is to provide income to support their family. If they do not do this they have failed as men. Just as with women trying to shake off restrictive predetermined societal roles, a small but increasing number of men are questioning this constraint which prevents them from defining themselves according to their own needs and aspirations. But if men do not go out to work they are in danger of becoming dependent on state benefits. If they pay for childcare while they work, it is argued that the children are at risk from lack of parental attention.

Many lone fathers, however, are better able to juggle work and childcare than their female counterparts and are less likely to become dependent on state benefits. This is because men can earn higher salaries than women (up to 30 per cent more) and the types of fathers who are awarded prime childcaring responsibilities tend to be better educated and higher wage earners (Greif 1992) than lone mothers. In studies, men have also been found to make more use of childcare support networks than women, e.g. using nurseries and childminders, parents of schoolfriends, grandmothers, etc. (Lamb 1986). This may be the result of the generally sympathetic view of them:

> Fathers felt that they were treated dichotomously – perceived on the one hand to be wonderful parents because they were male parenting alone, yet seen as being incompetent on the other. Despite this stress, like previous fathers studies, they were generally pleased with their parenting situation.
>
> (Greif 1992)

Their perceived incompetence may actually foster an indulgent and supportive attitude amongst the (mainly female) onlookers who can offer childcare.

As far as the state is concerned, the fact that lone fathers are not a major financial drain means that they are not seen as needing particular attention. The consequences for children are not really considered. Unlike fatherless families, motherless families are not seen as repositories of future delinquency – which suggests that it is not what mothers *do* that causes delinquency, but what fathers *do not do*.

Men pose a sexual threat to children

> The issues of sexuality, sexual activity and sexual orientation have been addressed in every case more explicitly than might have occurred with a single woman or a heterosexual couple. In two separate instances there was concern expressed by third parties during the assessment about the applicant's sexual activity. In one case a referee implied that the man has associations with local young men which might be of a sexual nature. The other man was the subject of a malicious allegation about his conduct with some children. This person cleared his name officially but felt he had been compromised and could no longer continue with his fostering plans.
>
> (Caine 1990)

We have already seen how allegations of sexual impropriety are used as a way of preventing access by fathers after parents have separated and for determining decisions about care of daughters and young children in particular. This is an underlying fear that society has of men as fathers involved in childcare. It is based on a widely held assumption that men are by their nature seething with barely controllable sexual urges which they will vent given any opportunity to satisfy their lust. It goes hand-in-hand with the deeply rooted belief in women as passive and self-sacrificing virgin mothers. It is a myth that has not been in the interests of men to debunk and perhaps women have been as responsible as men for encouraging it.

Much of the research into paedophilia has pointed to the fact that men who interfere sexually with children have themselves been interfered with and have not developed an understanding of the distinction between love and sex. Many claim that the children have seduced them and will go to great lengths to deny their coercion. Paedophiles exist and society demands that children be protected from them. They are however an example of a particular set of men with particular family histories – not of all men. One could argue that the more men that have experience of parenting, the more they will learn about other forms of relationship and the more they will pass on the nurturing aspect to their own sons. (A recent report has also uncovered the existence of female sexual abusers of children, which again undermines the case that only men are a sexual threat to children.)

The children of lone fathers will be stigmatised

That this expectation exists not just among lay people but amongst professionals such as teachers and social workers was powerfully demonstrated by a piece of research carried out by Fry and Eddington (1984). Three hundred professionals and three hundred lay people were each shown videotapes of four 10 year old boys in different day-to-day situations at home and school with other children. The viewers were divided into groups, each of which was told different stories about the children's backgrounds. One group was told that the boys came from two-parent families, another group that they were being looked after by divorced mothers alone, and the final group was informed that the boys were being looked after by divorced fathers alone. The viewers from each group were asked to judge the boys' behaviour.

The researchers found that viewers varied in their judgements of how well-adjusted the same set of boys were according to what they believed to be their family background: the boys thought to be from a two-parent family were believed to be the best adjusted, happiest and best at assuming responsibility, while boys from lone father-headed homes came out least well in these respects. They were also rated highest for delinquency, poorest in situations demanding obedience, the ability to cope with stress and cooperate with adults and other children. Same boys, completely different interpretations (Fry and Eddington 1984). The experiment highlighted the power of preconceived notions about the inherent disadvantages of lone-father families while at the same time suggesting that they were inappropriate. However, this stigma is dropping away as more men are seen to be sharing the childcaring role in two-parent households – it is not that easy to distinguish lone fathers at the school gates from other fathers who (because of unemployment or shift work or choice) are able to participate more fully in childcare.

Children need mothers

Until the 1970s men's role in childcare was seen as marginal. Society colluded with mothers to mock the competence of men in domestic or childcare tasks. It was seen as undesirable for a man to be doing such things – indicating effeminacy and lack of clear and distinct role models for the children. But times changed. As the feminist movement questioned the traditional roles, men were encouraged to become more sensitive and involved with their children. It has now not only become socially acceptable for men to share the care of children, it is something from which men can derive much kudos. Over the past few years women's magazines, baby goods catalogues and car commercials have increasingly focused on the man-with-cute-baby image to promote their products.

Child development experts now argue that what children need is 'mothering', and though women have traditionally been socialised to carry this out, men too can mother. So what is it that women provide that constitutes mothering?

A uterus – but surrogate mothers provide womb loans for infertile couples, so why not for single men?
Breastmilk – but babies can be, and frequently are, bottlefed.
Gentleness and selflessness – girls are undoubtedly more deliberately socialised to be gentle and selfless but the degree varies among women, and there are men who are capable of being gentle and selfless enough to care for children.

Mothering clearly also includes activities, knowledge and skills which it is taken for granted that a woman will learn as she grows up and then continue to learn on the job. Seeing how men are seen to struggle with or fall short of some of these qualities helps us to identify exactly what mothers are seen to do as parents.

- Provide continuity of nurturing relationship.
- Teach children social skills.
- Cook, clean and maintain day-to-day running of household.
- Deliver to and from school and monitor school activities.
- Organise children's social and leisure activities.
- Nurse children when ill.
- Shop for and clothe children.

It quickly becomes apparent that while the man's role is seen as being largely that of an outsider who provides income and status, the woman's is seen as arising from the intimate relationship she has with her children's lives and the home. It is thus more difficult for men to take over the 'absent' woman's role without a considerable shift from the norm of most men in society.

> Dealing with daily concerns of childhood, like establishing friendships, completing schoolwork, buying clothing, going through puberty and so on leave many fathers bewildered. They often have little knowledge about the range of behaviours that children may display. Other concerns may be loneliness, keeping the house clean and balancing work and childrearing.
>
> (Greif 1992)

It is assumed that women find these easier. There is undoubtedly a sense in which because society is geared up to expect women to be the prime carers and domestic controllers, women in this role are seen as less incongruent. They can thus seek information, advice and reassurance from a large number of sources without feeling that they will get labelled as incompetent or strange. Men on the other hand do not have as ready access to this congruence in their relationship with society. They may feel thus inhibited about participating in childcaring social events which are primarily populated by mothers such as parent–toddler groups. They may find other parents are reluctant to send their children to play with children without female supervision. Public facilities also marginalise lone fathers – a small example is the lack of nappy-changing facilities to be found outside of women's toilets. So, like many of the other marginalised groups they may miss out on the sources of support and information that other parents can and do take advantage of in their daily lives.

Most studies into how men care for children have been done with married fathers and compared their behaviour in contrast to their wives' – so men emerged as the providers of stimulation and rough play while mothers are essentially the care-givers. Less work has been done on how single men care for children. A recent study tested the hypothesis that 'single fathers will adopt parental behaviour that more closely resembles that of women who mother than that of married fathers', and found that the analysis confirmed this hypothesis and suggested that parenting behaviour is shaped not by biology and early socialisation experiences but rather by opportunities and access to social networks (Risman 1987, in Greif 1992).

Other studies suggest that men are no less able to do what has traditionally been regarded as mothering but that they may do so in different ways. This creates a problem if those that assess them are comparing them to traditional female ways of mothering (Hipgrave 1982). But as for the other deviant groups so far studied, there is a danger of expecting difference:

> Observational studies in the infancy and toddler period noted that although researchers often highlight the areas of difference between mothers and fathers, studies show many more variables on which a mother and a father do not differ significantly from one another. Moreover, although research of this nature focuses upon interesting central tendencies of behaviour, the results tend to draw attention away from the variability that different fathers show, the range of adaptations that exist within contemporary families.
>
> (Berman and Pedersen 1987)

It is tempting to suggest that the generally positive findings of the lone father by researchers is in part due to their sympathy for his predicament and a general personal desire among those researchers to encourage more egalitarian perspectives of gender roles. The findings are thus in keeping with trends in the social mores of the professional classes.

USEFUL POINTS TO NOTE FROM THE EXPERIENCES OF LONE FATHERS

- Men as well as women can take care of children – their success depends on their individual history and circumstances and on their financial security and support networks.

- Lone fathers are also opening up the boundaries around who can do childcare.
- There are many activities which if colonised by men, go up in status. Becoming a chef for example has more kudos than being a school cook. There is thus considerable hope that as men get more involved in daily childcare they will raise the status of parenting. Politics, transport, architecture, working patterns – all of which have largely been designed by men for other men – may finally start shifting to accommodate the reality of this breed of 'new men' and thus benefit all those involved in child-rearing.

WHAT ASSESSMENT OF LONE FATHERS TELLS US ABOUT FIT PARENTS

Ideal

- Only two-parent families are normal.
- A child needs two parents for correct role models.
- Children need two parents with clearly defined and complementary roles working in partnership. A father's role is to be the provider to and protector of his children. A mother's role is to nurture and care for them. A father's arena is the outside world of work and politics, the mother's is the home and the daily activities of her children.
- A father's role is to provide a role model as a worker and a warrior.

Actual

- Men's and women's roles are interchangeable.
- Men are as capable as women of nurturing children.
- Lone fathers resemble mothers more than they differ from them.
- Society needs carers as well as workers – more than it needs warriors.
- Men may have different styles of parenting to women but these need not be better or worse.
- Success depends on support networks and financial security.
- Stigmatisation depends on socioeconomic class.

14 Working mothers

MOTHER'S CHILDCARE 'UNSATISFACTORY' BECAUSE SHE WORKS

A judge has stirred up controversy over his refusal to certify as satisfactory a woman's arrangements for the care of her children on the sole ground that she is a working mother.

Judge Callman refused to grant a full certificate of satisfaction over the woman's childcare arrangements prior to her obtaining a decree nisi in her undefended divorce proceedings.

(Frances Gibb, *The Times* 13/3/89)

Employed mothers challenge some of the most fundamental beliefs about ideal family life: male–female gender role divisions, the exclusive and irreplaceable need of a child for its mother, the significance of childhood experiences to later life and so on. Science has been unable to come up with convincing arguments to keep mothers at home and financial necessity is increasingly dictating when women return to work after having children rather than whether they do so. Society remains ambivalent about whether it approves or disapproves. There is a general feeling that families should be financially self-reliant and if that means both parents, or a single parent alone, working, then so be it. But there are unresolved doubts about the effects on children – working mothers are blamed for neglecting their children, producing a generation of junk food and television addicts and delinquents, and for demoting the role of the housewife.

As with the previous chapters in this book it is interesting to note the difference between women and men in terms of labelling pathology: men are unfit if unemployed, women unfit if employed. (Unemployment benefit is only available to a father, not to a mother in a two-parent household.) Even when the working woman has a partner, she remains the one who is responsible for childcare arrangements both in practice and in the eyes of professionals and the state – women seeking adoption, prime care of children after divorce or fertility treatment are commonly expected to be stay-at-home women.

A BRIEF HISTORY OF WORKING MOTHERS

The beginning of the 'traditional' pattern of men going out to work to earn money and women running the home and raising children is ascribed in the West to the Industrial Revolution. Since that time many mothers have worked inside and outside the home but the real change we are witnessing over the past thirty years is the large-scale employment of middle-class mothers, increasingly those with very young children.

The state tends to oscillate in its support according to the needs for workers. During the Second World War while men went to fight, women were needed in the ammunition factories so nursery care was provided, the working woman was treated as a national heroine and no one worried about whether the children were being harmed by the daily separation. But with the men returning home in peacetime, the women's role was quickly redefined.

The 1950s witnessed a unique convergence of a number of new social, technological and scientific trends which combined to encourage women to stay at home and care for their children and their husbands. Post-war euphoria and the sense of optimism about British life raised the status of family life, and the emerging Freudian-based theories of childcare were used to promote the sanctity of the mother–child relationship alone responsible for a child's future well-being, not just physical but also psychological. In the 1950s there was considerable stigma attached to middle-class working mothers because it supposedly indicated the husband's inadequacy in providing for his family.

But in the 1960s mothers started to enter the workforce in greater numbers, and a new flurry of research began to study the possible effects this would have on the children. The research did not lead to any convincing reasons for keeping mothers at home and the emergence of the women's movement in the late 1960s made it more socially acceptable to acknowledge women's rights to 'equality' with their male peers.

Today, women are having children later into their childbearing years and have grown up expecting to be employed. Therefore many more will have worked and become accustomed to the financial and social gains that work brings prior to having children and wish to pursue these after their children are born. The statistics show that most will go back to part-time or full-time employment while the children are still young, increasingly while they are still babies. Whether or not the state actively supports her, the norm is no longer the mother who stays at home throughout her children's childhoods. Women show remarkable resourcefulness in creating the networks which enable them to work. Often it is the child's grandmother, aunt or neighbour who cares for the child while the mother works. It is rarely the father. Increasingly it is a succession of strangers who care for children in return for money and who will probably have no long-term relationship with the children after they stop being their paid carers.

The ambivalence towards working mothers highlights society's difficulties with handling two opposing ideologies: the need of the state to have economically productive citizens and the belief that children's needs are best served by their mothers. The fact that, throughout the western world, mothers are remaining in the workforce confirms that the ideology of economic independence is winning. As far as the state's needs are concerned, whether women are working for job satisfaction or personal development is irrelevant.

But there are also an increasing number who do have a choice, who weigh up the interests of their children with their own needs and choose to continue in or take up employment. As with chosen single parenthood, it is these mothers who have been accused of selfishness and irresponsibility. The role of their male partners' decisions to work after becoming fathers is never questioned. In fact, the only research into the role of employment in the parenting of men focuses on unemployment. Nowhere do researchers seem to be rushing to recognise the impact of high stress, business travel, long hours and the constant scramble up the career ladder on the ability of men to be involved in their children's upbringing.

Let's now look at the assumptions about working mothers and what these tell us about society's expectations of fit parents.

Working mothers are all the same

Researchers have seldom differentiated between motivations, yet these are crucial to understanding likely effects on parenting (Lamb 1982). Working mothers do not constitute a homogeneous group and will have different effects on family functioning and parenting according to their individual circumstances and motivations.

When working mothers are discussed it is rarely made clear whether the writer is talking about part-time or full-time employed mothers. Nor is there any mention of the type of work, its particular stress factors or rewards, or the sources of support to which they have access. There is also the assumption that working mothers have a choice about whether they go to work. The reality is that like men, most women work out of necessity as much as for potential personal satisfaction and social contact. Given the range of jobs and pay (UK: women's salaries are on average 75 per cent of men's salaries) the idea of the selfish career woman having a ball at work while her children suffer in a stranger's care is clearly a misleading view of the majority of working mothers. Many mothers who work do so under considerable stress of juggling their roles at home and work in order to best meet the needs of their children. For an increasing number of families, women are the only breadwinners (either because they are single mothers or because the father is unemployed). Despite the huge numbers of mothers in employment now, it is largely only the middle-class mothers whose experiences get regular publicity.

Working may be hazardous to the pregnant woman's foetus

A number of recent cases in the USA have highlighted discrimination against women in the workplace on the basis of their future possible childbearing. The justification has been foetal protection: that fertile women should not be working in hazardous environments as their employers do not wish to take responsibility for any possible defects that might result.

There is an implicit assumption that fetuses and children are best protected in a traditional setting with a stay at home mother. The picture is reminiscent of 19th century medical advice given to women that their 'natural' role was to be nurturing and unselfish, devote themselves to others, and eschew education and other forms of self-advancement . . . the risks to all workers, community residents, and consumers from the massive creation, use, transport, and disposal of toxic substances – are all obscured by the focus on the foetus, as if the problems would simply melt away if women didn't work.

(Bertin 1993)

There is an uneven assessment of risk when applied to working women – hazards such as toxic substances or radiation may be highlighted whereas others such as long hours, night shifts, heavy lifting, unhealthy atmosphere (e.g. infectious conditions in hospital wards or office smoking) are routinely ignored, even though they arguably affect more women.

Men's risks in the workplace in relation to their family responsibilities have not received such attention. At first glance this may seem justified – after all, it is women who have babies. But researchers have simply not devoted much attention to exploring the possible consequence of workplace hazards on men's reproductive health. One of the few exceptions is the association (identified by Gardner *et al.* 1990) between childhood cancers and paternal exposure to radiation at the Sellafield nuclear processing plant in Britain.

Men are regularly expected to take risks in the workplace which may affect their health but they are deemed capable of making the decisions for themselves. The stress at work for many fathers may significantly affect their future ability to provide for their children, and certainly the present quality of their parenting – but this does not stop employers hiring men and expecting them to comply with workplace requirements. Again the difference is clear: women's first duty is to care for their children and that means they should stay at home and nurture their babies and leave men to go out and take whatever risks they choose. They cannot be trusted to make the best decisions for their children, whereas men can.

However, many women do not have a choice about whether or not they work during pregnancy. Their economic survival (and perhaps that of the rest of their family) may depend on it. Often the hazardous workplace also offers better salary and benefits than other available employment. Women may thus decide to take the risk in the absence of good alternative choices.

In an important case relating to a major employer demanding medical confirmation of sterility in its female employees, the US Supreme Court recently upheld a woman's right to make her own decisions about the possible effects on the health of a potential or actual foetus:

It is no more appropriate for the courts than it is for individual employers to decide whether a woman's reproductive role is more important to herself and her family than her economic role.

(Bertin 1993)

The ruling was a reversal of the previous court decision in support of the employer's stance. The case received much publicity because, as a dissenting judge pointed out at the time, it could affect as many as twenty million jobs in the USA. He warned the employer not to assume 'that the interests of the next generation always trump the interests of living women and that the only acceptable level of risk is zero' (Easterbrook 1989).

This has so far been an important leitmotiv in my investigation of attitudes to assessment of mothers.

A child's needs are more important than a mother's needs

WOMEN'S EQUALITY 'HARMS' CHILDREN

Mothers who seek equality with men could be doing so at their children's expense, a leading social scientist claimed.

(Anthony Doran, *Daily Mail* 7/1/2/90)

Mothers who work are just selfish, says Paula Yates.

(Quoted by Edward Verity, *Daily Mail* 15/1/92)

These sorts of comments perhaps reflect more about the commentators' need to justify their own life-styles than they shed any useful light on how children's needs can best be met. They are rooted in the belief that only women have any responsibility towards their children's care. They mask a justifiable concern which is that, if two parents are in equally demanding jobs the chances of the children getting adequate attention are more precarious. This is a good argument for career breaks and more equitable sharing of childcare between men and women. Instead the arguments tend to go hand-in-hand with the following:

They would be better mothers if they stayed at home with the children

Simply being the woman who gave birth to a child is seen as the only qualification required to be the best carer for that child. This takes no note of previous life experiences or their motivation for becoming mothers and denies the importance of any other potential childcarer (e.g. the father). We cannot find direct answers to this by looking to social scientists. Most past research has been inadequate and again and again academic commentators (e.g. Lamb 1982) are reduced to suggesting common-sense but untestable propositions such as:

It seems unlikely that a child is materially better off with a dissatisfied full-time mother who would prefer to be working than with a part-time mother who is happy and fulfilled, assisted by a consistent, extrafamilial caretaker during working hours.

One of the secrets that has come out into the open with greater numbers of employed mothers is that many mothers do not enjoy being full-time carers of their children, nor do they feel that they alone are best equipped to do it well. Ann

Oakley's work (e.g. 1981) on the depression and frustration experienced by many mothers who do care for their own children at home should raise concerns about whether they can provide the best environment for growing children.

Clearly one of the benefits is seen to be more time and individual attention, but not all mothers at home can or do provide this so it cannot be assumed that merely remaining at home produces better parenting. (Some pieces of research have suggested that working mothers actually provide better parenting.) It is certainly the case that parenting style is independent of whether mothers work or not.

Separation from the mother will cause damage to a young child

In surveying the huge mountain of academic literature on this, one is left with an uncomfortable image of hundreds of moles determinedly burrowing down the same tunnel – how to demonstrate the effects on young children of their mothers' absence for a few hours each day. The research has not really been about the effects of employment on mothers' abilities to care adequately for their children – purely on whether her absence was detrimental. The popularity of nannies in wealthy households in the early part of the century suggests that the mere temporary daily absence of mothers would not be regarded as critical to a child's well-being, but it appears so.

To understand why this view arose and why it has so powerfully remained a part of popular belief, we need to look at the prevalent childcare philosophies that preceded the big surge in mothers' employment in the 1960s. The belief was launched by the rise of post-war psychoanalytical views of mothering – in particular the work of John Bowlby who asserted the need of a child under the age of 3 for 'a warm, intimate and continuous relationship with his mother' (Bowlby 1951). Bowlby's studies of children in institutional care were used as evidence to show that children suffered dreadful emotional deprivation if separated from mothers and that this could have lasting effects on their capacity to relate to others. The idea of 'maternal deprivation' thus entered the common vocabulary simultaneously with the idea that mothers were uniquely responsible for a child's future psychological well-being. It is this legacy that is still with us and which underlies the guilt that mothers who go out to work are supposed to feel.

This elevation of the importance of the mother to her children tied in well with the prevailing social and political attitudes of the 1950s. The views of Bowlby also tied in with what many middle-class mothers observed in their children's behaviour such as their preference to be with their mothers and their distress at their parting. (Since their previous experience was likely to have been of only having the exclusive care of their mother, the distress was hardly surprising.) Thus the desire to honour their responsibility to their children was easy to encourage.

However, as more mothers started to go out to work, they became the subject of research by psychoanalysts who naturally expected to see some disruption of the essential attachment bonds. In a large number of studies comparing children of mothers at home with children in out-of-home day care, there have been differences noted in some of the children's behaviour and interpretations made of the causes of these differences.

The chronicled correlates of extensive infant day care experience (i.e. avoidance, insecurity, aggression, noncompliance, withdrawal) have been found across a host of ecological niches and caregiving milieus . . . children of impoverished, middleclass, and upperclass families . . . children cared for in unstable family day care, high quality centres, and even in home, babysitter care . . . leads me to conclude that entry into care in the first year of life for 20 hours or more per week is a risk factor for the development of insecure attachment in infancy and heightened aggressiveness, noncompliance in preschool and early school years.

(Belsky 1988)

Critics have questioned the quality of the research and its ideological frameworks as well as the interpretation of the outcomes. Even if you accept the premises of attachment theory, the interpretation of the behaviours observed as being ascribable to day care *per se*, there is still a high proportion of children who do not seem to be adversely affected (50 per cent according to studies by Belsky). In fact the conclusion of most contemporary development experts is that present knowledge is insufficient for them to be able to advise on the matter of whether or not day care is harmful.

Saying we don't know is inconsistent with the developmentalists' desire to be authoritative and knowledgeable. But it removes a spurious aura of scientific credulity from the public policy debate concerning early day care and acknowledges other considerations that must legitimately play a role in this debate.

(Thompson 1988)

The mother–infant bond is uniquely important to the child's future well-being

Critics argue that while Bowlby's work was extremely valuable in identifying the need of very young children for continuity and stability from responsive and familiar care-givers, his mistake was to extrapolate from this and insist that mothers alone could fulfil this role and if the mother did not the child would surely suffer. Mary Ainsworth, a contemporary of Bowlby, postulated a theory of understanding the behaviour of a child in terms of the quality of its attachment relationship with its mother. But she went on to do research with infants in a Third World setting where the nuclear family is not the norm, and found that infants readily form multiple attachment relationships (Ainsworth 1967). So even within the bounds of attachment theory the mother–infant relationship is by no means exclusive. (Indeed, it is interesting to note that in cultures such as in India where the psychoanalytical model has not infiltrated, there has never been the same stigmatisation of working mothers.)

More recent studies have indicated that while the mother continues to be the primary care-giver in most western families, other people can be equally satisfactory as far as even a young baby is concerned (see Tizard 1991 for a review). Given the role that an increasing number of fathers are playing in the care of their children, this does not seem as surprising as it perhaps did thirty years ago. The myopic focus of researchers on the mother–infant bond has led to a failure of past research to acknowledge the role of, e.g. the father, siblings, peers, etc., as well as the wider constellation of relatives, neighbours, childminders or friends.

> It seems likely that because of the different kinds of relationships each forms with the child, each plays a distinctive role in the child's development. These relationships do not develop out of the child's relationship with her mother; rather, they seem to develop concurrently, and even independently.
>
> (Tizard 1991)

Undoubtedly for most children the mother is the sun in their solar system, but other planets can and do provide different social orbits in which they can freely move and there is now growing evidence that these other relationships can act as a buffer for children experiencing a difficult or absent maternal relationship.

The care the child receives up to the age of 3 will determine the course of his later life

There is a widespread belief that babies need their mothers until the age of 3 or else they will suffer lifelong damage. Work with adults who have been separated from their mothers and also suffered appalling experiences in childhood has shown that long-term problems are not inevitable. Children vary in their resilience and responses to social and physical environment and subsequent experiences may mitigate early problems – so the presence of full-time maternal care is not the only factor that needs to be examined. We clearly need to find out a lot more about what factors differentiate those who display resilience and those who do not, given differing care environments in their early childhood.

Other care is worse than mother care

A mother's employment does not prevent her from being her child's prime care-giver for the majority of time, i.e. outside work hours. Many other factors such as the continuity and stability of the home environment, the hours she works, the demands of her job and of her particular children, the support of her partner or others will all determine the quality of the care she provides. Whether or not she works, or whether the child is absent from her for a number of hours each day, will not of themselves determine the quality of parenting being provided.

What we are witnessing is a growing recognition that even young children can thrive in the care of a number of different adults. Many parents continue to believe that mothers alone are the best people for the job, since it minimises many of the practical problems, and for many it is a source of satisfaction. But this is no longer seen as the only solution. For the majority of mothers, sharing the care of their children is becoming the norm so the focus has shifted to what sort of other care is available to parents. The picture that exists in Britain is one of parents being left to their own devices, struggling to find care that suits their needs and their wallets. For many, a willing relative such as a mother or sister is the source of that childcare. Increasingly it is childminders and a variety of trained and untrained young women. There is for many parents with such arrangements the constant threat of the childcare disappearing and leaving them stranded, with no one else to call upon at short notice.

A number of recent headline stories in both the USA and Britain have focused on young children left alone while their mothers were at work because the childcarer had failed to turn up and they had no one else to turn to in the 'communities' in which they lived. It may be more difficult for working parents and their children to build social networks within their communities because of their absence from or inability to reciprocate in the social exchanges that take place. This may be taken as an argument for stable community-based childcare rather than workplace creches.

Certainly the consensus amongst those demanding more state-led provision of childcare is to establish day care centres. The focus of the research has again shifted now to how that childcare will fit in with the parental care.

> Instead of regarding day care as a substitute for home care with research focusing on whether this substitution harms children, day care can be seen as one of a number of care settings that contribute to children's total experience. Taking this approach, research can ask more subtle questions, focusing on how different care settings relate to each other, how day care fits in to the child's wider experience, and the specific contribution of day care to that experience.
>
> (Hennessy *et al.* 1992)

It is interesting to examine what criteria nurseries regarded as providing high-quality care have in common as this tells us about what the perceptions are of what children need (and hence what fit parents should be providing too):

- Should have high adult–child ratio.
- Carers should be responsive and sensitive to children and their stage of development and help to promote their further development.
- Should provide a stimulating environment with toys and activities which are tailored to the children's developmental stages.
- Trained and stable workforce with proper pay and conditions.
- Childcare environment should remain stable, be clean and secure.
- Should provide interaction with other children, because children enjoy this and because there is some evidence that it improves social skills.

(Hennessy *et al.* 1992)

For children who come from families which do not provide these at home, there is no doubt great potential for good nurseries to improve their level of care and experience. For children who come from loving and materially adequate backgrounds, the advantage of day centre care is less obvious. Many parents argue that being with other children helps to teach independence and to form relationships with their peers. But critics such as childcare author Penelope Leach argue that most young children are better off in the home environment, observing and sharing daily life with their families. Children are programmed to learn to adapt to the adult world through participation in daily activities – the more they are segregated, the less opportunity they have to do this.

There is also the danger that in the handover from parent to multiple care-givers the continuity of feedback from the child which informs the care-giver's responses and understanding of the child's behaviour is lost. This may not be so significant with older children who can talk, but for babies and toddlers whose communication arises as part of a two-way relationship, it could lead to problems. And what would be the legal liability of the day care centre? If a child dies as a result of food poisoning or an accident in the home no one would (yet!) sue the mother. But should the same happen to a child in a day care centre? Would we see a rush to the courts to prove negligence?

Even for those who accept that there is no scientific reason to disapprove of children entering regular day care, the likelihood of it being consistently adequate is a more real worry.

> My concern derives from how expensive it is to provide good quality infant care, the limitations experienced by many young families in the cost of day care that they can afford, the generally high turnover of staff, widespread social perceptions that caring for children is essentially 'unskilled' labor and the general unwillingness of governments to regulate the quality of early care or subsidise its expense.
>
> (Thompson 1988)

Looking at these sorts of concerns and the high standards that would be required for justifying wide-scale provision of childcare it is interesting to note how much society does expect of parents looking after their own children without actually acknowledging the skills and personal sacrifices that they have to make. It has been noted that to provide the best chances of high-quality childcare the right conditions need to be established and one of these is the way that staff are treated:

> To take just one link in the chain, children's experience and well-being in day care is affected by staff behaviour which in turn is affected by pay, conditions and training, which in turn again depends on the level of resourcing for services and training.
>
> (Hennessy *et al.* 1992)

One could argue that this applies as much to parents as to care staff.

Society will suffer

LATCHKEY LIFESTYLE ATTACKED

Inadequate and aggressive pupils are the victims of their working parents, teachers will be told this week.

(Fran Abrams, *Sunday Correspondent* 29/7/90)

Tyrant children of working wives – pampered youngsters exploit the guilt at home.

(Tracey Harrison, *Daily Mail* 28/12/90)

The economic and social backdrop to parental employment has undergone a remarkable change in the past thirty years, and discussion of working mothers seems to epitomise so many of the current discontents and anxieties with the pace of that change. Many of the objections against mothers going out to work appear to be a nostalgic longing for a time gone by when people had more time and were satisfied with the simple things in life, when the environment, politics and the understanding of the world were simpler. In this scenario, the ideal father was the reliable wage-earner, the mother was the loving and ever available maypole of family life, their mere joint presence prevented delinquency and immorality and promoted a healthy society. And then women were corrupted into wanting personal happiness and fulfilment outside their family roles and the rot set in. If only they had stayed at home.

Society is too ready to find easy scapegoats and it inevitably picks out those who do not conform to the prevailing social norms whether they be working mothers, single mothers or immigrants.

Many people point to the low crime rates of the 1950s and indicate that this coincided with a time when mothers did not work outside the home – therefore modern society's ills can be blamed on working mothers. This is a potent argument because it seemingly ties in with so many people's personal observations that children of today do not get as much time and attention from their mothers as they did in the halcyon days of the past. Studies have repeatedly shown that being in outside employment does not reduce the domestic burden on the woman. Men are no more likely to significantly share the domestic chores if their partners are working. The effects of this overload on the quality of parenting that a child receives has not yet been extensively studied but it is an argument for more social support of childcaring, not of returning women to the kitchen sink.

Working mothers demote the role of caring

CHILDREN: THE UNFAIR BURDEN ON MOTHERS

. . . . It is this major handicap which drastically reduces promotion prospects for women and keeps their wages at an average of 75 per cent of men's.

(Gill Swain, *Daily Mail* 28/6/88)

The notion that childcare is a burden unfairly shouldered by mothers is a source of genuine distress to many people, including mothers. The definition of work is that it is paid for, so all useful activity that is not paid for is devalued in a society which now rates working as more important than simply earning a living. The recognition that women do for nothing what would otherwise cost a considerable sum of money is undoubtedly significant. In Britain an insurance company recently calculated that £18,000 was the annual price tag for the work of a mother in the home. They break down the job as follows: nanny, cook, cleaner, laundress, shopper, dishwasher, driver, gardener, seamstress.

In recent years there have been many attempts such as this to put a price on the work that mothers do in the home and how much they lose in income by staying at home to look after children. This emphasis on costs and lost earnings and the view of childcare as an economic burden has arguably contributed to its reduction in status. Our society places a high value on wealth so it follows that anyone who chooses or is forced to forgo the greater financial benefits of childless employment by staying at home to look after children must be disadvantaged.

There is a sense in which because children are no longer seen as an investment for their parents' old age the rewards of child-rearing are down to whether parents enjoy it or not. So for many, child-rearing becomes a job that they will only do if it is paid for or if it can be supplemented with paid work. The taxes that the working parents pay to the state then go towards their own pensions in old age, thereby freeing them of any dependence on their adult children.

In other areas of life we are seeing caring being taken over by paid staff (e.g. the care of elderly people or of people with severe disabilities) so the caring role is increasingly seen as a job that could be done by any unskilled but financially motivated worker. This raises the question of how much emotional investment in a relationship is critical to caring. This process of treating the role of the mother at home as work has been part of an overall trend and many people argue that it fails to recognise the intrinsic importance of the parent–child relationship that underlies the variously listed tasks. Breaking it down into jobs that could be done by a number of separate people with no particular long-term commitment to the child demotes the importance of continuity and caring. It is interesting to note that Sweden (which has been held up as an example of the best state support of working mothers and the most comprehensive provision of childcare) is facing a shortage of childcare workers. This may be indicative of the workers absorbing the subliminal message that childcare is not a high-status occupation and should be avoided if at all possible.

But mothers at home have traditionally done more than just these tasks – they have fulfilled major roles as builders of community support networks which combine very naturally with caring for young children because there is an obvious benefit to getting to know neighbours, parents of other children, helping to run playgroups, looking after the frail – all these act as a strengthening buffer for the entire community, not just the family itself, and motivate a desire to preserve communities and protect them from adverse change. If mothers go out to work, their contribution in the community may be minimised. This is not an argument against working mothers – it is a call for the recognition of the value of the multiple roles that mothers do play in relation to their communities as well as to their children and that this may need to be replaced or augmented by others.

USEFUL POINTS TO NOTE FROM THE EXPERIENCES OF WORKING MOTHERS

- As working mothers become the norm rather than the exception, there has been a greater trend towards addressing the actual issues that concern them (i.e. childcare) rather than the issues that concern the critics (i.e. how the children will suffer from maternal deprivation). If this same pragmatism could be applied to other groups there might be a greater recognition of the commonality of the needs of modern parenting.
- The positive benefit of good-quality day care is that it opens up the suffocating and potentially dangerous domestic isolation of parenting in much of modern society, and that it also enchances the notion of childcare as being a communal responsibility. It also has the potential for standardising the care and stimulation that children from a wide range of social backgrounds receive. It could thus have a very democratic outcome, minimising the risk to the children of parental problems or poverty of home background.
- In two-parent households studies suggest that the level of the father's involvement with children is likely to increase if the mother is employed which it is also believed will have a positive effect on child development.
- Having strong relationships with other adults can help minimise problems following the loss or departure of a parent.

WHAT ASSESSMENT OF WORKING MOTHERS TELLS US ABOUT SOCIETY'S EXPECTATIONS OF FIT PARENTS

Ideal

- A woman is totally responsible for the health of her foetus.
- The mother is the best person to care for her children to ensure their future physical and psychological well-being.
- A child needs a twenty-four-hour-a-day mother at least up to school age and preferably after that.
- A mother who leaves her children to the care of others should feel guilty.
- A mother's duty is to the home and to her children – it is for fathers to support the family through paid work.
- The child's needs must come before the mother's need to work.
- The mother's role is to help the father to be a good worker so that he can provide for the family.
- The mother's role in society is to care for the vulnerable and to be a pillar of the community.
- The father's role in society is to be a good worker to promote the wealth of the country and, if the need arises, a defender of its security.
- Parents' rewards for child-rearing are their children's support of them in old age.

Actual

- The health of unborn children is the joint responsibility of society and parents.
- Parents share the responsibility of raising children with society.
- Parents are primarily responsible for ensuring that their children are adequately cared for.
- Carers other than the mother can look after a child – what is important is consistency and responsiveness of care provided by both parents and other childcarers.
- The quality of care a child receives depends on the care-giver's behaviour which in turn is affected by the reward, conditions and training the care-giver receives.
- A parent's self-esteem is important to the quality of care he or she provides.
- Parents' needs are as important as children's needs.
- Financial security and self-reliance are important to a family unit.
- Men's and women's roles in society are interchangeable.
- Parenting brings only emotional rewards – and for some, limited financial support. There are no long-term guarantees of support by the child.

15 Black parents

Herte Mariyam is a young mother. She is also a Rastafarian. When she was pregnant she spent five months in a mental institution with seriously ill patients. She still does not quite know why, except what are, for her, the most obvious reasons.

'These people (health professionals) think that because you've got dreadlocks in your hair, you're ignorant, dangerous. I had a bit of depression and no roof over my head. But I wasn't mad.'

(Alibhai 1988)

The assessment of black people as parents defines more clearly than any of the previous groups studied the dangers of focusing on one criterion of difference and making it the pivot for official assessment – see-sawing between whether or not it makes them bad parents. Black parents are commonly noted as problems in professional practice. The concerns about their fitness to parent arises in tangential ways: the notion that a disproportionate number of black children are received into care suggests that their parents must be seen to be providing less adequate care themselves, the heated debates about transracial adoption, the recurring negative stereotypes of black and Asian families living in western societies – all these suggest that being parents of a different race in a predominantly white society is still perceived as a problem.

I therefore felt it was worth exploring the issue of race in professional assessment of parents, but found my investigation frustrating. There is little published work on parenting by people of faiths and ethnic origins different to the majority, and most of what I did find related to the American experience, not the British. This chapter is thus perhaps more based on personal experiences than the previous ones but I have included it none the less because I hope it will it offer useful insights into how fit parenting is judged in western countries such as Britain.

WHAT IS BLACK?

Until very recently, stereotypes of black people abounded in the media: black-skinned people were depicted as aggressive, dangerous, criminal, sexually uncontrollable, childlike, immoral, unhygienic, drug abusers, generally untrustworthy and unintelligent. Over the decades charity posters of emaciated black and brown faces have cried out for 'white' pity and guilt. It is not surprising that, combined with the historic associations of slavery and colonial rule, so many western people have built up an unconscious picture of black people as uniformly inferior. The term 'western' is used here to denote the dominant culture of the industrialised countries of Europe, USA, Canada, Australia and New Zealand whose attitudes and behaviours with regard to parenting are regarded as more similar to each other and more different from the rest of the world. When viewed from within these countries, the term Black generally signifies a connection with distinctive cultures outside those national boundaries, such as those from the Caribbean islands.

In Britain the term Black is applied to people of a wide variety of religious and racial backgrounds, many of whom had come at the invitation of the British government, mostly from countries that had been colonised until their recent past. (In America Black usually signifies descendants of Africans brought over, often forcibly, by slave traders during the eighteenth and nineteenth centuries.) About half of all black people living in Britain were born here, so their cultural attachment to their ancestors' countries of origin cannot be assumed, nor can their connections to each other (e.g. between Caribbeans and Africans or between Pakistanis and Indians).

Since the development of the civil rights movement in the USA in the 1960s, the term Black has come to signify a political pride in belonging to a non-white ethnic group. It has come to include all who are discriminated against on the basis of the colour of their skin, regardless of their country or culture of origin. As a means of uniting forces to fight common oppression, the term is undoubtedly important but it has the disadvantage that it perpetuates the stereotype of all black people being the same as each other and more different from people with white skin – and of only white people as racist. It denies the commonality of needs, fears and aspirations of all human beings. It also discounts the very different individual experiences of black people living in western countries and perpetuates a view of all black people only in respect to their experience of racism. Many people do not like to be classified in this way, seeing it as a perpetuation of the blacks-as-victims portrayal of themselves. (This is also a common criticism of the use of the term Disabled.)

I cannot present here a comprehensive treatise on racism and its consequences for family life but I am interested in the similarities with the other 'deviant groups' so far considered, particularly in respect of pathology associated with sexuality, socio-economic position, lack of role models, crude labelling and lack of understanding of different social values leading to stigmatisation – and a deep-rooted fear that they will somehow displace the dominant culture by their very existence.

Blacks are promiscuous, over-sexed and immoral

Myths surrounding black sexuality have been around since western explorers and merchants first began to encounter black people in their native countries (see e.g.

Rogers 1968). Most have focused on the insatiable and uninhibited appetite for sex that both black men and women are supposed to display. Their observations probably tell us more about the sexually repressed backgrounds of the observers than they do about African-Caribbean people's sexuality but these views have had a powerful influence on how black sexuality, and therefore fertility, is perceived. There appears to be a complex mixture of fear and envy based on these assumptions which then defines the views of the dominant white culture towards black people. The stereotypes have no basis in any research which directly reflects black people's own observations or behaviour. (It is interesting to note that white Europeans and Americans travelling in non-western countries are commonly regarded as promiscuous and perverted in their sexual practices by local people.)

The perceived preponderance of pregnancy in Britain amongst black teenagers is seen as further confirmation of their lax moral standards. However, the rapid rise in white teenage pregnancy rates has diluted this particular line of attack. Studies of differences in the way that white parents and African-Caribbean parents treat their teenage daughter's pregnancy suggest that while both show strong disapproval, amongst the black parents there is usually a greater degree of reconciliation and subsequent support of the teenage mother (Gibson 1980). This is in contrast to the statutory support they may receive. For example, a study by the Commission for Racial Equality (CRE) of one London borough's allocation of local authority housing showed that non-white applicants received poorer-quality housing than white applicants (CRE 1984).

Black women breed like rabbits

There are many concerns in western countries with black immigrant populations about the fact that their fertility rates may be higher than the indigenous or white population's. The focus in many countries has been on pushing contraception, abortion and sterilisation on to black women, which is believed by many black people to be an attempt to preserve the dominant cultural position by minimising black population growth.

> The cultural theory of race difference holds that the family supplies the units, the building blocks from which the national community is constructed. This puts black women directly in the firing line. Firstly, they are seen as playing a key role in reproducing the alien culture, and secondly, because their fertility is seen as excessive and therefore threatening.
>
> (Gilroy 1990)

Planned parenthood measures funded by rich countries focus on controlling the population of non-white countries. The subconscious image of all black and Asian people is that they have no responsible attitudes to their fertility and have to be trained by western professionals. We have already seen in previous chapters the importance attached to planned pregnancy in western countries, so the notion of children appearing at will is seen as symptomatic of immature and irresponsible behaviour.

In most non-western countries, having many children is regarded as a blessing, a *raison d'être* of life, whose care can be shared with other adults and siblings but also who will become independent at a younger age and so not need caring for as long as in the West. The attitude to children is less sentimental but arguably less patronising because of their potential for future contribution to the wealth and security of the family. This attitude is shared by the peer group and so many children bring status to the parents. In such a cultural climate it is natural to want as many children as possible but even then the ideal number does shift according to the perceptions of the peer group and the cultural acceptability of family planning methods. (A popular Ghanaian saying is that a pot needs three legs to stand on – a woman with only one or two children has an unstable future. This is in direct contrast to western society where the parents' financial security is seen to be undermined by too many children and the fear is of children not having enough *parents* for their own security!)

When people from such cultures arrived in western countries the dominant attitudes did begin to impinge as their experience of bringing up children in a different environment made the disadvantages self-evident: e.g. the climate and dangers which prevent play outside; the premium on space which prevents accommodation of many relatives; the geographical isolation from peer group support; the difficulty of travelling with more than two children on public transport; the cultural messages which dictate 'small is beautiful' and which ask parents to put more effort and money into fewer children.

The fertility rate amongst immigrant groups falls within one or two generations to resemble that of the indigenous population, suggesting a cultural shift according to the realities of the new environment which does not accord status to mothers, enable childcare to be shared or guarantee wealth and security in old age.

A report commissioned by the Centre for Economic Policy Research (CEPR) which identified this fall in ethnic minority fertility rates noted that 'If the demographic dynamics behind this process of stabilisation were more generally appreciated, fears of swamping which feed racial prejudice and discrimination might be more effectively countered (CEPR 1989).

They have peculiar childcare practices which are unacceptable in a civilised society

A recent item on British Ceefax news (14/2/93) told the tale of a 2 year old in India who was rescued from a ritual religious killing by his father, supposedly guided by the goddess he worshipped. It was the only item of news from India that day, at a time when so much of world significance is happening there. The report did not put it in any context or hint at how such practices are regarded by the majority. It was just another example of the barbarism of foreigners. In the absence of a wider variety of coverage, these types of unpleasant peculiarities dominate in the minds of outside observers as being what is normal and acceptable in Asian society.

Similarly, western media coverage of bride-burning or of girls 'forced' into arranged marriages, children 'forced' to pray or study the Koran after school, presents a view of Asian parents which again tells us more about the commentator's view of what degree of influence parents should have over their children than it does about Asian families.

Black people are deficient as parents

How easy it has been to remove black children from their families and reward a white family by placing them for fostering and adoption, at the same time saying black families do not have the capacity to care for their own children.

(J. Small, *Community Care* 20/7/87)

Disproportionate numbers of black children are thought to come into the care of local authorities, and since this tends to be the only contact that most professionals such as social workers have with black families it appears to lead to a pathological view of all black parents. (Again, note the similarity with disabled parents.) However, it is the lack of familiarity with some of the different norms of black families that may be more to blame.

The focus again is largely on mothers. Black fathers are seen to fail for what they do not do – e.g. because they are absent or unemployed – whereas black mothers are seen as deficient because of what they do as parents. Large numbers of care orders in the past have been on the basis of neglect or physical punishment. There appears to be a common perception that black parents use too much physical punishment, do not show as much affection, use harsher language and expect children to take responsibility beyond their years (e.g. looking after younger siblings). Their lives are seen as less ordered and therefore dysfunctional. A recent study (by a mother who was born in Ghana and who is an experienced social worker) found that this is not the case but suggested the attitude is rooted in the confusion amongst social workers and other outside observers about how to understand behaviour which does not fit in with what is familiar to them.

There may be different cultural meanings attached to behaviours which appear the same. Take physical punishment as an example. In western middle-class culture it is becoming increasingly unacceptable as a form of disciplining children – the legacy of hordes of childcare experts and psychoanalysts shoring up piles of guilt at the doors of any parent who should dare to risk her child suffering lasting emotional damage. But for many other people, a smack can be a form of showing your children that you care enough to ensure that they learn right from wrong. A study of working-class mothers in Hackney found little difference between the African-Caribbean mothers and white British mothers in their attitudes to using physical discipline with their children and the majority in both groups felt they had benefited from being physically disciplined in their own childhood (Bartells-Ellis 1992).

Physical punishment, harsh language, a lack of kissing and hugging or saying 'I love you', do not necessarily indicate a lack of affection or caring. If we turn back to Vera Fahlberg's shopping list of how to encourage attachment (p. 26) or to the extract of Dora Black in Chapter 1, p. 25, and present it to most non-western parents, it might be dismissed as sentimental and patronising. The actual indicators of affection may well be invisible to a western observer or, more likely (as with sleeping in the same bed as parents, being allowed to take greater responsibility in household chores, or living at home beyond a certain age), dismissed as inappropriate. Psychoanalytical views of attachment and separation, of mother–infant bonds, of psychological guilt, have had no place in the cultural inheritance of most non-western families living in western societies. That does not, however, mean they do not care about their children's feelings.

There is also criticism about black children being given too much responsibility. It is an extension of the western idea of children as helpless and in need of protection from the harsh realities of adult life for as long as possible before being thrust out into a life of total independence. Children in non-western societies are expected to participate in the chores and activities of family life from as soon as they are walking. They are expected to be able to manage their own washing and dressing, to help with increasingly complex chores, with the care of siblings and thus to see that they play a useful role within their families as a model for their own future family lives. (Fiona Bartells-Ellis (1992) described how when a group of black and white social workers were asked to describe what tasks a 12, 14 and 16 year old would be doing, the black ones were very clear while the white ones dissembled.)

The purpose of presenting these 'cultural differences' is not to say one set is better than any other but to show that there are different and less pathological ways of interpreting the behaviours of parents with different cultural heritages to the dominant western one. How many of these distinctive characteristics are retained within a different dominant culture remains to be seen but the signs are that, as with family size, there is a shift away from the practices of the first-generation immigrants as a result of the daily exposure to the values and practices of the dominant culture.

Child assessment is carried out predominantly by professionals who are white and middle class. Some have argued that the over-representation of black children is not indicative of poorer parenting:

> For it is a reality that the black child may not just be a victim of child abuse, or at risk. She or he may be the victim of ignorance, dilemma, unawareness, subjective judgement, insensitivity and prejudices of the social work (and other) professions. She or he may be at the receiving end of personal and institutional racism.

> (Ahmad 1989)

To challenge stereotypes we clearly need more information about the realities of family life and to ask people from those groups to define themselves – which is why I have been so interested to read the findings of such research which concludes:

There is no evidence from this probably not unusual group of African-Caribbean respondents and the nitty gritty of what they do, of strange or dysfunctional parenting with characteristics attributed to numbers of their culture by the profession (of social work).

(Bartells-Ellis 1992)

There is a virtually total gap in understanding about the culture of different African-Caribbean families to the extent that they are frequently seen as without any cultural heritage, but for Asian families there appears to be the reverse situation. There is some respect for an older culture (helped by the fact that Asian families are seen as less dependent on the state than black families) but this can lead to a different set of stereotypes – ones which seem to suggest that too strong a cultural identification with the mother country is a bad thing. There appears to be a widespread belief that however acceptable their customs were in their original countries, here they have to conform to the western model of good parenting:

One Asian mother, for example, was given a long lecture on bonding because the health visitor felt that every time she came the baby was being held by the younger sister-in-law. The notion of a nuclear family 'owning' a child is often seen as the norm.

(Alibhai 1988)

Examples of this sort abound: Asian women being told that they are only allowed the support of their husbands in labour, the disapproval of hospital visiting by members of the extended family after the birth and so on. Shama Ahmed relates how

panic swept through one department's office when an extended Asian family arrived for an interview to be taken on as foster parents. Ahmed said 'They couldn't measure up to dominant attitudes to what is acceptable because they had not come as a couple or as single parents.'

(Ahmed 1987)

Yet the same author has criticised social workers for over-emphasising cultural differences without understanding what is considered normal and abnormal in cultures they do not belong to; for example, 'An Asian father was told that incest was "not acceptable in our society". It isn't in Asian society either.' This is a good indication that there needs to be more involvement of people from the same peer group of the family being assessed in the assessment process.

Black parents don't have the same need for outside help

The Public Inquiry into the death of Tyra Henry who had been killed by her father after being placed by social workers with her grandmother, Beatrice Henry, noted:

We believe that the assumption that Beatrice Henry would cope in the circumstances we have outlined was rooted in the perception of her as a type rather than as an individual. There is an everpresent danger in social work (and not only there) of believing that the poor are so accustomed to poverty that they can be expected to get by in conditions which no middle class family would be expected to tolerate. There is also a 'positive', but nevertheless false, stereotype in white British society of the Afro-Caribbean mother figure as endlessly resourceful, able to cope in great adversity, essentially unsinkable. In it are both a genuine recognition of the endurance of Afro-Caribbean peoples in conditions of great hardship and an evasive and guilty recognition that disproportionately, many such people live in poverty in modern Britain. We do not suppose for a second that anybody concerned with social services in Lambeth would have taken a conscious decision that a lower standard of social service support was appropriate for poor black clients than for others, but we do think that it may have been an unarticulated and unconscious sense that a woman like Beatrice Henry would find a way of coping, no matter what, that underlay the neglect of Area 5 social services to make adequate provision for her taking responsibility for Tyra.

(London Borough of Lambeth 1987)

There is an apparent paradox here about the stereotypes of black people as needy yet self-sufficient. It is often noted that black parents and Asian parents do not appear to use as many of the statutory services as would be expected in relation to their numbers. This has often been explained away as a cultural difference – that all black people have extended families to look after their own and are not interested in the help of outsiders. This may be true for the first-generation immigrants coming from countries where there is minimal state provision of social services, but not so ready an explanation for subsequent generations where the extended family is weaker or completely absent. There appears to be growing recognition that the information about available services simply does not reach these groups and often people are too proud to ask because they do not want to conform to the prevailing stereotype of Blacks as needy. Again there are many parallels with the previously examined deviant groups. There is often fear of scrutiny by people who might misunderstand and thus aggravate the situation instead of help solve it. The result is that many black and Asian families do not get the support that others have ready access to and which would minimise the stresses, perhaps preventing more serious later problems.

In Britain a number of recent studies of ethnic minority mothers describe their negative experiences within the health services when having their babies; I have been struck by the similarities with previous work interviewing disabled mothers (Campion 1990; Lewis 1991).

Asian women are observably denied equal access to the maternity services by the lack of proper interpreting services as well as through staff attitudes which equate lack of English with a lack of intelligence.

(Alibhai 1988)

If you substitute 'Asian' with 'deaf', and 'English' with 'hearing', it quickly becomes apparent that the issue is not simply one of race but a mismatch between the expectations of the dominant culture (i.e. in this example, English speaking and hearing) about the attributes necessary before being allowed access to the same standards of services available to other citizens. As with mentally handicapped parents there is a systematic marginalisation of non-English-speaking parents from the statutory institutions. Parents may avoid school parent meetings or social events in which other parents make and secure their networks – but which remain closed to those who do not speak the language confidently. Yet to learn the dominant language in a society which is characterised by its reserve and hostility towards 'foreigners' is not easy either. Many of those who need help in the English language work long hours and cannot get ready access to suitable tuition. A recent report by the Adult Literacy and Basic Skills Unit estimated that of the 500,000 people in Britain needing help to improve their English, only 44,000 received tuition. Fewer than 25 per cent had ever received any help with improving their English; 59 per cent were unaware of local schemes offering help (*Social Work Today* 5/2/90).

If black parents complain, they are once again in danger of being misunderstood and labelled difficult; stereotypes of African-Caribbeans as aggressive and Asian women as passive and compliant can prevent serious appraisal of their views. It is interesting to note however that, as with disabled parents and teenage mothers, 'There is some suggestion that [black mothers] have developed a pride in having to overcome the struggles of raising children without the support they wanted or needed' (Bartells-Ellis 1992).

Children of black parents do badly at school

For a long time it was believed that people from the darker-skinned races had intrinsically lower intelligence so poor performance at school was perhaps expected, but black parents were still often blamed for having low expectations of their children. However, research has shown that expectations of black parents are as high if not higher than those of white parents because they see education as a passport out of poverty and discrimination (Bartells-Ellis 1992).

Certainly racial discrimination is seen by many black parents as the reason for their children's underachievement.

'What I find going up to my son's school is that they don't expect very much from the black children . . .'

'By about the fourth year, they picked out certain kids who would take O-levels. And lo and behold this other black girl and myself weren't one of them. Although we were in the top stream of this class, we weren't picked out. But there was no chance of black children getting O-levels – you took CSE. That was it. . . . In the four years that I was there, there was never a black that had taken O-levels.'

(*The Voice* 26/5/87)

Many studies have highlighted the poor educational attainment of African-Caribbean children in British schools. In the absence of other fuller images of black people, the media coverage of these reports has arguably contributed to the popular stereotype that black people are incapable of becoming educated, and therefore civilised. Discrimination in employment reinforces this since even well-qualified black people are forced to take jobs of lower status than people who are white.

Recent commentators have started to refute these past studies. They argue that there is no clear evidence that black children do worse than white children at school. The statistical studies on which so many reports were based (e.g. Swann 1985) were frequently flawed.

> [In 1984 Troyna wrote] 'The greatest danger lies in the possibility that ill-conceived and poorly formulated studies will perpetuate the notion of black educational underachievement as a given rather than as a problematic that requires sensitive and systematic interrogation.' The dangers today are still as great as they were then.
>
> (Drew and Gray 1991)

By focusing on race as the main factor, it is possible that more significant factors have been overlooked. For example, since many black children live in poor inner city areas with poorer-quality schools, they may have less opportunity than most white children to develop their educational prowess. So the studies may have been highlighting the relationship between class (rather than race) and educational underachievement.

One such study, based on results from the National Youth Cohort Study which follows the progress of 50,000 young people in England and Wales, found that:

> Black young people are much more likely than white young people to come from working class backgrounds and for many reasons, particularly socio-economic disadvantage, this group does less well at school than the middle-class group. If the sample is controlled for social class, differences between ethnic groups decrease.
>
> (*Asian Times* 5/5/89)

This would certainly tie in with the findings that, while Asian children frequently appear to do very well academically, amongst the recent Bangladeshi immigrants children appear to do much more poorly. Even a cursory comparison between their relative economic conditions would indicate that race is not the defining factor as far as educational potential.

Other factors such as the relevance of what children are taught in relation to their lives outside school clearly also need to be considered. Emotions play a major role in how receptive a child is to being taught – children who are confident and feel accepted by their teachers and peers will be more inclined to learn than those who do not. If the environment, the school role models or the teaching materials seem to exclude and undermine them, there is a greater chance that they will not learn. This is true of all children but can clearly become more of a problem to children for whom there is a mismatch between their parental culture and that of the school.

The regular media coverage of the 'controversy' of Muslims seeking separate educational establishments is a good example of this. While Jewish and Catholic groups have long enjoyed separate denomination schools, the outcry against Islamic schools has been that they will form a barrier to effective race relations. Yet Muslims do not form a single racial or ethnic group.

> The objective of the campaigners for Muslim denomination schools is to produce confident and assured young Muslims who will be spiritually, mentally and physically prepared to contribute to the society in which they are living.
>
> (M. Sheriff quoted in the *Independent* 5/5/89)

The establishment of special schools by black parents for black children has success-fully shown that children can thrive in an environment which is supportive of who they are and where the authority figures are ones with which the pupils identify. Again this is not simply a matter of race – girls are found to do better in all-girl schools because they are not in competition with another group which is given preferential treatment and whose values are used to undermine them.

Black children will become delinquent because they lack fathers

The media coverage of race riots in British and American cities in recent years has highlighted the 'problem' of black youths. While liberal commentators asked for mitigating circumstances of poverty, racism and inappropriate policing tactics to be considered, the lasting images in the minds of the population at large are ones which reinforce the popular stereotype of the young black man as a fatherless and therefore out-of-control law-breaker threatening the security of the decent, white, law-abiding majority.

This overlooks the fact that those who suffer most from the conditions which produce a few law-breakers are largely other black families, living in the same overcrowded inner city council estates which architecturally and spiritually offer little hope of escape for their denizens and who are subjected to daily racist attacks on their security and self-regard. It also overlooks the fact that in Britain most black children live in two-parent families (Phoenix 1988) and, as amongst white people, of those living in single-parent households, the majority do not become delinquents.

As we have seen in Chapter 12, the perceived problems associated with 'absent' fathers in western society are to do with lack of a family wage-earner and lack of a law-abiding male role model for the children as well as the lack of a model relationship of loving husband and wife that the children will want to emulate when they grow up.

When we look at other cultures and observe men and women in their relation-ships to their children and each other there is a danger that we superimpose our own culture's view of what their roles and behaviours should be. The traditional model of a nuclear family with father, mother and children living in self-contained isolation is not a common feature of most non-western societies, although where these become more urbanised they are also witnessing a shift to this model. The differences between family patterns in different parts of the same African country or between different islands in the Caribbean warn against any generalisations. But perhaps it is worth pointing out other ways of looking at the 'problem' of absent fathers.

- In many non-western countries, the father's role may be looser and less well-defined than that of the mother and therefore the absence of the father *per se* is seen as less pathological. The care of children is seen as the work of women and marriage is commonly delayed until a man is able to provide income to support the family. The father may come and go, live in a separate house and still play an important role. Even the term 'household' may not signify the same stability of its residents as in the western model of the family home – this does not indicate instability of non-western modes of family life but instead a more fluid relationship between people (parents, siblings and other relatives), child-rearing roles and the buildings that individuals occupy. (Since this seems to match a growing and very similar trend in modern western societies there may be much that immigrant families have to offer in valuable experience.)
- An absent father does not necessarily mean a lone mother. Black mothers are more likely to have the support of other relatives such as grandmothers, cousins, aunts and sisters than their white counterparts.
- There are not enough men to go round. In many African and Caribbean countries there is a higher proportion of women to men. There are various explanations for the shortage of men. For example, there is a well-documented recognition that boys are statistically found to be more vulnerable than girls in terms of their health and tolerance of adversity so fewer survive to adulthood. Emigration to find work takes many of the marriageable and married men away from their communities and may destabilise married family life. This demographic legacy may in itself affect expectations of marriage and family life, even for people now living in western countries. Other factors of the new environment are superimposed on these.
- The differential discrimination against black men and women in white societies means that it is easier for women to get jobs than for men so it undermines their role as exclusive family wage-earners. Freed from dependency, women may be less willing to put up with men who cannot provide for them.
- A large proportion of men in the fathering age bracket are in prison or in psychiatric care. This may in part be due to the greater readiness of white society to label a black man as deviant, violent or criminal. But it may also be as a result of the particular combination of pressures on black men living in hostile societies. The marginalisation in every sphere of life prevents them from achieving any status in white society while at the same time they are not being allowed a role as head of black families.
- Many black men are married to or cohabiting with white women.
- The social and economic trends of western society that are determining the marriage and family lives of white people are also affecting people of

different races now living in it and resulting in a greater break-up of relationships, pregnancies out of wedlock and less certainty of long-term commitment. This may be the most important factor of all but is commonly overlooked in the search for differences.

All these explanations need to be seen in the light of a wider non-pathological picture of black families, a picture which is largely absent from the television screens or newspaper headlines or social workers' caselists. Black people living in Britain display a wide range of family patterns which match those of white people in their complexity and variety. Those who have been born and brought up here undoubtedly show more in common with white British parents than they show differences.

Black children should stick to parents of their own culture and white children should stick to theirs

Historically, European colonialism, American slavery and Nazi 'racial hygiene' programmes were all underpinned by the belief that 'lesser' races did not have the same intelligence or feelings as their white superiors and so could be treated like animals. Although science and experience have proven these beliefs to be completely erroneous, they have not been completely wiped out. In polite circles, a more common form of racism still prevails which is one that accepts the equality of races but prefers that they remain distinct.

> Only those belonging to the common 'stock' and forming part of the national 'kith and kin' are capable of sharing and contributing to its way of life. The rest are instinctively rejected by the national body as outsiders.
>
> (Parekh 1988)

Ironically, the latest, more liberal and well-intentioned professional practices are now colluding with their view of separateness – that children of different races need to maintain their own links to their ancestral past by only having parents of the same race in order to maintain their distinct identity.

> The critique of pathological views of black family life that were so prevalent in Social Services during the late 70s and early 80s has led directly to an extraordinary idealisation of black family forms. Anti-racist orthodoxy now sees them as the only effective repositories of authentic black culture and as a guaranteed means to transmit all the essential skills that black children will need if they are to 'survive' in a racist society without psychological damage. 'Same-race' adoption and fostering for 'minority ethnics' is presented as an unchallenged and seemingly unchallengeable benefit for all concerned.
>
> (Gilroy 1990)

The trans-racial adoption debate raises one important issue of whether a vital aspect of being a fit parent is to bring up a child to belong to one's own culture – perhaps at the expense of his birth family's culture. The philosophical issue is clouded by the practical reality, in most western countries, of there being more non-white children needing to find parents but more white adults seeking children. The argument in Britain and the USA of whether an African-Caribbean child is better off remaining in care until a suitable African-Caribbean family is found to foster him has caused heated debate and many media stories focus on the apparent lunacy of tearing a happily settled child away from white foster parents with only a vague hope of finding a same-race family.

There exist a large number of adults in western society who wish to care for children and a large number of children all over the world who need to be cared for. The barrier to solving this equation often appears to concern the ownership of the children – in particular whether a country or a race has some rights to its children. The initial acceptance of a simple relationship – disadvantaged black children going to more advantaged white homes where they will be wanted – is increasingly causing discomfort. In Britain, the campaigning of certain black social workers has led to a guilty change in policy amongst most local authorities regarding the placement of black children. The discovery of many unofficial traders in foreign babies has provoked fears for the safety of many children and cast doubts about the ethics of removing children from poor mothers. Increasingly, 'donor' countries are tightening controls on children leaving and suggesting that the wealthy countries should exercise their love of children by enabling them to be cared for in their home countries, preferably with their own families.

So, who will be the winners and losers in this change of thinking? The objections to different-race placements issues need to be clarified – is it discrimination of those around him that will cause the child to be disadvantaged or the difficulty in accepting that he 'belongs' to his different-race adoptive family? Will he miss out on aspects of the culture common to his race that will be vital to his adult well-being and sense of identity?

Recent studies have already begun to question the belief that mixed race children will suffer a confusion over identity.

MIX-RACE CHILDREN GET 'BEST OF BOTH WORLDS'

A University professor hit out yesterday at 'race industry' dogma surrounding adoptions. New evidence confounded the idea that children of black or mixed race should be placed with families of the same groups.

(B. Tizard quoted by Anthony Doran, *Daily Mail* 19/12/91)

In placing the individual child, the ideology has to be weighed up against the reality of what options do exist. That requires more detailed knowledge of what is important in the individual child's life and what the best chances are of providing him with security and stability.

In looking at the importance of passing on cultural identity as a factor of being a fit parent we have to ask:

1 How much do racial differences dictate cultural differences in a multiracial society? A black child from a poor estate may have more in common culturally with a white family on the same estate than he would with a wealthy black family. If both want to adopt him, where would he be better off? (A recent small-scale but detailed study of parenting behaviours and attitudes showed more similarity than differences between the current parenting practices of white working-class mothers and African-Caribbean mothers living in similar socioeconomic circumstances – despite the differences between their own parental backgrounds in different parts of the world.)

2 What value judgements are being used to dictate whether a child should be placed in a home which is racially similar to that of his birth parents or in one which offers something better (in the eyes of the agency involved)?

A crucial offshoot of this debate is whether it is implied that immigrant parents should be trying to bring up their children to conform to the norm of the host community or to their own culture as experienced in the country of their origin.

Race is the most important criterion

The issue of race and how it has been handled in recent years gives an interesting indication of how other groups who are presently discriminated against may fare in the future.

> It is becoming increasingly apparent that the caring professions, particularly social work, are operating at two extremes in relation to black children and their families. Either they seem to have a liberal or safe approach, anxious not to be labelled racist, so keen that they shy away from their duties of protecting the black child from abuse, or they do not hesitate to remove black children from their families, who according to them are not suitable parents or whose childcare practices are perceived as being substandard.
>
> (Ahmed 1989)

Either they ignore the cultural element or overplay it – both result from focusing on the criterion of blackness.

> We are unhappy at the use that was made of the Good Practice Guide in Area 5, at least in dealing with Tyra. It was stressed to us, and we accept, that it was not a manual of rules or procedures, but it contained some valuable insights. It represented in particular a considered attempt to deal responsibly and constructively with what had become a serious issue, the removal of black children from their families on grounds which had more to do with racial and cultural preconceptions than with the wellbeing or safety of the child.
>
> . . . We are troubled by the possibility that the existence of the Good Practice Guide and the knowledge of the reasons for its existence may have operated, quite wrongly, as a disincentive to embark on investigations which might lead to the removal of yet another black child from her family.
>
> (London Borough of Lambeth 1987)

There exists a great deal of professional confusion about how to assess African-Caribbean and Asian families, and it is the families who suffer.

> The families whom the social workers visit are totally at the mercy of policies of which they know nothing. The party line at present can be gleaned from a booklet entitled *The Good Practice Guide for Working with Black Families and Black Children in Care*. It tells social workers to 'encourage positive black identity in the child'.
>
> But what, one has to ask, is black identity? 'Black culture', taking in the African continent, the Caribbean, America North and South, Europe and Asia, is surely more diverse than 'white culture'. So how can something which cannot be defined be encouraged?
>
> (Zenga Longmore, *Independent* 23/12/87)

> . . . Another point made in the *Good Practice Guide* is that 'the black child must be provided with survival skills necessary for living in a racist society'. Survival skills sound to me like guidelines for North Pole explorers. What are these skills, and why are they assumed to be the innate knowledge with which every black family is endowed?
>
> (Zenga Longmore, *Independent* 23/12/87)

As with the previous 'deviant' groups, the most obvious factor may not be the most significant in the assessment of parenting – it may be relevant but there is danger that it is overplayed and obscures other more significant aspects. Also because people with non-white skin are expected to be more different in the current debate on race, people more readily find it, whereas difference in those with white skin is not sought.

FOSTER BOY TAKEN FROM 'EXTREME' CHRISTIANS

> Social workers have removed a nine-year-old boy from his foster parents after accusing the devoutly Christian couple of abuse by indoctrinating him with religious beliefs.
>
> Officials from the London borough of Southwark said the boy was 'emotionally abused' by having to spend 30 minutes a day praying and learning passages by heart.
>
> It is unlikely that anyone could have picked up the extent of that couple's religious beliefs or what an imposition they were going to be on the child.
>
> (*Sunday Times* 26/10/91)

Race is the most important variable in determining parenting behaviour

The focus on race or ethnicity can and does detract from the most important fact of all – that black parents have more in common with parents as a whole than they have differences. By looking at other cultures we see that there are various common objectives that they all share with respect to the upbringing of children:

- Physical care
- Healthcare
- Adequate nutrition
- Cognitive development
- Protection from environmental and social dangers
- Stability of close relationships
- Affection and trust
- Development of independent living skills
- Development of social skills
- Economic support
- Spiritual development
- Preparation to be an adult who contributes to the community
- Education
- Moral guidance
- Development of identity
- Teaching self-regulation
- Modelling of socially desirable adult behaviour

The specific ways in which they achieve these objectives may vary but it is important to understand the vast range of commonality in the basics. People from different cultures tend to have more in common with those in the indigenous society – particularly those in the same socioeconomic class – than they display differences. An interesting study of childcare and health amongst West Indian, Bangladeshi, Greek Cypriot and white indigenous mothers in inner London found that:

> mothers across all class groups started off with much the same ideas about children's health and much the same aims, with the primary objective of keeping them healthy. But as time went on, class differences in practices appeared and these can be linked to material resource problems. For instance, children in poor housing were especially difficult to manage. Controlling types of food intake became more difficult as children got older and entered a social world where sugary and fatty snacks were the norm.
>
> (Mayall 1991)

And in another study of thirty-three households which included parents from twenty countries all over the world:

> Mothers' accounts suggested very great similarities between them, whatever their background, as regards their aims and methods of childcare. Cultural differences sank into insignificance compared to their shared knowledge. Mothers also shared experience of the devaluing of their knowledge and morality by professionals. . . . As regards factors that differentiated between households, material affluence, years lived in the UK and the quality of social networks seemed important as factors affecting parents' ability to provide a healthy way of life for themselves and their children.
>
> (Mayall 1991)

The study noted many interesting cross-cutting factors such as the fact that most mothers in the sample wanted paid work and day care for their child.

> Among those women whose qualifications and experience characterise them as professional workers, it was the white indigenous, with their good knowledge and contacts, who had found a satisfactory mix of work and day-care; black indigenous women and immigrant women, whether white or not had been less successful.
>
> (Mayall 1991)

In another recent study of African-Caribbeans and white British mothers in East London the findings of similarity amongst childcare practices were very marked. Both these researchers have interesting comments about the research process itself in particular being treated with some suspicion by those they were interviewing. A number of points are worth noting:

> Interviewees gave us some forceful reminders that good data depends on taking people's perspectives into account. For instance, mothers commented to the interviewer that it was obvious she as a black woman must be working as a junior in a white dominated research project. Why otherwise would she be asking questions which lay at tangent to black women's concerns? Specifically, these women said that what concerned them was racism, housing, finding decent employment and day-care; their children's health and health care was not problematic.
>
> (Mayall 1991)

A further point concerned the unit of analysis:

> During our interviews, shared responsibility for and concern about child-rearing was demonstrated by two, three or more adults. Interviewees were thus proposing alternatives to the individual as the unit of analysis: both parents, the women of the household, or all adults interested enough to be present. Researchers who focus on individual mothers may be both missing something and reinforcing stereotypes.
>
> (Mayall 1991)

Finally, there is the point about labelling of groups which resonates with all the previous deviant groups studied so far.

> Two main problems were identified with the word 'group' and with assigning people to groups in a study. First it suggests that there are finite fixed sets of characteristics associated with that group, which can be described and then enlisted to understand a person's behaviour, beliefs and problems. Second, whilst the concept of the group may have some value in helping onlookers to understand people's self-identity, the concept devalues the idea of dynamic interactions and developments arising from people's contact with each other, at both individual and institutional levels. Indeed, the concept of ethnic minority groups complements the multi-cultural thesis, where people are

perceived as encapsulated within their social and cultural group and where these groups co-exist in plural society. Theory, politics and experience indicated that in order to get good data on people's experiences, we needed a design that broke out of the limiting and distorting framework imposed by the concept of ethnic groups.

(Mayall 1991)

This led me to the most important fallacy in assessing black parents.

Different race is synonymous with different culture

The Good Practice Guide goes on to say that the child must 'develop cultural and linguistic attributes necessary for functioning effectively in the black community'. The black community in Britain encompasses millions of people speaking hundreds of different languages. So what are these linguistic attributes? Ibo? Hausa? Yaroba or Jamaican patois? Is a black child who can speak only English at risk, and if so, what is it risking?

(Zenga Longmore in the *Independent* 23/12/87)

It seems from the preceding pages that there is a great deal of confusion between race and culture. My own experience as an Indian growing up in Britain convinced me that there is an inherent fallacy in the arguments which equate race with culture: it mistakenly defines culture as a biological phenomenon. It represents it as a product not of human choices and accidents of history but of racial characteristics of the British people (Parekh 1988).

It also treats culture as a homogenous entity, a once produced and precious inheritance to be protected from outside attack rather than something which is, and has always been, a diverse and dynamic range of values and experiences, constantly shifting at the margins where it encounters others, and from within as people absorb different ideas and develop with the passage of time.

Culture is not a pure substance to be preserved unadulterated through time and migration – even 'traditional' British culture is a complex amalgam of different race invasions and cultural exchange brought about through trading, colonialism and missionary activity in distant parts of the globe. All immigrant people in Britain, irrespective of racism, experience changes from the culture of their country of origin. Different climate, geography, transport, architecture as much as different social mores, contribute to this. Although culture is not a biological phenomenon, the biological analogy of species evolution is a useful one – it reminds us that the homeland culture is also constantly shifting and that geographical separation inevitably brings about separate evolution, to a greater or lesser extent, according to the extent of difference of the new environment from the previous one. This is a process which in a culturally 'fair' world would advance at its own pace – immigrant cultures exchanging what is valuable with indigenous cultures rather than one forcibly swamping others with its own beliefs. This is nowhere more true of parenting and family life. No culture anywhere in the world has a perfect solution for all time to the riddle of what family practices are ideal. The more options a society has access to the more solutions it can try out as the environment changes around and within it. Cultures that try to remain completely cut off from outside influence (like the Amish or Shakers in middle America) can only hold out for so long before the environmental change becomes so great that it wipes them out.

In the past the tendency has been to believe that non-western cultures are more 'primitive' and uncivilised because they are always contrasted with what is seen as the dominant western ideology of progress – those who try to question that dominance often fall into the trap of romanticising other cultures and comparing them with an almost nostalgic view of pre-industrial Europe when everything was simpler and the extended family was the answer to everything.

There is thus more interest in studying customs of isolated tribes in remote parts of the world than there is in looking at other non-western mainstream cultures. We have a very partial view of how other people confronted with similar challenges view those challenges and how they then tackle them. This inevitably leads to tunnel vision when viewing people from other cultures who have moved into western societies.

But to allow different cultures to jostle side by side and find commonality in their shared environment also requires taking seriously those that are different from the dominant culture, without a fear of being swamped. And should anyone be under any illusion that Britain has not already been colonised by another culture without witnessing any mass immigration of a different race of people? The impact of the United States of America on the rest of western (and increasingly, non-western) culture has been phenomenal over the past thirty years. Through the media of its films, television, books and advertising, its social mores and values have pervaded the thoughts and aspirations of the British people. It is no accident that so many of the quotations and expertise I have used in this book have come from the USA. Despite being such a different country geographically and historically, as far as its social trends are concerned, where the USA leads other countries inevitably seem to follow, for good and for bad.

What factors are significant to child-rearing practices in other cultures and how that has evolved amongst immigrants to the West may help us crystallise what modern objectives in the West should be. At present there is a complete failure to mine this rich vein of experience in society's midst.

USEFUL POINTS TO NOTE FROM THE EXPERIENCES OF BLACK PARENTS IN BRITAIN

By examining the experiences of black parents in Britain we can all learn how a dominant culture views differences and ascribes positive or negative value judgements on the basis of 'neutral' attributes such as skin colour or maternal behaviour. The many parallels with the previous chapters indicate that this can teach us much about how any society accommodates, or fails to accommodate, differences on the basis of other 'neutral' attributes such as gender, sexuality, physical and intellectual functioning.

I began Part II with the metaphor of parents and the professional assessing parents as dancing to a frenzy of music whose different themes were unclear. This metaphor may provide a useful way of looking at the findings of this chapter. In raising their children, all parents dance to the rhythms of the environment in which they live. By environment I mean all the different aspects of it: physical, spiritual, economic, social and political. In their early years children dance the steps they learn from their closest care-givers, using the rhythms that they are born with and combining them with those to which they are daily exposed. As children get older they are exposed to a wider variety of music and rhythms, they watch how their own previous dance steps match with those of their new models: those they see at school, on television and elsewhere. Depending on the value judgements they pick up from these wider groups, they may discard their homespun steps and take up the new ones or they may combine and enrich their own and those of others. They will scrutinise how society at large values their parents' dance steps – if society seems to reject these then the child may learn to despise them too – even though they may be so deeply ingrained in his own body's rhythms that to do so causes a temporary or lasting loss of personal harmony.

The bigger the difference between the dominant culture's dance steps and the child's own, the greater the potential for painful culture-clash. Through understanding the variety of reasons and expressions of culture-clash, of the consequences of a lack of a match between the values a child is receiving from his home and those he is receiving from his peers at school, from the media and other societal show-cases of its own norms, we can understand some very valuable things about the importance of congruence to an individual child's healthy development, but so far this does not appear to have been recognised: 'The fact that an individual's sense of identity depends not only on how the child's parents valued him or her, but also on how the parents were valued by society, is not acknowledged' (Ahmed 1989).

What appears to be significant is the congruence of the individual's cultural make-up with the dominant cultural behaviours and expectations. The more these match the more chances are of good enough functioning both for the child and her parents. The degree of congruence is affected not only by the individual's willingness to conform to the dominant culture but the willingness of the dominant culture to adapt and enable a good enough match to occur. By focusing on race or colour of skin (or indeed gender, disability, sexual orientation) there is a danger that the natural shifting of boundaries between the dominant and other cultures over generations does not take place and actually impedes the possibility of genuine sharing of valuable experience. The result can be that children and parents are handicapped in their own healthy development but also in the contribution they are able to make to the society in which they live.

WHAT THE ASSESSMENT OF BLACK PARENTS IN BRITAIN TELLS US ABOUT FIT PARENTS

Ideal

- There are absolutes in what childcare practices are best.
- Parents should conform to the psychoanalytically derived normative model of the nuclear family.
- Parental influence alone determines children's behaviour.
- Men and women play a unique and inviolable role in relation to their children.
- It is parents' duty and exclusive power to pass on their own culture and its values intact to their children.
- Effective child-rearing is dependent on the parents' continuous shared occupation of the same home.

Actual

- There exist a wide variety of childcare practices that children can thrive on but value judgements determine which any particular social group deems suitable to its needs.
- Cultural beliefs about fit parenting are dynamic in time and space.
- The skills deemed necessary to raise children will depend on the nature and complexity of the environmental and social demands to which both parents and children are exposed.
- Effective child-rearing is not inextricably linked to the parental occupation of the same household.
- Men and women can successfully play a wide variety of roles in relation to their own children depending on the cultural norms of their peer groups.
- Each culture invests different meanings in terms such as motherhood, fatherhood and childhood which may not be the same as every other culture but in the same society have more in common with other cultures than differences.
- Parents play an important but not exclusive role in guiding their children's absorption of other cultural values.
- Good parenting is made easier if there is a congruence between personal beliefs, beliefs of the family unit and that of the wider social groups. Absence of this congruence can be a stress factor to the lives of families.
- Class rather than race is the most important factor affecting parenting practices in a particular society.

16 Key themes from Part II

This examination of parents who are labelled deviant lays bare the cultural values of current western society and acts as a barometer of how those values have been shifting in recent times. What quickly becomes apparent when these groups are put side by side is that they are labelled on the basis of a single trait which is not the most significant one in relation to their parenting behaviours but which often becomes the main axis around which all assessment revolves. The arguments against most of them come down to the notions that both society and their children will suffer because a) the parents show a particular deviant trait, and b) they might become dependent on the state.

Why can't they be more like us? The pre-eminence of middle-class values

Throughout Part I it became clear that those of a lower socioeconomic status are scrutinised more by professionals with regard to their parenting and are more likely to be found wanting. In Part II I looked at many of the groups that are deemed unsuitable as parents and found that the majority fall outside the middle classes. It is significant that those from the middle class who display the deviant trait such as being gay, black, disabled, single or working mothers do not face the same stigmatisation as those from the lower classes.

As more of the middle classes enter the 'deviant' groups, they are beginning to openly question the assumptions that negate or devalue their own experiences with regard to their children and the stigmatisation is falling away. This is not the case for those groups which have not yet been colonised by the middle classes (e.g. parents with learning difficulties and middle-class parents are mutually exclusive by virtue of the distinguishing criteria: learning and intelligence and professional status).

If we look at the recurring characteristics of what is deemed necessary for fit parenting, i.e.:

- physical fitness
- education – in particular a shared knowledge base
- choice and control over one's life
- secure employment

- domestic permanency
- wide support networks
- congruence with the dominant culture

we see that these are precisely the attributes of the middle classes. If we look at the people who compose the groups considered least fit we see that they are the ones least likely to be able to fulfil these requirements. We live in a society which still disadvantages a large proportion of its population by discrimination in access to adequate housing, education and secure jobs. Society therefore creates an impossible catch-22 situation: you need to have a secure home and a secure job to have children; many people from the deviant groups cannot get these, therefore they should not have children.

> A family doctor in Norfolk, Dr Richard Wyndham, has proposed that child benefit payable to families on welfare 'should be reduced by a set amount every time a new baby is produced'. This revolutionary suggestion comes from his experience with one of the families on his books. 'They are six in all, two parents and four children. Their combined IQ, I guess, is just into three figures. The father cannot work because of his "bad back" but despite this, he seems able to copulate effectively as he has fathered a second family of five children by another lady in the city. He says he likes children.'
>
> (© The Telegraph plc, London, 24/1/93)

The overall impression is that all people on state welfare are lazy, immoral, stupid and irresponsible and therefore should be prevented from having children. People are thus only fit to be parents if they conform to middle-class values such as the need to be financially secure before having a few carefully planned babies – if you cannot be productive through employment you should not be productive in children either.

> If this no-hope family and the many like it produce no-hope children in the quantities they do, if they never make any contribution to society in which they live, and if each generation increases in near-geometrical progression as they seem to, how long can the chain letter of social security payments continue?
>
> (Reported by James Le Fanu, © The Telegraph plc, London, 24/1/93)

This article which first appeared in *General Practitioner* – a professional paper aimed at family doctors in the UK – stated openly a belief held by many but usually kept under wraps for fear of accusations of political incorrectness. It echoes the sentiments of Keith Joseph's speech nearly twenty years earlier (see p. 131). It is still essentially an issue of class but, like race, it is no longer acceptable for the professional classes to talk of the lower classes even if they continue to be treated as such. The solution he offers is not a revolutionary one – family planning policies all over the world have targeted the poor. Educated professionals are widely preferred as parents by the state (this is more explicit in countries such as Singapore where the state has long being actively encouraging professional women to marry and have more children, even to the extent of organising matchmaking holidays for professional singles).

What has also become evident in the course of Parts I and II is the conflict over how professional classes prescribe to and judge lower-class parents. And 'parents', as I have shown, largely means 'mothers'.

> In part the conflict results from the socially legitimated remit of sets of paid workers (health visitors, doctors, social workers) to oversee and modify mothers' childcare work; both their remit and their training indicate to them that their knowledge is superior to mothers'. But more fundamentally the problem lies in the power of the socio-political majority . . . to define and authorise knowledge.
>
> (Mayall 1991)

The above author identifies professional men as the culprits in this conflict but it appears to be a particular group of professional men whose beliefs and values are based on a very narrow experience of other walks of life and who are able to perpetuate a limited and academic knowledge base:

> In the case of childcare, knowledge consists of prescriptions backed with explanatory theories that a man may muster from a textbook. Men have been telling women how to do childcare for hundreds of years. But mothers' knowledge of childcare does not fit the male-stream paradigm; it is experiential, learned on the job, sensitive to the individual child's changing moods, growth and development, and subject to contexts surrounding mother and child. It is not reducible to generalisable prescriptions, based on universal psychological theories.
>
> (Mayall 1991)

What is normal?

Every culture invests different meaning to the events and processes it observes and what it therefore decides is normal and what is deviant. In western cultures the dominant framework through which parent–child relationships are observed has been the psychodynamic one. It is dominant in that it pervades the middle-class professional view of parenting which is all-influential – it has not necessarily been taken up by those with no time for, or interest in, intellectual frameworks, but they are none the less equally likely to be judged accordingly.

> Popular and professional adaptation of psychoanalytic ideas between the 1920s and the 1960s has led to some problematic developments in relation to gender, sex and sexuality. What has evolved is a normative view of the family, gender relations, masculinity and femininity and normal psychosexual development, which excludes and pathologises certain groups.
>
> (Wilson 1977)

The deviant parents' lack of compliance with what psychoanalytical theories have constructed as normal sexual and family relationships is taken to mean that this will invariably lead to suffering or deviancy in the children and so the parents are to blame for inflicting the deviance on them and causing havoc with the stability of society.

As we have seen, psychiatrists' and psychotherapists' views are regularly requested as expertise on normality and deviancy – but this expertise is based on a diverse range of theories, not a single body of proven or provable facts. It is a framework which can be very useful in certain contexts but as a body of expertise on what should be regarded as normal it does not stand up to much scrutiny.

The title of a paper I came across in my research was 'Patterns of attachment in two and three year olds in normal families and families with parental depression'. This was published not long after another piece of research which reported that a large proportion of mothers of pre-school children are depressed. If it is so widespread, how can it be abnormal? Again and again the term normal is used to describe the absence of a single criterion that has been labelled deviant by psychiatrists or social science researchers, and fails to acknowledge the contextual circumstances that affect parents' lives.

All of the groups have had a similar trajectory through time in terms of their public reception. To begin with they did not just feature as parents; when only a few existed there was widespread condemnation, but as numbers have increased more optimistic views of them as groups are beginning to emerge.

Poor-quality research

The poor quality of research to date makes it almost impossible to define the quality of parenting of the hitherto pathologised groups except to suggest that their label is in itself not indicative of their fitness to parent – good research should help ascertain how different types of parenting and family situation can work, so offering a broader range of solutions for everyone.

However, Part II further highlights the paucity of good research methods in the study of parenting. The starting point of research into all of the labelled groups has almost always been focused on what might be wrong with them and then ascribing any problems to the label, so there has been a tendency to confirm prevailing prejudices. I find I am now always trying to glean information about the background and values of the researcher so that I can put the research into some sort of perspective before I look at the findings. Should their own previous backgrounds and views not be made explicit in order to provide a fuller context for their judgement on others?

It would be easy to dismiss scientific attempts at understanding parenting as a task doomed to failure, given the complexity of the issues, but perhaps that would be rash:

Good science never promises certainty or consensus. Rather it promises a way of informing wisdom; it offers tools for refining controversy and for deepening our understanding of complex human endeavours. Because the study of consequential social problems is never easy or straightforward, researchers and practitioners need to ponder the uncertainties of field research, the nature of evidence and constraints surrounding the inferences permitted by a given body of data. If research has been found wanting what will fix it?

(Fein and Fox 1988)

I would argue that one of the key failings of most research into parenting to date is the failure of social scientists to involve their subjects, i.e. parents and children, in helping define the goals of the research. (Nearly all the studies ignore the role of children – yet there is good reason to believe that age, sex, position and temperament of children influence the quality of parenting that children receive.)

Too often the subjects are studied within unsuitable parameters by remote outsiders using questionable methodological and ideological principles – all of which fail to recognise the full range of the experiences and expertise of the people being studied. The resulting findings – because they have supposedly been produced by 'experts' – are then invariably used to further stigmatise the subjects of their research. Stigma caused by negative research findings further isolates those who have been scrutinised – I repeatedly came across examples of this in all the groups: mothers under stress who had to prove themselves to be doubly fit and so felt that they have to spend more on dressing their children well, paying for expensive toys or rejecting help so as to compensate for any perceived lack in them as parents.

There is a tendency to treat all such parents as guilty until proven innocent and to keep ascribing society's problems to their deviancy. But this has no basis in logic: you cannot prove that something is true by repeatedly saying it is true – however often you say it does not make it any more true. However, a single example which breaks the rule does, in logic, prove it to be false. We should be starting to recognise that there are many exceptions that disprove the rule that says gay/disabled/single parents cannot be fit parents. Once the rule has been thrown out, more useful information can emerge. In the past the rarity of parents from such groups ensured that the stigma kept them in check. They could not afford to stick their heads above the parapet and ask for approval, so remained invisible – and therefore the ones that disproved the rule could never be identified. Now there are too many parents from each of these groups to ignore their breadth of experience.

Little research has been done by people from the deviant groups – when it does happen it tends to be more positive and also reflect greater variety of experience. The need to value experiential accounts as much as, if not more than, quantitative and analytical research is often derided. But it is the only opportunity for hearing the full story unedited by the researchers' parameters and frameworks.

The importance of self-definition

It is only when members of those groups start speaking up for themselves that an important and distinctive view emerges: one which suggests that parents from all these groups have more in common with all parents than they have differences. But it is notoriously difficult for their voices to be heard: the groups which they come from – poor, black, female, young, old, gay – usually have little influence through the media or professional or academic literature. If you look back at the quotes I have used from the media it becomes apparent that the pathological views of the groups deemed deviant are found entirely in the (largely middle-class-controlled) channels of mass media and in the academic and professional media. The quotations reflecting the reality of being a parent in one of those groups comes largely from tiny-circulation, marginal and non-professional media which have little influence on the perceptions of the general population. This difference is very significant because it maintains an image of pathology rather than normality amongst the wider society but also specifically amongst professionals who are responsible for assessing those parents.

Accommodating difference

Much of the true picture has emerged despite the system rather than because of it. What it reveals is that many of the parents from the deviant groups do have specific difficulties and strengths but that these are obscured by the stereotypical labelling – either they are seen as all bad, or more recently, no different from anyone else. It is as if their differences are either over-magnified or ignored but never addressed properly.

It is not enough to suggest that every family needs to be treated simply as individuals. It is necessary to dispossess ourselves of the belief that there is only one way of looking at parenting by exposing ourselves in an open and learning way to the variety of other ways of being. The variety of self-help groups and voluntary organisations springing up in Britain are beginning to play a major part in getting recognition of parents from the marginalised groups.

Part II has shown that assumptions which are made about those regarded as abnormal act as a mirror reflecting back the values of the observer rather than providing useful information about those who are being observed. That is why it is so essential to evaluate those assumptions. The dominant cultural model is no longer one that reflects the reality of the majority of people's lives. Despite the ambivalence towards working mothers the model of normality has shifted to accommodate the fact that most mothers do return to the world of employment. They are no longer regarded as so abnormal – perhaps in time we will see the same accommodation of other groups presently considered deviant. Then, as with working mothers, perhaps we will begin to address the specific problems of parenting that they highlight for all parents.

In the meantime what this examination has revealed is how slowly the deeply entrenched bias against parents on the basis of age, gender, sexuality, sexual orientation, disability, race and class is shifting. My investigation strongly confirms that none of these factors in themselves preclude good-enough parenting, but the labels obscure the real problems: of poverty, isolation, poor role models, low self-esteem and the poor recognition of the worth of parenting. Yet it is not all a matter of problems. Their experiences also reflect a wide spectrum of success and fulfilment. What most of the deviant groups are doing is opening up the boundaries of family life and the boundaries between home and the outside world, between childcare and employment. All of these could provide much needed ideas for how to solve the many difficult problems facing children, parents and society today.

Part III

The job description

In this final part of the book I would like to attempt to put together the pieces of the jigsaw acquired in Parts I and II. A picture of what it is to be a fit parent in contemporary British society should thus emerge which may enable us to see if a job description could be drawn up to describe what a fit parent is supposed to do.

As we have seen, there are currently two models of fit parents implicit in the values of society and the criteria of those professionals involved in assessing parents. These are what I have termed the *Ideal* and the *Actual*. The Ideal Model appears to represent the values that society and professionals ascribe to how they believe most 'traditional' parents once were and how many would wish all modern parents to be. The Actual Model is the emerging reality based on the actual experiences of parents who do not conform to the Ideal Model as well as on more recent professional views and academic research concerning children's development in different family situations.

The examination of how parents are assessed has revealed as much about the relationship between parents and society as about the relationship of parents and children. I have therefore assembled the criteria in groups which relate to parents, parents in relationship to their children and parents in relationship to society. ('Society' is the term I have chosen to represent the totality of the influences outside the parent–child unit which determine the physical and social environment in which parents bring up their children – this includes the state, e.g. through its economic, education, welfare, employment, housing, transport policies; professional expertise; science and technology; religion; peer groups; the workplace; the media; and the local community of friends, neighbours and family services.)

17 The Ideal Model and the Actual Model of fit parenting

IDEAL MODEL

Parental characteristics

Those with a blood bond to the children are the fittest to be their parents.

Parents should love their children and naturally do what is in the best interests of each child.

Parents should conform as closely as possible to society's perceived norm of the traditional married couple and avoid eccentric behaviour.

Middle-class parents are better than those of lower educational and socioeconomic status.

Parents need to be healthy and without physical or mental disability.

People from different religious or ethnic backgrounds can only be fit parents if they can adopt all the dominant cultural attributes of western society in which they live.

Parents should lead morally virtuous lives.

Parents should have control over their behaviour.

Parents should be capable of putting their children's needs and happiness before their own.

Once a fit parent always a fit parent.

Parents should conform to the professional expectations of their behaviour with regard to their children.

ACTUAL MODEL

Parental characteristics

A blood bond with the child is neither necessary for fit parenting nor does it automatically result in fit parenting.

Parents' own personal histories are significant to their parenting styles and behaviours.

The gender, age, race, employment, class, sexuality, physical condition or intelligence of the parents are not in themselves indicators of the quality of parenting the children will receive.

Financial security and self-reliance are important but not essential.

Lifelong health cannot be guaranteed for any parent or child. While it may be desirable, it need not be essential to successful parenting.

Parents can be fallible.

Parents may need help to become good enough parents.

Self-knowledge, self-esteem and the respect of society help promote good parenting but may fluctuate over time.

Parents need to feel empowered in their own decision making regarding their child-rearing – not undermined by the expertise of professionals.

IDEAL MODEL	ACTUAL MODEL

Before becoming parents

Should conform to the dominant culture.

Should conform to society's expectations of normal-looking parents.

Should be over 20 and under 36 when they start a family.

Should be emotionally mature before becoming parents.

Should be financially secure before becoming parents.

Should be young enough to be able to cope with the physical demands of child-rearing and old enough to understand the responsibility it entails.

Should only have children if they are physically healthy and if they have no reason to expect a short lifespan.

Should do everything in their power to have healthy, able-bodied children.

Should recognise that children are a blessing, not an entitlement.

Should not want to have children as accessories or to fulfil their own unmet needs (e.g. for affection or acceptance in society).

Before becoming parents

People can successfully challenge dominant cultural expectations of parenting without harming their children.

Parents' physical health, emotional maturity and financial security are desirable but cannot be guaranteed at any age, so they may need support in their parenting.

There is a balance to be struck between the ideal time in terms of physical fitness and the ideal time in terms of emotional and economic readiness. If people believe they have made the choice at the right time for them it is more likely to be so.

People are themselves the best judges of whether and when to become parents and need accurate information to enable them to make informed choices. Society should play a more significant role in preparing people for parenting.

It is all right to have children to satisfy one's own needs if that means a greater commitment to the job of parenting. Becoming a parent is a normalising process and can be a valid means for personal rehabilitation.

Becoming parents

Conception of children should follow marriage and a period of setting up home.

Parenthood should be a carefully exercised choice, not an accident.

Parenthood is a biologically and socially constructed activity that begins with the marriage of a man and a woman and results from sexual intercourse between them. The baby is carried in the mother's womb until birth and is thereafter nurtured by her with the support of her husband.

A man and a woman need to have sexual intercourse to produce a child. This act leads to a pooling of genetic material to create a baby which gives those two people rights and responsibilities to that child as well as a natural bond.

Becoming parents

Parenthood may begin at any time: pregnancy, birth, after birth, in later childhood.

Social acceptance of an individual on becoming a parent – whether by accident or choice – helps good parenting, while censure can hamper it.

Becoming a parent is a socially created role more than a biological one.

Sex is not essential to procreation.

Providing the genes or womb does not necessarily confer responsibility for rearing the child.

Pregnancy and birth are desirable but not essential experiences of parenthood, nor are they necessary for a full bond with the child.

IDEAL MODEL

ACTUAL MODEL

The family unit is based on shared genetic material.

A fit mother nurtures her baby in pregnancy by not engaging in any harmful activity and consuming only substances that will promote the baby's well-being.

Women carry the sole responsibility for producing healthy babies.

Women should submit to the expertise of professionals to determine what is in the baby's best interests.

A family unit can be successful without genetic bonds between parent(s) and children.

There are no guarantees in life; disability and illness may affect children whatever the age, health or behaviour of the mother.

Promoting the health of a new baby is a desirable goal for every parent but also the responsibility of wider society (e.g. employers, food manufacturers).

Self-confidence and a sense of control over one's own life are important aspects of becoming good parents and caring for children's needs.

Parents' personal relationships and roles

Parents' personal relationships and roles

Should be two parents of opposite sex and sharing a sexual relationship.

A man and woman living together in a loving and supportive relationship are most likely to provide good parenting.

However poor the parental relationship, children's needs are best met if the parents stay together.

Effective child-rearing is dependent on the parents' continuous sharing occupation of the same home.

The parents' relationship should ensure continuity and stability in the daily domestic routines for their children.

A father's duty is to financially support the mother so that she can fulfil her duty to the home and to her children. The mother's duty is to support the father to be a good worker so that he can provide the family with both income and a good role model for his sons.

The mother is the best person to care for her children to ensure their physical and psychological well-being and their socialisation as future mothers. The father is the best person to socialise his children's aggressive behaviour and provide a role model for his sons as future fathers.

The existence and nature of a sexual relationship between parents is not necessarily significant to the child–parent relationship.

The quality of the parents' affective relationships is more important than the form of those relationships.

Ongoing conflict between parents may be more harmful for children than their parents' separation.

Effective child-rearing is not inextricably linked to the parental occupation of the same household.

Parents need to do their best to ensure as short a period of conflict/uncertainty as possible in the event of a break down of parental relationship.

Men and women can successfully play a wide variety of roles in relation to their own children depending on the cultural norms of their peer groups.

Men's and women's roles in relationship to their children can be interchangeable. Single parents may be preferable for certain children.

IDEAL MODEL

Parents in relationship to their children

Parents are solely responsible for how their children turn out.

Parents' care for their children determines their healthy development and protects them from physical danger.

Parents should conform to the psychoanalytically derived normative model of the nuclear family.

Parents should not place any emotional burden on their own children, nor should they expect children to help too much in domestic chores or in any physical care of parents.

A fit parent to one child would be a fit parent to any other child.

Caring for children should be a reward in itself.

Parents should put the security and future needs of their children before their own personal happiness.

Parents should not draw undue attention to their sexuality but should behave in such a way as to ensure that their children grow up to be heterosexual.

Children need two parents – no more and no less.

A mother who leaves her children to the care of others should feel guilty and a father who abandons his children's upkeep should feel guilty.

Even when parents are under stress they should put their children's needs first.

Parents have rights and duties to their children which are inseparable – when parents become old and frail, their adult children reciprocate by caring for them.

Parents are for ever.

Parents are constants in their children's lives.

Parents should follow professionally prescribed ways of childcare.

ACTUAL MODEL

Parents in relationship to their children

Parents alone do not determine children's behaviour or their adult outcome.

Children are active contributors to how they are parented – the age, health, personality, history of children as well as their other sources of support, determine how care-givers respond to them and affect how they turn out.

Children can receive successful parenting in a wide variety of non-conventional as well as conventional family and domestic situations.

Children are resilient creatures. However, the prevention of excessive emotional and physical stresses may require the help of outsiders.

A person may be more fit to parent one child than another. All parents and all children have some weaknesses and some strengths. Some adults may have more strengths than others which may make them more suitable for a wider range of children. Others may have a lot of weaknesses but just the right strengths for particular children.

The quality of care a child receives depends on the care-giver's behaviour which in turn is affected by the reward, conditions and training the care-giver receives.

It is preferable that parents place a high priority on their children's needs but these cannot be exclusive to their own needs.

Care-givers need to facilitate the development of a secure sexuality in their children whether they develop into hetero-, bi- or homosexual adults.

It is not the quantity but quality of parenting that is important to a child. Carers other than the mother can look after a child – what is important is consistency and responsiveness of care provided by both parents and other childcarers.

Parents need to try to provide stability, and reassurance for their children even when under stress, but they may need outside help to do this.

IDEAL MODEL

ACTUAL MODEL

Parents have responsibilities and privileges with regard to their children, not rights. In old age parents cannot depend on their children's care.

The parent–child role changes and evolves with time; in particular the closeness with different parent figures may vary.

Parenting requires continuous adjustment to external circumstances and to individual needs.

There exist a wide variety of childcare practices that children can thrive on.

Parents' skills

Mothers need to have instinctively and independently acquired the following skills by the time they have children:

Show affection, interest and trust in their children.

Provide adequately nutritious foods.

Organise daily household routines.

Make judgements about safety.

Provide reasonable and consistent discipline with minimal use of physical punishment and praise for child's compliance.

Control anxiety and anger in face of difficult or irritating child behaviours.

Recognise and respond to dangerous or high-risk situations.

Play responsively.

Make frequent positive remarks to child.

Be open to learning and developing.

Apply rules flexibly to meet their children's developmental needs.

Provide cognitive stimulation appropriate to their children's developmental stage.

Help with formal education of child.

Supervise homework.

Participate in school activities.

Fathers should have skills which enable them to keep the family self-sufficient and to discipline their children in what is socially acceptable behaviour.

Parents' skills

Parents' essential role lies in the moral, intellectual and spiritual guidance they give to their children throughout life, not in their physical skills of childcare.

Neither the mother's nor the father's physical skills are made explicit but may in any case be shared between a number of care-givers. The precise skills required depend on the complexity of the social and physical environment in which the parents live. For parents or other care-givers who are deemed inadequate, training by professionals may be required to teach e.g. running a home, organising daily routines, playing responsively, using appropriate discipline and having a knowledge of child development.

Parents' (or those acting in lieu of parents) essential role is to coordinate the involvement of as many different care-givers as necessary to ensure that children are adequately looked after.

IDEAL MODEL

Parents in relationship to society

It is the parents' duty – and not that of the state – to ensure their children's welfare.

Parents bring up their children in such a way that they are not a burden or threat to society.

Decisions relating to children are the responsibility of their parents.

Parents are for ever, but if they die or separate it is their responsibility to ensure that the children are cared for and do not require state help.

Parents should ensure a wide range of support networks in the community so as to minimise the vulnerability of their families.

Parents should conform to the dominant culture.

It is parents' duty and exclusive power to pass on their own culture and its values intact to their children.

Mothers and fathers have distinct and complementary roles in society – mothers to care for the vulnerable and to promote the well-being of their local communities, and fathers to work and if necessary fight to promote the wealth and security of the nation of which they are citizens.

Parents have obligations to produce children who fulfil similar roles in society to themselves.

Good parenting is made more possible by the recognition of its importance by society at large.

Good parenting is made easier if there is a congruence between parents' values, beliefs and practices with those of their peer groups and those of society at large.

ACTUAL MODEL

Parents in relationship to society

Parents share responsibility of raising children with society. Society at large plays an important role in how children turn out and how parents are able to care for their children.

There is a need for society at large to temper the myths of romance and parenthood with information about and support for the reality of adult relationships and parenthood. Society also has a responsibility to ensure that people have access to accurate information about the effects of their life-style on their children before they become parents.

Society may need to provide expert treatment and support to enable parents to provide good enough parenting. Parents under stress benefit most from help that is therapeutic, not judgemental.

Strong and varied support networks can make a big difference to the success of every parent. Society needs to help in the establishment and continued existence of support networks for families.

Parents may require training so that they can be seen to be good enough parents on the terms of the dominant culture but the dominant culture needs to adapt according to the needs of different groups within it.

Society plays a greater role than parents in guiding their children's absorption of cultural values.

Parents' roles are profoundly influenced by the social, physical, spiritual, economic and political environment in which parents and their children have to function.

Apart from obeying the law, parents have no explicit duties or obligations to society.

There are no clear guidelines about the roles children should play in society other than that they be law-abiding and self-sufficient when they grow up.

Good parenting is made more possible by the recognition of its importance by society at large.

Good parenting is made easier if there is a congruence between parents' values, beliefs and practices with those of their peer groups and those of society at large.

OBSERVATIONS ON THE IDEAL MODEL OF FIT PARENTING

The Ideal corresponds to what is commonly referred to as the 'traditional' family. The traditional family is seen by many as the essential unit of a healthy society: father, mother and children living in a lifelong mutually supportive and self-reliant unit. It is seen as the most productive economic unit: the father going out to work and paying taxes to the state, the mother's productivity in bearing and rearing children and caring for the weaker members of the extended family – so minimising the need for state support for anyone who cannot fend for themselves.

It represents the family as a very self-contained and closed unit within the confines of the home environment. Although the model of the nuclear family living in a home built for individual privacy stems from the eighteenth century, its particular attributes appear to stem from the 1950s when there was a widespread consensus over the role of state and individuals with regard to family life. This could be explained in terms of the post-war euphoria of having survived outside invasion and thus ushering in a time of turning inwards and rebuilding that which had come closest to being completely shattered: the family, the home, the country.

The sanctity of the home and traditional family life was reinforced at every level by the state's institutions: the Church, the Royal Family, professionals such as social workers and the emerging panoply of psychoanalytical perspectives. Full employment, the newly constructed welfare state and National Health Service, low rates of crime and a high degree of social stability all combined to support the traditional family and promote it to an all-time peak. The family became a very private institution enclosed within the four walls of the home – the Englishman's castle where his 'queen' dutifully performed her role as housewife and mother while the husband commuted to work, dutifully serving the nation in rebuilding industry. For the first time manufacturers focused on the family as a consumer unit, bringing in labour-saving devices and foodstuffs to reduce the burden of housework so that the mother could get on with the important task of raising happy and healthy children. The home came to represent all that was safe and secure.

Children and parents had mutual duties and obligations and so did wives and husbands. This closed and hierarchical pattern to family life was echoed by the state, institutions and the workplace. The paternalism and values (such as unquestioning respect towards authority, duty to one's family and to one's country, self-discipline, conformity) were seemingly reproduced at every level of mainstream life, producing a remarkable congruence between child, parent and state.

For those who could fit in within those very clear and rigid boundaries it was, on the surface at least, a time when families had never had it so good. For me, the picture it conjures up is one of three logs that have drifted separately and randomly along a river, coming together, tied by shared values and historical accident to produce a raft of stability – a platform for family life which simultaneously offered a course of least hardship to parents, children and society, but (and here's the catch) only for as long as they remained dependent on each other, fulfilling their mutual obligations. And for those who did not conform to those shared values there was no place on the raft. It was a time of harsh judgement for anyone who deviated from the strongly evident norms: unmarried mothers, gays, the new immigrants, all felt the full force of a united society's prejudice. The proscribed style of that period was noticeable in attitudes to class, race, gender and sexuality. People were expected to stick very closely within the norms of their own particular group be it working-class men or aristocratic women. There was little exchange between different groups except to fulfil specific obligations. Anyone who did dare to cross their group boundaries for any other reason was immediately pathologised, for example those few who dared to enter mixed-race marriages or reverse gender role division of labour. Deviancy from the norm resulted in very sharp retribution by immediate ostracism. The strength of societal stigmatisation demanded secrecy – any deviancy that emerged was kept forcibly under cover within the confines of the home and the family but, if this was not possible, the alternative was a total rejection of the individual who had contravened the norm.

Given these closed belief systems of the 1950s it was entirely appropriate that professionals (who were also operating in closed systems themselves) assessing parents could discriminate simply on the basis of non-conformity and behave in a paternalistic way towards those whom they were assessing, accountable to no one. Their values were entirely in keeping with those of state and family life of the time.

But this consensus did not last long. Mass conformity to a single model of family life could only be maintained as long as the dominant culture could remain homogeneous and sealed from other ways of being. As soon as the raft became even a little porous to external influences, cracks appeared and major channels of heterogeneity began to permeate the hitherto homogeneous facade. So what caused the cracks to appear? Returning to my metaphor of logs representing the needs of children, parents and society drifting along the river of time, over the ensuing decade the unified raft was to be buffeted with such intensity from all sides it was inevitable that it would come apart. Social, cultural, economic and technological trends operating during the 1950s all had built-in obsolescence as far as stability of traditional family life was concerned. Although these are too numerous to discuss here, some in particular stand out as having combined to ensure the most lasting effect on the break-up of that raft.

The promotion of the goal of personal happiness. Since psychodynamic ideas such as those espoused by Bowlby had been used to persuade mothers to nurture psychological well-being in their children, it was perhaps inevitable that the children raised under this ideology would expect personal happiness and fulfilment as a right when they reached adolescence and adulthood. The emphasis in western societies on children's entitlement to happiness has profoundly affected our view of how parents should behave and of how adults pursue their lives in search of personal fulfilment. The notions of duty, self-sacrifice and lifelong commitment have only a tentative hold on society today.

The media opened up the cracks from the outside by getting into people's homes in an unprecedented way. They played a critical role for those who were seeking a way out in showing other choices and legitimising the value of exploring those choices. Radio, the Press, advertising and television in particular brought new ideas and direct evidence of alternative ways of being with a new enthusiasm for consumerism, particularly from the USA whose economy was booming, unbattered by the effects of war, and thus had a head start on Britain in the emergence of its iconoclastic culture. The glamour and excitement of its music, films, products and ideas were rapidly being transferred around the world and found a ready audience amongst the young people who had grown up in the lacklustre conformity of post-war Britain. The media brought news of American social trends such as the rise of liberation movements representing Blacks, women, gays, and disabled people and thus began to uncover people whose voices had been stifled in the 1950s but who were no longer prepared to be ignored and excluded.

While society's cultural ethos had remained homogeneous, it could get away without defending its values – any heretics could quickly be silenced simply by ostracism. But as the number of heretics grew, this became impracticable. The media took over from the Church in guiding public opinion about morality and values, but unlike the Church they questioned everything and demanded scientifically based or logical answers. The media played an increasingly independent and less reverential role towards the great institutions of British life – for example, they were no longer willing to keep quiet about the misdeeds of public figures or the extramarital liaisons of royalty. Satirical television shows openly ridiculed public figures and created a climate of greater questioning. They were nonchalantly throwing open previously closed doors and asking the public to make their own judgements about what they saw – there could no longer be an automatic acceptance of the status quo.

The dominant culture had to defend itself and justify its values on the basis of logic. As we have seen in Part II, few stand up well to such scrutiny. Thus by the mid-to-late 1960s Britain was witnessing an increasing rejection of traditional institutions and values about family life and an inexorable move towards the more open and fluid belief systems which we see today.

The economic situation had also begun to change – conforming to traditional patterns of behaviour was no longer enough to guarantee a job. The cycle of strikes and economic recessions began again in the 1970s and created disillusionment about the state's ability to deliver its part of the deal to those who had conformed. The combined effects of socioeconomic changes, of the ingress of psychoanalytical ideas and of the impact of the media had profound effects on how people perceived their own parents and made it acceptable to question the validity of one's upbringing and if it did not result in personal happiness then the parents were clearly to blame.

They fxxx you up, your mum and dad

(Philip Larkin 1974)

If we look at most western societies today we would be hard pushed to find many parents who fit the Ideal Model for any significant period of their parenting lives:

divorce, poverty, isolation, lack of social support, unemployment, are so wide-spread as to make the Ideal a virtual fantasy. Yet it is a very powerful fantasy and one which informs most people's personal aspirations when embarking on parenthood or trying to cope with the consequences of the reality.

OBSERVATIONS ON THE ACTUAL MODEL OF FIT PARENTING

The Actual Model of fit parenting which is now emerging from the flux of the past thirty years is a more open and fluid one, with few clear-cut rules or boundaries. The vast majority of parents today are thus raising their children in very different circumstances to the ones in which they were raised themselves. Children are no longer guaranteed the care of either one or both of their bio-logical parents. The household is no longer the sole workplace for the job of parenting and a variety of individuals and state agencies may now be involved in sharing the parenting roles. Individual people are less stigmatised when they choose to pursue a particular form of family life because the norm from which they are supposed to be deviating is one that is being thrown out by so many other people that it cannot be enforced. Words that describe the Ideal Model such as duty, obligation, conformity, have been replaced with words such as needs, rights and personal choice in the Actual Model.

This Actual Model represents more accurately the reality of people's family lives today. However, as we have seen from Parts I and II, the tremendous inertia of the state and many institutions in their view of family life has produced a reluctance to adjust to the new reality for fear of encouraging it – they have remained closed while popular culture has opened up. As yet we do not have congruence between societal values and actual family lives. But it may well come as previous bastions of the Ideal Model of family life such as royalty and the middle classes fall prey to the same vicissitudes and flux as those of the less influential classes.

There are many potential benefits of the Actual Model: a less prejudiced society, more opportunity to focus on the aspects of child-rearing that really matter, a wider input which prevents child-rearing from becoming a suffocating and housebound activity – and perhaps a greater opportunity for personal fulfil-ment for a wider variety of people than has hitherto been the case. But these potential benefits will only become real if there is a recognition that the new trends need to be accommodated in a more imaginative way than at present.

18 Implications of the Actual Model of fit parenting to assessment

The more open system clearly demands a different approach to assessment of parents and children. While in the 1950s it was entirely appropriate to view parents as having sole charge of their children's future physical and psychological well-being and therefore simply to assess them, today the greater range of influences on children is being recognised and that means looking at what parents *do*, not who *they are*.

The previous sections emphasise the shift away from assessing *parents* to assessing *parenting*. The very terminology is significant; until recently all you had to do was to be a parent – it was a passive verb embodying a biological relationship. Now society requires us to *parent* our children – an active verb denoting conscious management of an activity. Modern society tends to compartmentalise all aspects of daily life that were once integrated: educating ourselves, earning a living, pursuing leisure activities, having sex, taking exercise, relating to partners, socialising with friends, parenting our children and so on. These are increasingly treated as mutually exclusive activities – unpicking the tapestry of our existence with the individual strands pulling us in different directions. We can thus no longer expect the activity of child-rearing to be automatically integrated into daily life. Once it has been separated off, it can be (and increasingly is) farmed out to people other than the biological parents.

Examining the open model of fit parenting entails not only looking at parents but also at the wider context in which the parenting is occurring:

- The child's age, personality, health and history (parents may be able to look after some children in a family but not those who are more demanding – e.g. premature or crying babies).
- The parent's background, upbringing, close relationships, health, income, life-skills and his/her expectations and understanding of children in general and of the particular child.
- The physical and social environment – secure and safe adequate housing, supportive networks, accessible transport, schools, employment, assistance with childcare, etc.

All three criteria interact and contribute to whether good parenting can take place. Yet most professional advice that parents receive (including that from childcare manuals) focuses on the parent–child relationship as if in isolation and as if it is the total responsibility of the parent.

As gene research reveals more about what factors affect children's responses to their environment, health and personality development, and social science and experience reveal more about the factors of the environment which determine how children turn out, perhaps society will treat them as more active participants in their own development rather than as passive recipients of whatever is thrown at them. We could then be fairer in our dealings of both parents and children: not trying to polarise their rights or needs as being mutually exclusive or inextricably tied to each other. Parents can no longer be seen as owners of children, solely responsible for moulding them as they choose. The view of children has begun to shift to see them as individuals with needs and rights – but it needs to go further to see them as making a significant contribution of their own.

This multifactorial approach to assessment is much more complex and requires a lot of information about factors that influence how children turn out, information that we do not yet have, in part at least because we have not bothered to look, having been so distracted by looking at the parents' deviancy. We need to know more about individual differences and mitigating circumstances that make one child more resistant to lasting damage than others. To do this we need to look at children who have emerged well at different stages and to see what they have in common but also to involve parents from a wide range of backgrounds to guide the focus of research – valuable expertise that is largely ignored.

What we would come up with is a system based on probabilities – not certainties. Some factors will emerge as more conducive to development and others as more risky. This would give those who are assessing parents a sounder base from which to work but would also provide information on how to promote better child-rearing amongst all those who become involved.

The need for a new framework

The new open system requires a different framework from the psychodynamic one that has predominated over the past half-century, one which acknowledges the general trends of the increased openness and fluidity of modern parenting that have been repeatedly identified in Parts I and II. Family life evolves according to external circumstances and the frameworks for understanding them need to do the same. For example, until this century, the religious framework was the one that determined how people's family lives were interpreted. This was entirely appropriate when the Church was central to people's lives. Similarly the psychodynamic framework was perhaps an appropriate tool for interpreting family life when and where the nuclear family was central to people's lives. But the lifelong nuclear family is no longer the source of all support so the value we attach to the family unit is changing – all this now has to be thrown into the mix when assessing parents. In constructing a new framework we need to look at what is now central to people's lives – what has replaced the Church and the nuclear family?

From Parts I and II three main indicators of successful parenting emerged: self-esteem, support networks and socioeconomic status, so it seems appropriate to see whether they provide any pointers towards a new framework.

Self-esteem

If we look at self-esteem and how it arises it is striking how it is related to feeling that you have a respected and accepted role as part of a wider group of people. For many non-western cultures this comes from being a part of a large family group and having a well-defined role and life course through it. In western cultures, smaller families and houses long ago demoted the extended family group as a source of status for the majority but this was replaced by other socially coherent groups brought together by beliefs (i.e. through the local church) and activities. Churches no longer have that magnetic pull and the only surviving major source of lifelong group participation has been employment. Having a job in a paternalistic organisation that paid money but also promised lifetime security and rewarded loyalty and years of service by progressively increasing status replaced the family group as a source of self-esteem first for men and, by the 1970s, increasingly for women. As citizens, we have become valued for the jobs we hold, not for the families we nurture and guide.

Support networks

Greater social mobility and greater participation in the workplace by men and women away from their homes has taken its toll on the availability of social support networks, and the state is paying the cost. The importance of support from the wider society that has appeared again and again is clearly critical to the success of producing children who value and are valued by others. Yet the growing division between the world of work and local community has eroded the traditional sources of such support. This suggests the need for a concentrated effort to reknit the increasingly threadbare fabric of community life with that of the world of work, to turn the disintegration of the cohesion of family life into a new integration. The state needs to support this not just through new employment practices but other social groupings which bring people together over long periods of time and build a sense of mutual dependency. The solutions must lie in a greater opening up of the boundaries between work and family life.

Socioeconomic status

Lack of adequate income is the single most important deterrent to the adequate provision of basic physical childcare needs: food, shelter and security. But it is also a powerful factor in eroding emotional and psychological well-being for the parent and the child for it signifies a lack of status and control. The socio-economic status of a family is determined by the parents' access to jobs whose conditions and rewards make them accessible to all who are willing and able to work. At present there are large numbers of people who work too much – men in particular whose attachment to their work has marginalised them as fathers. But, as we have seen, there are still large sections of the parent population who cannot work – either because employers won't give them the opportunity, or because they do not have the right qualifications for the jobs available, or because they cannot find suitable childcare. Yet it is precisely these parents whom the state is forced to support through welfare payments, to an extent which is rapidly becoming unmanageable.

The solutions to these imbalances are political but require a greater consultation with those who are presently marginalised but doing the most important job of all – raising the next generation whose economic productivity will pay for the pensions of the present generation. In the absence of spiritual and moral convictions, this is the most powerful argument of all for supporting the job of parenting, raising its status and conditions so that people can do it well.

The relationship between employment and parenting

During the course of writing this book I have become very interested in the parallels between parenting and employment: the similarity in the tasks facing employers and employees and parents and children in terms of obligation, development and serving a due to society. The availability of employment and the nature of employment practices closely define and are defined by parenting practices.

For example, we have seen over the past century an interesting parallel between the nature of employment ideologies and parenting ones – e.g. like the Victorian parent, the Victorian employer was answerable to no one but himself. Gradually the state became more involved through legislation to protect employees and to help industry. In the 1950s and early 1960s the heyday of full employment parallels the heyday of the traditional nuclear family with its clearly defined hierarchical roles. There was consensus about the type of self-disciplined and compliant worker who was required for the production line or bureaucratic work. The state took a very paternalistic role towards industry (e.g. through nationalisation) and its citizens (the establishment of the Welfare State); employers similarly took a very paternalistic role – employers had a duty to their workers for lifelong employment and had to conform to the expectations laid down. The more or less reciprocal arrangement of duty and obligation was paralleled in parenting practices – between fathers and mothers, and between parents and children.

Since the 1970s we have seen an inexorable decline in the success of traditional models of employment and also of traditional parenting. More and more, it is personal happiness and satisfaction that we seek through both our jobs and our roles as parents. Labour-intensive industry has been eroded to the point of virtual extinction, completely upturning the foundations of working-class family life. There has been a major shift away from work that involves simply labour to work that is based on information management and personal skills. Currently the bureaucratic middle-class enclaves are being subject to the most massive reorganisations since they came into existence – the media, civil service, the law, the health and welfare systems, all are attempting to become more open, accountable and 'customer-led'. There is at present a lack of clear direction to those who want to work, with an accompanying erosion on the part of employers to any lifelong commitment to their employees. And so it is for parents and their children.

The lack of clear obligations noted in the Actual Model of fit parents has far-reaching consequences on the sort of employees parents and society are now producing. Novelist Fay Weldon recently described what she termed her 'open fridge door' style of child-rearing by which her children (and most of their generation) have been raised: to be able to eat when and what they choose, to come and go as they please and not have to adhere to rigid timetables or to comply unquestioningly to authority. It is not surprising as these young people now approach their twenties that they are unemployable in most of the traditional nine to five jobs. Increasingly they look for jobs in which they can do what interests them and not just what someone else wants them to do.

For those who find such jobs or are able to create their own, there may be satisfaction, but for an increasing number there will be disaffection and long periods of unemployment. Yet the type of workers needed now is different from the 1950s. There is a call for more self-starters with a wide range of transferable skills including creativity and adaptability, for those who can create jobs, not just await them. The sort of parenting and education available to children of today needs to match the new job environment.

What is absent is any clear vision of the state in its expectations of parenting. I would suggest that the vision could be the same as it appeared to be in the heyday of the traditional nuclear family: to produce a platform for family life that brings greatest benefit to all citizens and to the state in which they live.

By making the vision clear we can see that the role of the state is very significant in achieving those objectives for the job of raising the next generation. The similarity with recruitment and selection for a job may offer a useful framework for how to pursue the assessment of parents in the new climate.

But is parenting a job?

I started this book by saying I was interested in trying to find out whether there exists a job description for parenting – it is increasingly being treated as a job that may or may not be done by biological parents. Throughout the book I have noted the occurrence of parallels between the selection of parents and the selection of employees. Parents fulfil a role for society in producing its future workers and as such they act as employees of the state and managers in relationship to the children.

The Ideal Model constraints of duty and obligation – of parents to children, of children to parents, of parents to society and of society to parents – have crumbled away. The result is that there no longer exist any clear guidelines as to what is required – of individual children, parents or of society. And yet, precisely because of the greater number of people and places involved, there is even more reason to have clear guidelines so that the 'shared responsibility' does not become an abandoned responsibility. What is missing for parents today (and interestingly, for those who are assessing them) is a clear job description.

That most parents and those assessing them are doing their respective jobs well enough is suggested only by the fact that most do not come under scrutiny – not because we have any clear idea of what they do. Both are undermined in their effectiveness by lack of clear objectives. For example, there are many similarities between parents and social workers:

- Professionalisation of what was previously a vocational and intuitive role.
- Anxiety in the face of an increasingly complex and demanding job.
- Risk assessment of their charges.
- Lack of clear guidance from society.
- Lack of wider support and agreed knowledge base.

As more and more other people become involved (be they foster parents, child-minders, nursery staff, step-parents, local authority professionals) the need for an explicit description of what is required becomes even more critical.

It is only in recent times that the role of the manager in an organisation has been recognised as one that requires specialist training and an identifiable knowl-edge base. In the past it was just something that you picked up – just like parenting. Yet, because virtually anyone can become a parent, parenting con-tinues to be seen as an unskilled job requiring no formal qualifications or expertise. This was perhaps appropriate in the days when children's welfare was seen as less important but also when the complexity of the external environment did not require such sophisticated management skills or detailed knowledge base.

As with a manager, the parent's role is to provide leadership and guidance so as to achieve a complex task. This requires sophisticated skills: dealing with conflicting demands, managing budgets, assessing risks and thinking ahead, problem solving in a wide range of situations, assessing complex information, making judgements about the contributions of outside experts, managing a team of people through life's ups and downs and so on. All these are skills which can be developed – as the burgeoning field of management training suggests.

The parallels between the job of parents and managers are becoming more obvious in the light of the new developments towards a more open management ideology that underlies the notion of what has become known as *Total Quality Management*. Their essential role is no longer that of supervisors, policing their employees' timekeeping and conformity to the organisation's rules about how to do things. Managers instead are seen as facilitators creating the environment in which the employee can develop the skills to be able to address any problem that arises independently and effectively. Prevention, not detection of poor-quality performance, is seen to be the key and continuous development is seen to be the ultimate goal (Wilkinson *et al.* 1992). Compare this with the facilitating environment that Winnicott (1964) described as being provided by good enough parents for their children and think too of how the state as a 'manager' to its 'employees' (parents) can facilitate an environment which aims for excellence through continuous development of all its citizens.

The new organisational framework addresses parenting not simply in terms of the parent–child relationship, but also of the relationship between children and society, and of that between parents and society.

Children and society

The first step to understanding the job of parenting is to ask what the general objectives are for a society in relationship to its children. Looking at cultures around the world we see that there are an array of general objectives which appear to be universal (see Figure 18.1).

The specific objectives vary from culture to culture, e.g. education may mean teaching children to read and write; it may also mean teaching children to tend sheep or fetch water. The age at which different skills need to be developed also varies – for example, development of independent living skills varies enormously according to the environmental demands and social norms of each culture.

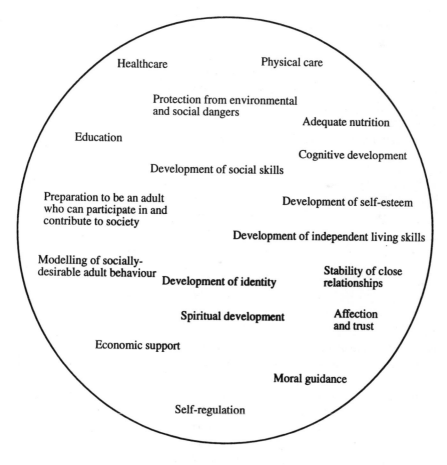

Figure 18.1 General objectives for the job of parenting a child

In Britain, we need to promote a public debate about the objectives of raising children for both society and parents. To some extent there is already an attempt to make explicit the objectives of education (hence the development of the National Curriculum), and healthcare has also been addressed the same way (e.g. inoculations and developmental tests). But what is needed is a much more wide-ranging debate about the values and skills associated with child-rearing. I believe it is important to look at these in terms not just of what children's needs are but of what society's needs are of the adults who those children will become.

At present there is a worrying trend towards greater sentimentalisation of children. Everyone talks with great fervour about the pre-eminence of the rights and interests of children without acknowledging why or how it is to be achieved. The growing use of pathetic pictures of abused or neglected children by children's charities to raise money for their care is an interesting example of this. As with black people and disabled people in the past, such charity images underline their inferiority and difference when what they need is an acceptance of their equality and importance to society. 'Rights Not Charity' is the phrase used by the disability movement. The right is to be respected as an equal member of society – not as an inferior one but nor as a more important one. This can only be made clear by looking at the duties and expectations of children (as future adults) and recognising their importance to fulfilling the needs of society. At present they seem to serve no useful purpose other than (possibly) to bring their parents some emotional reward and so charities can only appeal to people's pity. Society needs to be reminded of the value of children. It can then be more clear-headed about what it requires parenting to achieve.

The following might form a basis for debate.

Duties of society (through government, statutory policies and services, and through the media):
- To provide democratic leadership that represents the views and needs of all its citizens.
- To ensure national and domestic security.
- To promote economic prosperity.
- To promote a safe environment.
- To endorse and support the task of child-rearing by valuing those who undertake it.
- To provide moral guidance and to model desired behaviour.

Duties of all those undertaking parenting roles:
- To protect and nurture children until an agreed age.
- To contribute to the economic prosperity of the nation.
- To abide by the law and contribute to the security and safety of the environment.
- To model desired behaviours as agreed and modelled by society.
- To teach certain agreed skills.

Duties of children:

- To contribute to family and community life in ways appropriate to their age and talents.
- To abide by the law.
- To aim for an adult life in which they contribute to their families, communities and humanity.

Addressing the duties of children forces us to examine the issues of children's rights and parents' rights in a more equitable way.

Parenting and society

Parenting is the job done by members of a society to bring up the next generation who will ensure the society's perpetuation. In this broad way the job is the same everywhere in the world but the ways in which it is carved up and shared out vary enormously from one culture to another. What has varied in time and space is who does the job – how many people and in what relationship to each other and to the child.

In the Ideal Model (Figure 18.2) the job description for mothers, fathers and society is self-evident and the boundaries between their respective roles clearly defined. In the Actual Model (Figure 18.3) the job may be shared at different stages in a wide variety of ways through childhood and amongst several different people but without a clear statement of the obligations or expectations of different parties involved, or of who is in charge of coordinating their efforts as a team. The danger for many children is that there are aspects of the job that may not be done at all or done inadequately either because no one knows what they are supposed to be doing or because they are unable to since they do not have the resources and/or skills.

The answer would appear to be to analyse the job of every person involved in relation to each child. What competencies do people need to have – which skills and knowledge are required to fulfil their objectives? What resources and training do they need? What set of performance indicators can be used to track and measure whether the objectives are being achieved? This new language of the workplace – which will be familiar to many professionals and academics reading this book from their own current work environments – may seem cold and inappropriate to something as complex and supposedly intuitive as parenting, yet just as the psychodynamic models of family life have until now directed our approach to parenting by focusing on the family as a closed unit, this framework may provide a useful model for the new open style of fit parenting that is now emerging. Of course, frameworks should simply be a tool for greater understanding and support of families, not a means to erect walls that exclude and pathologise certain groups (as both the religious and psychodynamic frameworks have done).

The literature on employee selection provides some very useful pointers in how to go about developing a job description for people undertaking any aspect

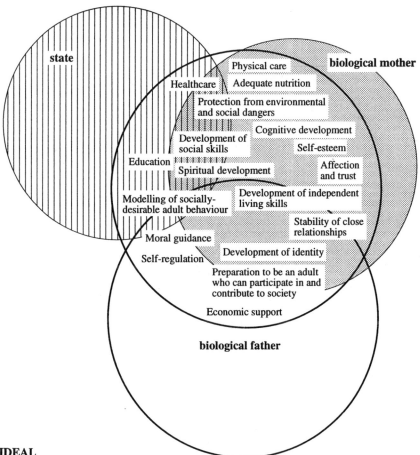

IDEAL

Involvement limited to small socially-prescribed team with clearly defined
boundaries between them as to who is responsible for achieving the different
objectives of parenting. This diagram shows the unique configuration which
remains stable throughout childhood.

Figure 18.2 Ideal Model

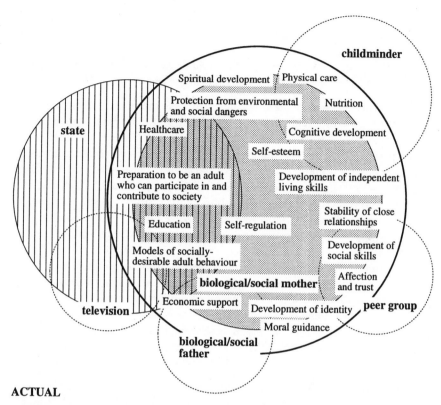

ACTUAL

Multiple involvement but unclear boundaries between the various people as to who is responsible for achieving the different objectives of parenting. This diagram shows just one example. Many variations are likely during course of childhood.

Figure 18.3 Actual Model

of the parenting task. As we have seen, there have been some attempts by psychologists and social workers to do this but these appear to have suffered from being too partial in their approach – concentrating solely on the needs of children for example, or in danger of being too reductionist in their final form. This is exactly the same sort of problem facing those involved in traditional approaches to employee selection.

Note for example the following in the light of the various procedures used by professionals in the assessment of parenting at present:

> It is possible to follow the procedure, but miss the point. 'Identify the job; understand its important features; and recognize the relevant human aspects of its successful performance' can easily become 'Take a job title; list its components; and itemize the characteristics of an acceptable candidate.' If this is the case, important elements of the analysis have been omitted. These are the ones that give the selector the 'feel' for the job. Questions that need to be answered such as 'How is the job more than just a collection of tasks?', 'What do incumbents actually like and dislike about it?', 'Are we willing and able to develop the shortcomings in otherwise good candidates?' remain unresolved.
>
> In essence this is a warning against the over-mechanistic approach to job analysis. A highly structured and detailed form on which job/person specifications are drafted can produce this effect. Filling in the form accurately can become the overriding objective rather than conveying a real understanding of the job. Also the problem can arise if those writing the specifications are different people from those who will be using them to make selection decisions.
>
> (Lewis 1985)

Some recognition has already been made of the dangers of undefined objectives being shared out amongst many people. For example, a recent panel of highly respected professionals came together to develop what could be described as a framework to assess whether the requirements of children in local authority care are being met (Parker 1991). They addressed the very relevant problem of how to ensure that the numerous carers cover all the children's needs between them and proposed a formal ongoing monitoring of such children and their needs with specific reference to who was responsible for addressing these needs.

Various attempts are currently being made to define what constitutes high-quality day care:

> Perhaps it is more useful to proceed by dropping the term 'quality' or agreeing to use it specifically in relation to promoting children's cognitive, language, social and emotional development. In its place, or supplementing this specific definition, we can refer to objectives; a good daycare setting would be one which achieved its agreed objectives. The task then becomes to define objectives for day care (which may cover a potentially wide range of aims concerning children, parents, the local community, and so on), and to use research

skills to understand how best to achieve defined objectives as well as to develop methods for monitoring the achievement of objectives.

(Hennessy 1992)

This author has clearly recognised the need for wider objectives but still sees them relating only to day care, not the overall care of children.

Yet all these attempts, while laudable, are incomplete and doomed to only partial success in the absence of a clearly defined societal goal as to what the desired objectives for all children should be. The value of making such objectives openly known is so that everyone would have knowledge of them before they became parents. The role of professionals would be made easier and less subject to the vagaries of individual opinion on what constitutes fit parenting and the 'hiring and firing' of parents would become less arbitrary.

The following Job Analysis Checklist (adapted from Lewis 1985, p.110) may help in understanding the nature of the job as well as for drawing up an accurate job description.

Job title	
Job context	
Main duties	
Most difficult duties	
Most distasteful duties	Job description
Features of the work	
Features of the workplace:	
a) Physical	
b) Social	
Criteria used in evaluating performance	
Attainments	
Aptitudes	
Physical requirements	Person description
Personality characteristics	
Interests	
External constraints	

- *Job title* – e.g. foster parent, step-parent, childminder.
- *Job context* – how does the job relate to other jobs that are connected to it (e.g. to that of another parent-figure, social worker, teacher, etc.)?
- *Main duties* – a list of duties can be compiled by looking at other people doing similar jobs and analysing the specific requirements of the particular child in question. These duties need to be detailed – particularly if there is a large number of other people involved. So these might include monitoring the health of the child (talking to the doctor, ensuring inoculations, etc.), and

supervision of education (taking child to school, helping with homework, meeting child's teachers). For each child the duties may need to be weighted in order of importance.

- *Most difficult duties* – these need to be examined together with the applicant so that it becomes self-evident where extra support or training might be necessary. So if, for example, a child needs intensive physiotherapy every day, could the applicant do this?
- *Most distasteful duties* – again, these can be suggested by others doing similar jobs and matching these to the individual applicant's own feelings about particular aspects of the job in question. An example for many substitute parents may be maintaining contact with birth parents. If this is identified then it lays open the possibility of discussing how to handle such aspects of the job.
- *Features of the work* – this is an opportunity to identify any unusual or unexpected aspects of the job. An example might be that the child requires a weekly visit to a hospital for treatment on a long-term basis.
- *Features of the workplace* – physical and social aspects of the conditions under which the job will be taking place. This might mean considering the home circumstances of a parent after divorce, or the venue for weekly access visits, or the conditions of a nursery. The social aspects would include the nature of other people in the workplace such as other adults and children, and their relationship to each other in relation to the person proposing to do the job.
- *Criteria used in evaluating performance* – the performance indicators need to be shared with the applicant so that they are able to assess how they are doing themselves and how to improve their own performance in relation to the job.
- *Attainments* – what skills, knowledge and experience does the candidate have already which are relevant to the job in question? Thus an applicant with prior experience of looking after children, or experience of working under difficult conditions, may have specific resources to bring to the job.
- *Aptitudes* – what competencies do they display which show that they are capable of development or training for the job?
- *Physical requirements* – age, sex and physical abilities may be relevant to recruitment for certain jobs, e.g. caring for a very small baby or an older disabled child who needs frequent lifting. It is critical to evaluate the specific requirements of the job – not to say that this aspect of the job can only be done by someone who is a strong young man. Candidates would then have the opportunity to discuss how they would envisage managing the particular physical requirements and to what extent they might need special equipment or help with specific tasks.
- *Personality characteristics* – again this is in danger of abuse if not related specifically to the child's job requirements. It is intended as an opportunity to examine enduring traits such as outgoing personality, being open to the ideas and suggestions of others – which may be specifically useful to the child's circumstances.
- *Interests* – outside interests can point to useful skills and opportunities for the

child. So being a Sunday school teacher or an amateur football player or a poet may all offer specific children just what they need to develop their own interests and sense of belonging, but also point to sources of support for the parent.

- *External constraints* – what external constraints must the candidate be free from? For example, having other employment which would take him away from this one for long periods or care of other children which would detract from the needs of the one under consideration. (We have already seen the growing recognition of the single person as a foster parent – free of the external constraint of a competing adult relationship.)

To compile such a job analysis would require the participation of parents who are doing a similar job already, but also the development of a knowledge base about the factors that indicate when the job is being done well. As we have seen in Part I, there is some existing knowledge in this area which may need to be re-evaluated in the light of this new framework and then developed further. One of the key aspects of new research would be to look at children who are successfully achieving the objectives laid down by society and to examine the nature of their parenting and environment and individual traits. We could then build up a body of knowledge on what constitutes effective parenting – not who makes a good parent.

While the process could start now it has to be recognised as one which will be continuously refined as new knowledge becomes available. At present we do not have a sufficient knowledge base from which to establish accurate performance indicators. What is needed is a serious attempt at data collection across the whole population rather than an assortment of biased and misleading information about a few unfairly targeted groups. There may be a case for looking at large numbers of children in a few particular geographical districts and following their progress closely – monitoring them against a wide range of criteria such as birth circumstances, family, income, parental occupation, health and sexuality, support networks and so on. Parental skills such as coping with stress, managing anxiety, negotiating, assessing products and services for their children could all be correlated. The task is a complex one but with information technology it is certainly feasible – if the public could be persuaded to participate. To do this it is vital that it be seen as a collaborative process which not only observes and analyses but is supportive.

There would be a value in setting up some form of national institute to address these issues:

1 To collate and assess existing information from whatever sources that exist – this means looking at any field of expertise that might pertain to the understanding of child-rearing.
2 To guide new research and vet its methodology.
3 To gather and impart accurate information on what constitutes desirable parenting and what risks are associated with undesirable parenting – while remaining open to its dynamic nature.

4   To organise a wide-ranging debate on what underlying values the state is trying to promote.
5   To help formulate a set of objectives which would form a part of a contract between state and parents as to what care and education children need to have.
6   To work with state departments such as social services, education, health and employment to ensure the best use of resources to fulfil the state's side of the contract and to support parents in fulfilling theirs.

Many would shy away from the idea of a centralised body producing edicts on what parents should be doing. That is why it is so important that it is a two-way process: not just to address what parents need to do but what the state needs to do as well – above all it needs to be responsive to the input of ordinary people, not just experts.

The importance of such work is that it may be the first attempt to recognise problems before they become unmanageable. As a society we cannot continue to leave parenting to chance – an increasing number of families are going to become dependent on the state if action is not taken to address the underlying changes that have already taken place. But more importantly such measures would be a very practical recognition of the need to invest in society's most important resource: its citizens.

Using the job analysis

There are two ways in which I can see such a job analysis of parenting being of use.

1   To direct the state's policies with regard to family life. Once the value of children has been acknowledged as central to the future stability and prosperity of a society, then the fundamental aim of government policies would need to shift away from the current marginalisation of children and the job of parenting.
2   The second would be to use the job analysis as a basis for the selection, assessment and training of anyone who wishes to undertake any aspect of the parenting job. This includes all prospective parents but also people such as childminders, childcare staff, social workers and foster parents, grandparents, step-parents and so on.

The experience of employee selection parallels much that professionals assessing parents are being asked to do:

• To predict the future:

> You look into the future to see what sort of employee behaviour is necessary and judge how well applicants perform in terms of this required behaviour. Selection is largely a prediction business.
>
> (Lewis 1985)

• To acknowledge the paramount necessity for unambiguous selection criteria.
• To incorporate a commitment to equal opportunities in the selection procedures and criteria.

If the objectives were explicit and widely accepted, society could be more relaxed about the variety of ways in which they might be achieved. We would no longer worry about whether two men make better parents than a man and a woman but look instead at whether the child was being ably cared for by indicators that could be measured. The competencies needed for the particular job under consideration (e.g. fostering a child with special needs) could be matched up to the applicant's set of particular competencies. These might cover such areas as dealing with unpredictability, ability to work in a team and so on. Past attainments (such as already having fostered a child with special needs) would be taken into account. Aptitudes (such as a willingness to develop one's own knowledge base) would be considered. The final selection would thus be based on more clearly defined criteria – ones which would leave the applicant in no doubt about the nature of the job requirements. And the job appointment would not be the end of the matter. In-service training and ongoing support may be critical to some parents depending both on the needs of the job and their own needs. In the past, just as with managers, the need for training was never recognised (except perhaps as a resource for those who were failing). In the new, more complex environment, it is increasingly being realised that all parent-figures can be offered tools to enhance the quality of the parenting, not just to correct incompetence.

The parenting-as-a-job framework might also be a sounder basis for refusing people the option of, or continued involvement in, a parenting role. The notion of licensing parents has been provocatively put by the philosopher Hugh LaFollette. Licensing parenthood has been proposed on the basis that society regulates other potentially harmful activities and so, just as we accept that drivers and doctors need to be trained and regulated before being let loose on the public, so we should with prospective parents.

> A parent must be competent if he is to avoid harming his children; even greater competence is required if he is to do the job well. But not everyone has this minimal competence. Many people lack the knowledge needed to rear children adequately. Many others lack the requisite energy, temperament or stability . . . . Consequently there is good reason to believe that all parents should be licensed.
>
> (LaFollette 1980)

It is an idea that I suspect (as with licensing social workers) will gain increasing currency in years to come, so is worth looking at in the light of the parenting-as-a-job framework. It appears that unlike driving a car, parenting is very specifically related to the individual child being parented and the social and physical aspects of the workplace. So the licensing procedures would have to be tailored to recognise this. But there are other factors to be considered.

At present, as I have shown, there is already arbitrary licensing of parents and prospective parents by the variety of selection procedures and ideologies that they are put through by the regulatory professionals.

No one is allowed to adopt a child until administrators can reasonably predict that the person will be an adequate parent. The results of these procedures are impressive. Despite the trauma children often face before they are finally adopted, they are five times less likely to be abused than children reared by their biological parents . . . . Consequently if we think it is so important to protect adopted children, even though people who want to adopt are less likely than biological parents to maltreat their children, then we should likewise afford the same protection to children reared by their biological parents.

(LaFollette 1980)

How much more effective would any such licensing process be if it were based on a clear statement of the objectives, and candidates were able to share the body of knowledge on which the competence tests were based? Furthermore, if they did not get a license then there would be an opportunity to appeal and re-apply after getting the necessary training or after a change in personal circumstances. Licensing seems like a radical option but it would encourage more societal consideration of the importance of training all those responsible for any aspect of the child-rearing job and for evaluating the skills that make parenting more likely to succeed.

If it can be established that a person is incapable of doing any part of the job effectively or safely then it would be necessary to consider how much formal training and support they might require to be able to do the job better. If some candidates were still to fail, it would then be appropriate to refuse them a license. It would not be a matter of saying you are a good or bad person (as at present), just as failing a driving test does not label the driver a good or bad human being. For this sort of assessment there would need to be a clear evaluation of the role society – the community and relatives, as well as the state – would play in supporting a parent who cannot fulfil the agreed objectives.

Frisch (1981) suggests that societies should operate licensing systems only if there is reason to believe that the licensing process will exert some control over specific risks; in the field of parenting he believes that this would not be possible. He identifies the categories of risk as those arising out of ignorance, arising out of physical or mental incapacity, from wilful misconduct, through negligence or inability to exert self-control. Risks associated with ignorance could be minimised by more explicit training and information related to the agreed objectives. Risks associated as arising out of physical or mental incapacity could be minimised by ensuring adequate social support of parents. But risks arising out of wilful misconduct or negligence are more difficult to minimise – unless the societal culture has shifted to ensure that shared values about what constitutes appropriate child-rearing have been agreed.

The trends in adoption procedures suggest that the way to pursue the notion of licensing is not as a process of policing but as a therapeutic tool which empowers people and helps them understand the job as it relates to their individual circumstances and the particular children involved. I cannot envisage licensing of parents being fair to parents or children unless the general culture were changed to be more supportive of childrearing.

Most of those who would not deny the sense of licensing childminders or residential social workers (which is now beginning to happen) might balk at the idea of parents being licensed to care for their 'own' children. Yet, while a biological relationship between a parent and child is obviously relevant, if that person cannot fulfil the agreed objectives, then in a society that recognises the rights of children, it cannot be reason alone for allowing a parent to continue in the job. If we recognise that a number of adults and statutory authorities are now sharing what was traditionally regarded as the biological parents' role, it is no longer unjustified to question parental authority. The recent spate of well-reported cases of children 'divorcing' their parents suggests that children's right to having a say in how and where they are brought up is being recognised by the courts. Those rights to do as one pleases with one's children have been eroded over the course of this century and appear to be doomed to being discarded completely at some point in the not-so-distant future. Just as with women and slaves in the past, equality of rights is not compatible with being owned by someone else.

This is a problematic development only if the objectives are not clear – children should not be given any more rights to happiness than any other citizen, but they should certainly be offered the same scope for personal development and to become contributing members of society as everyone else. At present they remain, like other marginalised groups, subject to more talk about rights than action.

My conclusion is that while licensing parents is not an appropriate response as long as its primary aim is to prevent potentially incompetent parents, if it were to be done in a society which promoted continuous development in all its citizens, the job analysis and performance indicators could be used to ensure the effective care and support for both children and the people who were involved in their development. If we want a society in which we wish parents to raise healthy children with high self-esteem and who care about others we need to ensure that their parents are treated the same way by professionals and society – that means all statutory services should follow the model of fitness that parents are expected to fulfil. That means professionals feeling well-supported, valued and working in conditions which encourage openness to learn and taking a pride in the quality of service they provide. There is no value to having professionals who are battered by their own bureaucracies in charge of battered parents of battered children. The idea of modelling desirable behaviour starts from the top – how politicians and public figures behave, as well as social workers and other professionals charged with monitoring parents.

19 Looking forward

As I hope this book has shown, the 'new types' of parents may pose a challenge to traditional models of family life but they also offer a new range of options on how to care for children and how alternative economic units of western society may function. If the industrial revolution heralded standardisation and conformity, then post-industrial societies may yet witness a celebration of individuality and variety. As we move away from needing workers who are allocated lifelong jobs fulfilling uniform roles on a production line and instead increasingly call upon the intellectual and creative resources of the individuals in our society to produce the wealth of the nation, the new family styles may actually be more suited to the needs of the state.

If we wish to address the financial and social spiralling of costs we have to be imaginative in looking at how to make the new models work well, not just to bemoan the passing of an outdated model. It is not a matter of whether one model was better than another but that evolution and change are inevitable, bringing good and bad outcomes which need to be accommodated.

The essential issue is one of what I have termed congruity. The reason why the 1950s were seen as such a golden era for family life was not because there were less single, teenage or working mothers, but because everything was pulling in the same direction: the perceived needs of children, parents and society were all complementary. The state of the nation, the policies of government and professionals, the state's requirement for certain types of workers, the childcare beliefs and women's role, the lack of media contradicting the dominant ideologies of parents or state – all reinforced each other to promote the nuclear family. It is easy to look back with nostalgia and say if only we could push women back into the home, strengthen the Church, stifle the media – we could go back to order and social morality.

But that is not only not possible – it would be unacceptable for the vast majority of people who have struggled to shake off the oppressive shackles of conformity. Here then is the crux: what we need to do is to find a way of realigning on a different plane to achieve a similar congruity but this time on the basis of a different set of knowledge and values.

If we look at the Actual Model we see a lot of incongruities – between what the knowledge base is telling us about children and parents needing to be seen in terms of their individual contexts and their need for wider support networks, while state policies such as the Children Act 1989 are emphasising that children are the primary responsibility of the parents – at a time when parents can no longer have the degree of exclusive influence they 'enjoyed' in the 1950s. The external environment in the form of physical, social and technological influences is moving rapidly out of the control of the individuals who live in it – and yet parents are being called upon to exercise more exclusive control over their children's lives. Children are spending less time with their parents as they go to be cared for in different homes and nurseries and are subject to a much wider range of conflicting influences, yet their discipline remains the responsibility of parents:

> If the socialisation of children is a more pronounced wider society activity, shouldn't their correction be too?
> . . . It seems to me that in this country some parents have, to their own and their children's and society's detriment, remained entrenched in the view that the behaviour of children is the sole responsibility of parents. The Children Act promotes this view and is bound to create real difficulties for parents. This is because it is out of sync with reality and social trends and parental attitudes that have evolved as a result of these.
>
> (Bartells-Ellis 1992)

Parents are being asked to take responsibility for turning out conforming, un-demanding workers when the jobs do not exist. They are being asked to teach morals and discipline when schools and politicians cannot seem to do so. The degree of incongruity is becoming great for every parent but particularly for those who remain stigmatised. I would argue that the degree of mismatch between expectations of child, parent and state are at the heart of most parenting problems today. Parents are being asked to do a job without any job description, with uncertain rewards and no job security by an employer who largely treats us as unskilled yet expects an increasingly professional level of service.

The new approach I would advocate is one which promotes excellence in the job of parenting, which shares the definitions of excellence with a team approach to making it happen. This can only develop if we see a substantial change in the culture of those in bastions of power and control that stand in the way of more openness. The culture of excellence has been referred to as the goal of the quality revolution – heralded by management gurus as equivalent in its importance to the industrial revolution. Within the framework of Total Quality Management (TQM) there appear important parallels between organisations and nations.

> TQM has implications which can affect the organisation's traditional power culture because it is about empowering people to improve systems: quality is about power sharing – about giving power to subordinates.
>
> (Wilkinson *et al.* 1992)

As with organisations, prosperity and stable development of a society depends on achieving congruity between its parenting styles and the way society works. For this analogy to bear fruit there needs to be a greater involvement by parents and children from all walks of life in the decision making which affects society. They can no longer be marginalised:

> It is necessary to change behaviour and attitudes throughout the organisation. Key features of Total Quality Management are employee involvement and development and a teamwork approach to dealing with improvement activities.
>
> (Wilkinson *et al.* 1992)

I would like to leave you with one final image I have found recurring in writing the latter parts of this book and that is of how western society will open up to accommodate the growing heterogeneity of its family life in the twenty-first century. What I see is that battered raft of logs representing the needs of children, parents and society, barely holding together as its forty-year-old ropes fall away in tatters. The river of time is flowing faster and faster, tossing it this way and that as it approaches a chaotic set of rapids.

The raft is steered by the same closed elitist group which believes that 1950s values provide the unique ropes that can hold the raft of stable family life together. So they try and steer upstream, against the flow of time, battling with the currents of social, economic and technological change. They are surrounded by frightened but helpless passengers whose own family lives have become increasingly confused. Hanging on to the sides of the raft and some clambering on board, are those whose parenting has been labelled deviant but who have none the less got on and achieved stability. They are offering new ideas and experience on how to rebuild the raft with new values that accommodate a wide spectrum of differences, not rejecting it. They are saying they need to be included in the crew to help change the direction and avert societal chaos, that their experience has taught them the resilience and expertise needed to negotiate the rapids. The crew don't want to hear. They grimly hold on to the steering wheel, unwilling to let anyone else near. But other passengers are beginning to listen, wondering if there might be another way through. The rapids approach. . . .

Bibliography

Adcock, M. and White, R. (eds) (1985) *Good Enough Parenting – A Framework for Assessment*. British Agencies for Adoption and Fostering.

Adcock, M. and White, R. (eds) (1992) *Significant Harm*, Significant Publications.

Ahmad, B. (1989) Protecting black children from abuse. *Social Work Today* 8 June.

Ahmed, S. (1987) Reports can oversimplify cultural issues. *Community Care* 20 July, 6.

Ahmed, S. (1989) 'Children in care: the racial dimension', in Morgan, S. and Righton, P. (eds) *Social Work Assessment in Child Care: Concerns and Conflicts*. Hodder and Stoughton.

Ainsworth, M. (1967) *Infancy in Uganda*. Johns Hopkins University Press.

Alibhai, Y. (1988) Maternity care: black women speak out. *New Society* 1 April.

Allen-Meares, P. (1991) Educating adolescents on the dangers of premature childbearing and drug use: a focus on prevention. *Child and Adolescent Social Work* Vol. 8, No. 4, August.

Arditti, R., Klein, R.D. and Minden, S. (1984) *Test Tube Women*. Pandora.

Bartells-Ellis, F. (1992) Issues in parenting (unpublished MSc thesis). Cranfield Institute of Technology.

Bebbington, A. and Miles, J. (1989) The background of children who enter local authority care. *British Journal of Social Work* 19, 349–68.

Belsky, J. (1988) The 'effects' of infant day care reconsidered. *Early Childhood Research Quarterly* Vol. 3, 227–34.

Berkowitz, G.S. *et al.* (1990) Delayed childbearing and the outcome of pregnancy. *New England Journal of Medicine* Vol. 322, No. 10, 659–64.

Berman, P.W. and Pedersen, F.A. (1987) *Men's Transitions to Parenthood*. Lawrence Erlbaum Associates.

Berryman, J.C. and Windridge, K. (1991) Having a baby after 40: I and II. *Journal of Reproductive and Infant Psychology* Vol. 9, 3–18 and 19–33.

Bertin, J.E. (1993) 'Pregnancy and social control', in Katz Rothman, B. (ed.) *Encyclopaedia of Childbearing*. Oryx Press.

Bilsborrow, S. (1992) You grow up fast as well. . . Barnardo's.

Bingol, N. *et al.* (1987) The influence of socioeconomic factors on the occurrence of Fetal Alcohol Syndrome. *Advances in Alcohol and Substance Abuse*, 105–18.

Black, D. (1990) What do children need from parents? *Adoption and Fostering* Vol. 14, No. 1, 43–51.

Black, D., Wolkind, S. and Hendriks, J. (eds) (1989) *Child Psychiatry and the Law*. Royal College of Psychiatrists.

Blunden, G. (1988) Becoming a single foster parent. *Adoption and Fostering* Vol. 12, No. 1, 44–7.

Booth, T. and Booth, W. (1992) An ordinary family life. *Community Care* 23 April 1992, 15–17.

Boswell, J. (1991) *The Kindness of Strangers.* Penguin.

Bowlby, J. (1951) *Maternal Care and Mental Health.* World Health Organisation, Geneva.

Bozett, F.W. (1981) Gay fathers: evolution of the gay father identity. *American Journal of Orthopsychiatry* Vol. 51, No. 3, 552–59.

Budd, K. and Greenspan, S. (1981) 'Mental retarded women as parents', in Blechman, E. (ed.) *Behaviour Modification with Women.* Guilford Press.

Caine, H. (1990) *What Sort of Family?* Barnardo's London Homefinding Project.

Campion, M.J. (1990) *The Baby Challenge.* Routledge.

Carey, J.S. (1991) I am not yet born – but that won't stop me suing you. *New Statesman and Society* 15 November 1991.

Carson, D. (1989) The sexuality of people with learning difficulties. *Journal of Social Welfare Law* No. 6, 355–72.

Centre for Economic Policy Research (1989) *The Changing Population of Britain.* Basil Blackwell.

Chesler, P. (1990) *Sacred Bond: The Legacy of Baby M.* Virago.

Clarke, J. (1990) Fit for a family. *Community Care* 5 April 1990.

Clulow, C. (1989) Child applications and contested divorce. *Family Law* Vol. 19, May, 198–200.

Clulow, C. and Vincent, C. (1987) *In the Child's Best Interests? Tavistock Press.*

Collins, R. and Macleod, A. (1991) Children first? Welfare reports in unmarried parent cases. *Journal of Social Welfare and Family Law* No. 6, 440–53.

Collis, G.H. (1991) Children of parents with sensory disabilities. *Scottish Concern* May 1991, 30–9.

Commission for Racial Equality (1984) Race and council housing in Hackney. Report of a formal investigation. CRE.

Cosis Brown, H. (1991) Competent child-focused practice: working with lesbian and gay carers. *Adoption and Fostering* Vol. 15, No. 2, 11–17.

Cosis Brown, H. (1992) Gender, sex and sexuality in the assessment of prospective carers. *Adoption and Fostering* Vol. 16, No. 2 1992, 30–4.

Cotton, K. and Winn, D. (1985) *Baby Cotton – For Love and Money.* Dorling Kindersley.

Craft, A. (1987) *Mental Handicap and Sexuality.* Costello.

Culp, R. *et al.* (1991) Adolescent and older mothers' interaction with their six month old infants. *Journal of Adolescence and Youth* Vol. 14, 195–200.

Darwin, C. (1871/1937) *The Descent of Man.* The Thinker's Library.

Davis, K.C. (1969) *Discretionary Justice.* University of Louisiana Press.

De'Ath, E. (1992) Stepping into family life. *Health Visitor* Vol. 65, No.1, 15–17.

DeJoseph, J.F. (1993) 'Pregnancy and work', in Katz Rothman, B. (ed.) *Encyclopaedia of Childbearing.* Oryx Press.

Department of Health (1988) *Working Together: A guide to inter-agency cooperation for the protection of children from abuse.* HMSO.

Department of Health (1989) *Protecting Children: A guide for social workers undertaking a comprehensive assessment.* HMSO.

D'Souza, S.W., Rivlin, E., Buck, P. and Lieberman, B.A. (1990) 'Children conceived by in vitro fertilisation', in Matson, P.L. and Lieberman, B.A. (eds) *Clinical IVF Forum: Current Views in Assisted Reproduction.* Manchester University Press.

Douglas, J.W.B., Ross, J.M. and Simpson, H.R. (1968) *All Our Future.* Peter Davies.

Dowdney, L. and Skuse, D. (1993) Parenting provided by adults with mental retardation. *Journal of Child Psychology and Psychiatry* Vol. 34, No. 1, 25–47.

Drew, D. and Gray, J. (1991) The black–white gap in examination results: a statistical critique of a decade's research. *New Community* Vol. 17, No. 2, 159–72.

Dubble, C., Dun, E., Aldridge, T. and Kearney, P. (1987) Registering concern. *Community Care* 12 March, 20–2.

Easterbrook, F. (1989) Dissenting opinion. *International Union, UAW v. Johnson Controls, 886 F.2d (7th Cir.).*

Eekelar, J. (1991) Parental responsibility: state of nature or nature of state. *Journal of Social Welfare and Family Law* November.

Eekelar, J. and Dingwall, R. (1990) *The Reform of Child Care Law*. Routledge.

Egerton, J. (1990) Nothing natural. *New Statesman and Society* 16 November.

Fahlberg, V. (1985) 'Checklists on attachment', in Adcock, M. and White, R. (eds) *Good-enough Parenting*. British Agencies for Adoption and Fostering.

Fein, G. and Fox, N. (1988) Infant day care: a special issue. *Early Childhood Research Quarterly* 3, 227.

Finger, A. (1988) *Past Due*. The Women's Press.

Finger, A. (1992) Forbidden fruit. *New Internationalist* July.

Fricker, N. and Coates, L. (1989) Conciliation and a conciliatory approach in welfare reporting. *Family Law* Vol. 19, February, 58–60.

Frisch, L.F. (1981) On licentious licensing: a reply to Hugh Follette *Philosophy and Public Affairs* Vol. 11, No. 2.

Fry, P.S. and Eddington, J. (1984) Professionals' negative expectations of boys from father-headed single parent families: implications for the training of childcare professionals. *British Journal of Developmental Psychology* 2, 337–46.

Furnell, J. (1991) Evidence of significant emotional harm. *Adoption and Fostering* Vol. 15, No. 4, 116–18.

Furstenberg, F.F. *et al.* (1987) *Adolescent Mothers in Later Life*. Cambridge University Press.

Gardner, M.J. *et al.* (1990) Results of case-control study of leukaemia and lymphoma among young people near Sellafield nuclear plant in west Cumbria. *British Medical Journal* 300, 423–29.

Gelman, D. (1990) A much riskier passage. *Newsweek* 10–16 June.

Gibbons, F. (1989) A framework for court welfare reports. *Family Law* Vol. 19, February, 60–1.

Gibson, A. (1980) *Pregnancy among Unmarried West Indian Teenagers*. Report by the Centre for Caribbean Studies.

Gilroy, P. (1990) The end of anti-racism. *New Community* Vol. 17, No. 1, 71–83.

Glover, J. *et al.* (1989) *Fertility and the Family: The Glover Report on Reproductive Technologies to the European Commission*. Fourth Estate.

Goldstein, J., Freud, A. and Solnit, A. (1973/1980) *Beyond the Best Interests of the Child*. Burnett Books.

Golombok, S. Spencer, A. and Rutter, M. (1983) Children in lesbian and single parent households: psychosexual and psychiatric appraisal. *Journal of Child Psychology and Psychiatry* Vol. 24, No. 4.

Graham Hall, J. and Martin, D.F. (1991) Is Article 8 out of date? *Practitioners' Child Law Bulletin* Vol. 4 No. 1, 10–11.

Green, R. (1978) Sexual identity of 37 children raised by homosexual or transsexual parents. *American Journal of Psychiatry* Vol. 135, No. 6, 692–7.

Greif, G. (1992) Lone fathers in the United States. *British Journal of Social Work* 22, 565–74.

Grimshaw, R. (1991) From negative to positive: interpretations of children having a parent with complex disabilities. *Scottish Concern* May, 41–53.

Grimshaw, R. (1992) *Children of Parents with Parkinson's Disease*. National Children's Bureau.

Hanmer, J. (1991) The wider implications of NRTS. *Royal Society Forum on Maternity and the Newborn* 14 February.

Hanscombe, G. and Foster, J. (1982) *Rocking the Cradle: Lesbian Mothers; a Challenge in Family Living*. Sheba.

Hartman, A. (1979) *Finding Families: An Ecological Approach to Assessment*. Sage Publications.

Hebenton, B. and Thomas, T. (1990) Approved households: checking criminal records. *Adoption and Fostering* Vol. 14, No. 2, 27–9.

Hennessy, E. *et al.* (1992) *Children and Day Care*. Chapman and Paul.

Henwood, M. *et al.* (1987) *Inside the Family: Changing Roles of Men and Women*. Family Policy Studies Centre.

Heywood, J.S. (1978) *Children in Care*. Routledge & Kegan Paul.

Higginson, S. (1990) Under the influence. *Social Work Today* 20 November.

Hipgrave, T. (1982) 'The lone father', in McKee, L. and O'Brien, M. (eds) *The Father Figure*. Tavistock Publications.

Hoeffer, B. (1981) Children's acquisition of sex role behaviour in lesbian-mother families. *American Journal of Orthopsychiatry* Vol. 15, No. 3, 536–44.

Howard, J. and Shepherd, G. (1987) *Conciliation, Children and Divorce*. Batsford Academic.

Human Fertilisation and Embryology Authority (1991) HFEA Code of Practice.

Hurst, R. (1992) The definition of disability: the right to define ourselves *Vox Nostra* Vol. 5, No. 4.

Inglis, R. (1978) *Sins of the Fathers*. Peter Owen.

Jakobson, M. (1988) Rights of disabled parents. *Parenting with a Disability* Vol. 1, No. 1, 4.

James, A. (1990) Conciliation welfare reports and the Children Act 1989. *Journal of Social Welfare and Family Law* No. 4, 235–44.

James, A. and Dingwall, R. (1989) Social work ideologies in the probation service. *Journal of Social Welfare Law* No. 6, 323–38.

James, A.L. and Wilson, K. (1984) Reports for the court: the work of the divorce court wefare officer. *Journal of Social Welfare* March, 89–103.

Johnson, A. (1990) Access – The basics. *Family Law* Vol. 20, December, 483–85.

Johnson, A. (1991) Practical guide to contact. *Family Law* December, 536–37.

Kenny, M. (1990) Spelling out the facts of life to the gay community. *Daily Telegraph* 9 June.

King, M.B. and Pattison, P. (1991) Homosexuality and parenthood. *British Medical Journal* Vol. 303, August.

Kingsley, J.R.K (1990) The best interests of the child? The role of the divorce court welfare officer. *Children and Society* Vol. 4, No. 3, 284–92.

Kirshbaum, M. (1988) Parents with physical disabilities and their babies. *Zero to Three* June.

Kissman, K. (1988) Factors associated with competence, well-being and parenting attitude among teen mothers. *International Journal of Adolescence and Youth* Vol. 1.

Koren, G. *et al.* (1989) Bias against the Null hypothesis: the reproductive hazards of cocaine. *Lancet* 2 (8677), 1440–2.

LaFollette, H. (1980) Licensing parents. *Philosophy and Public Affairs* Vol. 9, No. 2.

Lamb, M.E. (1982) 'Maternal employment and child development', in Lamb, M.E. (ed.) *Nontraditional Families: Parenting and Child Development*. Lawrence Erlbaum Associates.

Lamb, M.E. (1986) *The Father's Role: Applied Perspectives*. Wiley.

Larkin, P. (1974) 'This be the verse', in *High Windows*. Faber and Faber.

Lasker, J. and Borg, S. (1987) *In Search of Parenthood. Coping with Infertility and High Tech Conception*. Pandora.

Lewis, C. (1985) *Employee Selection*. Hutchinson & Co, London.

Lewis, V. (1991) *A Good Sign Goes a Long Way*. Royal National Institute for the Deaf.

London Borough of Lambeth (1987) *Whose Child? The Report of the Public Inquiry into the Death of Tyra Henry*. London Borough of Lambeth.

Longmore, Z. (1987) Why social work isn't working for black families. *The Independent* 23 December.

Macaskill, C. (1982) Adoption of mentally handicapped children (unpublished MSc Thesis). Cranfield Institute of Technology.

Maidment, S. (1984) *Child Custody and Divorce. The Law in Social Context*. Croom Helm.

Mansfield, P.K. (1988) Midlife childbearing: strategies for informed decision making. *Psychology of Women Quarterly*, Special Issue: Women's Health, Our Minds, Our Bodies 12, 445–60.

Mason, M. (1992) 'A nineteen parent family', in Morris, Jenny (ed.) *Alone Together*. The Women's Press.

Mathews, J. (1992) *A Mother's Touch: The Tiffany Callo Story*. Henry Holt.

Mayall, B. (1991) Researching childcare in a multi-ethnic society. *New Community* Vol. 17, No. 4, 553–68.

Melhuish, E. and Phoenix, A. (1988) Motherhood under twenty: prevailing ideologies and research. *Children and Society* No. 4, 288–98.

Miles, M. (1992) Concepts of mental retardation in Pakistan: toward cross-cultural and historical perspectives. *Disability, Handicap and Society* Vol. 7, No. 3.

Mitchell, A. (1985) *Children In The Middle: Living Through Divorce*. Tavistock Publications.

Morgan, D. and Lee, R. (1991) *Guide to the Human Fertilization and Embryology Act*. Blackstone Press.

Morris, J. (ed.) (1992) *Alone Together – Voices of Single Mothers*. The Women's Press.

Murch, M. (1980) *Justice and Welfare in Divorce*. Sweet & Maxwell.

Nordhaus, B.F. and Solnit, A.J. (1990) Adoption 1990. *Zero to Three*. Vol. X, No. 5.

Oakley, A. (1981) *From Here to Maternity*. Penguin.

Oates, M. (1984) 'Assessing fitness to parent', in *Taking a Stand*. BAAF.

Parekh, B. (1988) The new racism. *New Statesman and Society* 22 January.

Parker, R. (ed.) (1991) *Looking After Children: Assessing Outcomes in Child Care*. HMSO.

Parton, N. (1991) *Governing the Family – Child Care, Child Protection and the State*. Macmillan Education.

Phillips, E. (1990) 'Bringing up Ella', in Morris, J. (ed.) *Alone Together*. The Women's Press.

Phoenix, A. (1988) The Afro-Caribbean myth. *New Society* 4 March, 10–13.

Phoenix, A. (1991) *Young Mothers?* Polity Press.

Pomerantz, P., Pomerantz, D. and Colca, L. (1990) A case study: service delivery and parents with disabilities. *Child Welfare* Vol. LXIX, No. 1, 65–73.

Richards, M.P.M. (1989) Joint custody revisited. *Family Law*, 83–5.

Rickford, F. (1991) Teenage mothers: too much too young? *Social Work Today* 31 October.

Risman, J.B. (1987) Intimate relationships from a microstructural perspective: men who mother. *Gender and Society* Vol. 35, 95–102.

Roche, J. (1991) The Children Act 1989: Once a parent always a parent? *Journal of Social Welfare and Family Law* No. 5.

Rogers, J.A. (1968) *From Superman to Man*. Rogers.

Rowe, J. (1966) *Parents, Children and Adoption*. Routledge & Kegan Paul.

Roy, R. (1990–1) Consequences of parental illness on children: a review. *Social Work and Social Sciences Review* Vol. 2, No. 2, 109–21.

Rutter, M. and Madge, N. (1983) 'Parenting in two generations', in Madge, N. (ed.) *Families at Risk*. Heinemann Educational Books.

Ryburn, M. (1991 The myth of assessment. *Adoption and Fostering* Vol. 15, No. 1, 20–7.

Sacks, O. (1990) *Seeing Voices*. Pan Books.

Salholz, E. (1990) *Newsweek* 12 March.

Saxe, J.G. (1980) 'The blind men and the elephant', in Doan, Eleanor (ed.) *The Child's Treasury of Verse*. Hodder & Stoughton.

Schaffer, H.R. (1990) *Making Decisions about Children*. Blackwell.

Segal, J. and Simkins, J. (1993) *My Mum Needs Me*. Penguin.

Selwyn, J. (1991) Applying to adopt: the experience of rejection. *Adoption and Fostering* Vol. 15, No. 3, 26–9.

Sheridan, Mary D. (1960) The Developmental Progress of Infants and Young Children. DHSS, Reports on Public Health and Medical Subjects, No. 102.

Smart, C. and Sevenhuijsen, S. (eds) (1989) *Child Custody and the Politics of Gender.* Routledge.

Smart, D. (1991) A chance for gay people. *Community Care* 24 January.

Snowden, R. (1981) *The Artificial Family.* George Allen & Unwin.

Steinhauer, P.D. (1983) Assessing for parenting capacity. *American Journal of Orthopsychiatry* Vol. 53, No. 3, 468–81.

Stevenson, P. (1991) A model of self-assessment for prospective adopters. *Adoption and Fostering* Vol. 15, No. 3, 30–4.

Stone, L. (1990) *The Road To Divorce.* Oxford University Press.

Swann, M. (1985) Education for All – The Report of the Committee of Inquiry into the Education of Children from Ethnic Minority Groups. Department of Education and Science.

Tasker, F. and Golombok, S. (1991) Children raised by lesbian mothers – the empirical evidence. *Family Law* May, 184–7.

Thomas, T. and Hebenton, W. (1991) Checking a person's criminal record before infertility treatment. *The Health Service Journal* 8 August.

Thompson, R. (1988) Infant day care and attachment theory. *Early Childhood Research Quarterly* 3, 281.

Tizard, B. (1977) *Adoption: a Second Chance.* Open Books.

Tizard, B. (1991) 'Employed mothers and the care of children', in Phoenix, A. *et al.* (eds) *Motherhood and Society.* Sage Publications.

Triselotis, J. (1970) *Evaluation of Adoption Policy and Practice.* University of Edinburgh.

Trombley, S. (1988) *The Right to Reproduce?* Weidenfeld & Nicolson.

Tymchuk, A. (1992) Predicting adequacy of parenting by people with mental retardation. *Child Abuse and Neglect* Vol. 16, 165–78.

Tymchuk, A.J. and Andron, L. (1990) Mothers with mental retardation who do or do not abuse or neglect their children. *Child Abuse and Neglect* Vol. 14, 313–23.

United Nations (UN) (1971) *Declaration of the Rights of the Mentally Retarded Person.*

Valentine, D.P. (1990) Double jeopardy: child maltreatment and mental retardation. *Child and Adolescent Social Work* Vol. 7, No. 6, 487–99.

Walker, B. (1992) 'A woman's right to choose', in Morris, J. (ed.) *Alone Together.* The Women's Press.

Wallerstein, J. and Blakeslee, S. (1989) *Second Chances.* Bantam Press.

Waters, E.G. and Wager, H.P. (1950) Pregnancy and labour experiences of elderly primigravidas. *American Journal of Obstetrics and Gynaecology* Vol. 59, 296–304.

Wates, M. (1993) Images of disabled parents. *Disability, Pregnancy and Parenthood International* No. 2 April.

Wates, M. (1991) Able parents – disability, pregnancy and motherhood. *Maternity Action* No. 52, 9.

Whitfield, R. (1991) Don't give in to pressure. *Community Care* 24 January.

Whitman, B. and Accardo, P.J. (1990) *When a Parent is Mentally Retarded.* Paul H. Brookes.

Whitman, B., Graves, B. and Accardo, P. (1989) Training in parenting skills for adults with mental retardation. *Social Work* September, 431–3.

Wilkinson, A., Marchington, M., Goodman, J. and Ackers, P. (1992) Total Quality Management and employee involvement. *Human Resource Management Journal* Vol. 2, No. 4.

Wilson, E. (1977) *Women and the Welfare State.* Tavistock.

Winnicott, D. (1964) *The Child, the Family, the Outside World.* Penguin.

Wolff, S.(1987) Prediction in child care. *Adoption and Fostering* Vol. 11, No. 1, 11–17.

Wolff, S. (1991) Children under stress in a disabled family. *Scottish Concern* May, 8–18.

Index